Praise for *Grown Woman Talk*

"In *Grown Woman Talk,* Dr. Sharon Malone offers straightforward advice on how to structure your healthcare experience, manage your personal health, understand menopause, and so much more. For Dr. Sharon, this isn't just about how to live longer; it's about how to live healthier—and happier."

—**Michelle Obama,**
former first lady and *New York Times*
bestselling author of *Becoming*

"With an extraordinary combination of lived wisdom, professional expertise, insider perspective, warm sisterly love, and honesty, *Grown Woman Talk* offers a timely guide to truly taking control of our health, our healthcare, and our quality of life. Dr. Sharon Malone has filled every page with the vital information and the inspiration that we need to improve our health and extend our health spans—immediately!"

—**Kerry Washington,**
Emmy-nominated actress and *New York Times*
bestselling author of *Thicker Than Water*

"For every woman who has ever felt unheard or marginalized by the healthcare system, Dr. Sharon Malone's voice resonates with compassion, clarity, and an unyielding commitment to driving change. *Grown Woman Talk* is a must-read for women of all ages seeking validation and agency in a world that often denies them both."

—**Naomi Watts,**
Academy Award–nominated actress

"*Grown Woman Talk* is a beacon of insight and grace, helping women navigate their health journeys with confidence and knowledge. A must-read!"

—**Lisa Mosconi,**
New York Times bestselling
author of *The XX Brain*

T0356713

"Dr. Sharon Malone's visionary approach sheds light on the intricate path of women's health through the aging process. She offers not just advice but also a lifeline. As healthcare systems, therapeutics, and technology evolve, her timely wisdom serves as a guiding star. This invaluable book reveals the life-saving importance of informed choices and empowers every woman, especially Black women, to practice self-care and navigate the healthcare maze with grace and confidence."

—Linda Goler Blount,
president and CEO of the
Black Women's Health Imperative

"*Grown Woman Talk* is a compulsively readable page-turner, packed with equal doses of science and sagacity, humor and history, plus practical advice galore. Dr. Sharon Malone is the compassionate doctor, soulful storyteller, surrogate sister, friend—and DJ extraordinaire—we all need and deserve in our lives. This book is an extraordinary public service to women of every age."

—Jennifer Weiss-Wolf,
executive director of the Birnbaum Women's
Leadership Center at NYU School of Law

GROWN WOMAN TALK

Your Essential Companion
for Healthy Living

Sharon Malone, M.D.

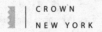

CROWN
NEW YORK

CROWN

An imprint of the Crown Publishing Group
A division of Penguin Random House LLC
crownpublishing.com

2025 Crown Trade Paperback Edition
Copyright © 2024 by Sharon D. Malone, M.D.

Penguin Random House values and supports copyright. Copyright fuels creativity, encourages diverse voices, promotes free speech, and creates a vibrant culture. Thank you for buying an authorized edition of this book and for complying with copyright laws by not reproducing, scanning, or distributing any part of it in any form without permission. You are supporting writers and allowing Penguin Random House to continue to publish books for every reader. Please note that no part of this book may be used or reproduced in any manner for the purpose of training artificial intelligence technologies or systems.

CROWN and the Crown colophon are registered trademarks of Penguin Random House LLC.

Library of Congress Cataloging-in-Publication Data
Names: Malone, Sharon, author.
Title: Grown woman talk / Sharon Malone, M.D.
Description: First edition. | New York: Crown, 2024 |
Includes bibliographical references and index.
Identifiers: LCCN 2023048707 (print) | LCCN 2023048708 (ebook) |
ISBN 9780593593882 (trade paper) | ISBN 9780593593875 (ebook)
Subjects: LCSH: African American women—Health and hygiene—Popular works. |
African American women—Medical care—Popular works. | African American women—
Diseases—Treatment—Popular works. | Women—Health and hygiene—
United States—Popular works. | Women—Medical care—United States—
Popular works. | Women—Diseases—Treatment—Popular works. |
Malone, Sharon, 1959– —Health. | Malone, Sharon, 1959– —Family.
Classification: LCC RA778.4.A36 M35 2024 (print) | LCC RA778.4.A36 (ebook) |
DDC 362.1089/96073—dc23/eng/20231208
LC record available at https://lccn.loc.gov/2023048707
LC ebook record available at https://lccn.loc.gov/2023048708

ISBN 978-0-593-59388-2
Ebook ISBN 978-0-593-59387-5

Originally published in hardcover in the United States by Crown, an imprint of the Crown Publishing Group, a division of Penguin Random House LLC, in 2024.

Editor: Madhulika Sikka | Assistant editor: Fariza Hawke |
Production editor: Ashley Pierce | Text designer: Ralph Fowler | Production: Alison Kaitcer |
Publicist: Lindsay Cook | Marketer: Julie Cepler

Manufactured in the United States of America

9 8 7 6 5 4 3 2 1

First Paperback Edition

The authorized representative in the EU for product safety and compliance is Penguin Random House Ireland, Morrison Chambers, 32 Nassau Street, Dublin D02 YH68, Ireland, https://eu-contact.penguin.ie.

This book is dedicated
to my mother, Bertha Davis Malone,
and to my sisters Vivian Malone Jones and
Gwendolyn Malone Moseby, who did not
live long enough to impart the wisdom
that comes with old age.

I write for those women who do not speak, for those who do not have a voice because they were so terrified, because we are taught to respect fear more than ourselves. We've been taught that silence would save us, but it won't.

—Audre Lorde

Dear Reader,

Dr. Sharon Malone is one of the smartest, funniest, and most charismatic women I know, and I've relied on her wisdom through good times and tough times. Over the years, she has become the first person I turn to for a whole host of issues, especially my health. In *Grown Woman Talk,* she'll become your confidante, too. Dr. Sharon offers straightforward advice on how to structure your healthcare experience, manage your personal health, understand menopause, and so much more. With her signature wit and charm, she threads together stories and tips that are interesting, approachable, and educational, all at the same time. For me, reading *Grown Woman Talk* felt just like one of our candid discussions—informative and a whole lot of fun. While the book is geared toward women of color, there's something in it for every woman, no matter their background. It's a must-read for anyone who cares about their quality of life, because for Dr. Sharon, this isn't just about how to live longer; it's about how to live healthier—and happier.

Michelle Obama

CONTENTS

INTRODUCTION

As women, we are called upon to be many things to many people. In my life, I have been a daughter, a sister, a friend, a doctor, a wife, and a mother. Given that I lost my parents early, my role as a daughter was cut short, but thankfully I have inhabited the roles of sister and friend for far longer than any of the others. I am writing to you as both. I have also imagined myself an ersatz deejay (here is where my kids start rolling their eyes). Those who know me well know that I have a song for every occasion—but more on that later.

As you read this book, at times I may sound more like your auntie or your mother than a doctor, because sometimes you need both. When it comes to our health, we can and must do better. But I am not here to admonish you (okay, perhaps just a little bit). This book is meant to empower you to wrest back some confidence and control around your health, your vitality, and your future. And you need to know that every piece of advice I give and every story I share is here for a reason—and that reason is, I care about your well-being [♪ "Nuttin' But Love"].

Thirty years as an OB/GYN in our nation's capital has given me a unique vantage point on our healthcare system and the women it serves. I have taken care of VIPs and housekeepers, octogenarians and high schoolers, and I have done my level best to give each of them the care and respect they deserved, regardless of station or age. I know what it is to be privileged and have access to the talent, information, and resources that privilege affords. But as a Black woman raised in the South by parents and siblings who endured the worst of what Jim Crow had to offer, I also know what it is to have none of that [♪ "Both Sides Now"].

My parents, Bertha and Willie Malone, grew up on small Alabama farms. They had no more than eighth-grade educations, but they were surefooted, wise, and devoted to our large family. I was the youngest of eight, so by the time I came along, my mom was 45 and old enough to be my grandmother. Given that I am seven years younger than my next sibling, I'm certain that my mother was hoping for menopause and got me instead. If you know anyone who's had an unplanned late-in-life baby, you know that once the shock passes, that bonus baby ends up being a beautiful surprise [♪ **"Beautiful Surprise"**].

Mom didn't smoke or drink and she stayed fit and trim. She routinely said things like, "Don't eat too much pork, it will make you slow," or "Eat more fish and nuts because that's brain food." Even after my parents moved to the "big city" of Mobile, my father grew vegetables in the vacant lot next to our house and my mother canned figs and pears grown in our backyard. So, note to the Michelin restaurant folks, my family ate farm-to-table before it was a thing.

Yet, despite all of her clean living and healthy eating, my precious mother—who had never missed a day from her job cleaning the officers' quarters at Brookley Air Force Base—got colon cancer at 57 and died. I was only 12, yet I instinctively knew that my mother's death was caused by more than her disease. It was somehow connected to her race, her gender and age, and an unjust system that gave rise to few options and an abundance of fear.

Bertha Malone died because she never had a real relationship with a doctor. She never even saw one unless there was an urgent problem. She died because she could neither trust nor afford medical care. She died because she didn't know the early warning signs of cancer and because she had no sense of her own medical history or its importance. She died because she had never had a cancer screening of any kind. Any of these could have made all the difference in the world for my mom and our family.

Once she was gone, my grief was raw, angry, and suppressed. I felt like my mother, this strong, wise woman who literally made a way out of no way for her entire life, didn't have the information or tools she needed to save herself. And when she most needed compassion and care from the medical profession, I felt she got neither. I am certain that my journey to medicine, and this moment here with you, began there.

I have come to see that, even at 57, my capable, stoic mother felt she had no more agency over her own healthcare than I, her baby girl, did. In the decades since, I've treated more women than I can count and am grateful that, together, we have scored more victories than losses. I've had a front row seat to what works for us and against us over the course of our lifelong journeys with sickness and health. I share many of those stories in these pages in the hope that my patients' and my family's experiences will positively inform yours. I have used pseudonyms when necessary and real names only with express consent. And lest anyone worry about privacy concerns, these stories are based on real-life situations but are not intended to be exact representations of any one patient's medical history.

I also want you to see that, no matter where you are or what you're facing in your journey with aging and your health, you are not alone [♪ "You Are Not Alone"].

The purpose of this book is to help you become your own best primary caregiver, so that my mother's experience will not be yours. You matter. And whether you realize it or not, you need this.

It's neither easy nor instinctual to advocate for yourself medically. And over the next several years, the challenges you'll confront in doing so will be complex and ever changing. The medical system is broken, and it didn't just now get broken, it always has been—especially for women, people of color, people who live in rural America, and those of limited means. The COVID pandemic laid bare the inequities that have always been percolating just below the surface. Finally, the magnitude of those disparities is being discussed in the public square.

I know what you're thinking: *Conversation alone is not a solution.* You're right, but it's a start. So, I invite you to join me in this much-needed talk about you, your health, and the agency you must exercise to have the life and get the care you deserve.

The first step is to realize that the foundation of modern medicine was never built with you in mind. Women's healthcare as a legitimate field of study did not even exist before the mid-nineteenth century, and it was deeply problematic from the start.

You probably have never heard of Dr. J. Marion Sims and, to be honest, I only learned the name because he is credited as being the Father of Gynecology. To this day, we have surgical instruments and procedures named for him even though we now know that he "invented" the field of gynecology and practiced many of his surgical techniques by operating and experimenting on enslaved women . . . without anesthesia, even when it was available. And they were certainly in no position to give their consent.

For generations, throughout the world, women's bodies were considered unclean and contemptible. As females, we were deemed emotionally, physically, and intellectually inferior to men. So, our concerns—even about our own bodies—were regarded as unworthy or frivolous, and our value was tied almost exclusively to our ability to reproduce. Medical research did not routinely include women in clinical trials until 1993. Just two years prior, the first woman to lead the National Institutes of Health (NIH), Dr. Bernadine Healy, commissioned the Women's Health Initiative, the largest and most expensive study ever to investigate health in menopausal women. Dr. Healy was not at the NIH long enough to participate in the interpretation of the data or make the decisions about how the results were communicated. We are all left to wonder how, had she been there, things might have turned out differently. Unfortunately, even with the best of intentions, the results of this study have not only been misinterpreted, they have also hobbled further research in this area for more than twenty years. Good luck if you happen to lie at the intersection of sexism, racism, ageism, and poverty, where a persistent lack of inclusive research cripples an adequate understanding of disease prevention, diagnoses, and treatment outcomes.

Many of the solutions to these issues lie far beyond the scope of this book. To be sure, medicine and research need a fundamental overhaul, but I wouldn't hold my breath on that one. In the words of the late, great musician Bill Withers, "While you're on the way to wonderful, you better take a good look at just alright, because that may be as far as you get." In other words, as broken as it is today, this system is what we've got. The good news is that while we are waiting on legislation, policy changes, and a real and substantive discussion of healthcare disparities, there is still a lot within your control. So, I want to shift the focus to where it belongs—on *you* and how you can effectively navigate a deeply flawed system.

We are far more than our reproductive parts. We will spend a third of our lives in our menopausal (also known as our "postmenopausal") years. The quality of those years would be greatly enhanced if we routinely leveraged more knowledge and preventative practices in the decades before this milestone. But it's never too late to learn and do better. And I am here to cheer you on, not to chastise.

This book is intended to give you the tools you need—a road map, if you will—to encourage more efficient and more satisfying interactions with the healthcare system. It offers an opportunity for you to become not just a better caregiver (and we women shoulder a disproportionate share of that load) but a better health consumer and advocate as well. You'll learn some of the basic facts and nuances of a system that too often fails you, so that you're equipped to maneuver through that system with greater confidence and success. I also want you to understand how your own history, susceptibilities, and behaviors may get in the way of being your best self as you age.

With all my heart, I wish for you what I wish for myself, my sisters, and my friends. I want you to cultivate greater self-awareness and resiliency as you age. I want you to slow, even prevent, premature decline. You should become familiar with the term *health span,* which is not just how long you live, but how long you live healthfully. I want you to heed the other Spock (of original *Star Trek* fame), who said, "Live long and prosper." I would add to that, protect your peace of mind.

So, find a calm, cool spot (because, girl, those hot flashes!). Sit back, take a deep breath [♪ "Breathe"], and affirm yourself as you begin this journey to a stronger, better, healthier you. This is *Grown Woman Talk,* and the topic of our conversation is you, so keep reading. Oh, and in case you're wondering what's up with the musical references and play-lists, I told you about my fantasy side hustle up top, and when we're done here, I want you to be able to truthfully say—*last night a deejay saved my life* [♪ **"Last Night a DJ Saved My Life"**]!

GROWN
WOMAN
TALK

CHAPTER 1

Solid♪

It's Time to Establish a Dependable Medical Home

Dear Sis,

Quick: What's your internist's name? When was the last time you went to the gynecologist? Have you had a bone density test? Did you get and keep the results of your most recent colonoscopy? How? And when was that?

You should know the answers to these questions cold! If you don't, we're going to get you there—and everywhere else you need to be to have better control of your health and a better life.

First, you need a team of sound and reliable healthcare professionals, and that's about their having more than board certifications and a decent bedside manner, although both are important. It's also about convenience. If your doctors are hard to get to, you won't go as often as you should. And you'll be better served if your doctors know one another and are affiliated with the same hospital system.

At this stage of your life, lots of things can get in the way of good care, from your socioeconomic status and politics to your gender and race. You cannot ignore that but you also can't control that.

That said, *you* are your primary caregiver! Not your significant other, your BFF, your parent, or your grown child. Not even your primary care physician.

No one is going to care more about your health than you do. No one is in a better position to do more about your health than you are. And no one has more to gain when you handle your business than you!

xo, Dr. Sharon

We know that whatever, whomever, and wherever we come from shapes us. But it also shapes our relationships with our bodies, with food and fitness, and with health-care and self-care. Even as a doctor, I am no exception. Care*giving*, I got. But, like most of us, I have a complicated relationship with care-getting. And that's rooted in how and where I grew up [♪ "**Home**"].

It is hard to describe my hometown. It is neither a small town nor a big city. It is urban without being urbane. Mobile, Alabama, sits at the mouth of the Mobile Bay and at the anus of the Mobile River. It marks both the beginning and the end of things.

For those fleeing the oppressive poverty and lack of opportunity of the state's interior farmlands, as my parents did, Mobile was a beacon of hope. As a way station, it served its purpose. But for many, Mobile was just a rest stop on the way to a better life.

In 1944, shortly before the end of World War II, my parents left the Black Belt, a large swath of rural Alabama named not only for its rich, dark soil but also for the preponderance of descendants of the enslaved who toiled there for generations.

I have often wondered what made my parents, Bertha and Willie Malone, leave "the country," which is what city folk called the 95 percent of Alabama that didn't have streetlights or paved roads. I mean, what makes a man and woman with no money, little education, and four babies uproot their lives in the midst of a war to move to the giant and scary unknown? Were the crops failing? Was there unspeakable violence? I can only speculate, because my parents never spoke of it, but the answer must lie in the notion that whatever they were leaving was intolerable and whatever lay ahead could be no worse.

Like millions of other Black people who fled the South during the Great Migration, they may have simply been searching for a better life for their growing family. And, to them, Mobile was The Big City—a mecca of possibility unlike anything they'd ever known.

Ultimately, they found jobs at Brookley Air Force Base—Mom as a maid and Dad in maintenance—and, indeed, they were able to create for us what had been denied to them. By 1949, they had managed to buy our two-bedroom house at 760 St. Anthony Street. They filled it with three more kids and my paternal grandfather, aunties, and a host of cousins who needed a place to stay until they got on their feet. How ironic that they made a home there, on the street named for the patron saint of lost and stolen things. How many things had my parents lost or had stolen away? I will never know, but I know that they moved there with the sincere hope of finding them.

Our neighborhood was unique. Although segregation was de rigueur in Mobile, it had once been white. I knew this because there were remnants of that whiteness all around.

We lived next door to the old Marine hospital, which during the Civil War supposedly treated both Union and Confederate soldiers, although I have my doubts about how many Union soldiers were treated there before the city was taken. By the time my family moved in beside it, the once-grand Greek Revival building had been repurposed into a tuberculosis asylum, never mind that a cure for tuberculosis had already been discovered. And who thought it was a good idea to put a TB hospital directly across the street from an elementary school in the middle of a residential area? As a child, I watched TB patients scale the six-foot brick wall that was supposed to keep them in. Then I watched them blend seamlessly into the neighborhood, only to return by nightfall.

One block to our west was the city hospital, Old Mobile General. Another approximation of neoclassical architecture, Old Mobile General provided a lovely facade for the completely separate and unequal medical care it delivered inside. Black patients entered through the "colored only" entrances in the rear and were attended by white doctors and white staff in segregated wards. In the 130 years of its existence, no Black doctors were allowed to admit patients there.

I say all of this to illustrate how much has changed in our orientation to medical care and its orientation toward us—and how much has not.

Too many of the geographic, economic, and cultural barriers that shaped healthcare in the Jim Crow South of my childhood persist throughout the country to this day. The world's most recent pandemic refocused our attention on preexisting inadequacies and biases in our healthcare system but offered no new solutions. And the same issues that have disfigured the system since its inception have given rise to our often-dysfunctional relationships with it.

Case in point: My four oldest siblings were born at home on the farm in my mother's tiny birthplace, a town so small and rural it didn't have a proper name. It shouldn't surprise you to know it didn't have a hospital either. After my family moved to the city, my parents' fifth child was born in a "colored" maternity hospital run by Catholic nuns. Surely my mother expected the care there would be at least marginally better than a home delivery—but it must not have been, because baby number six was born at home.

My mother delivered her next child at Old Mobile General, the segregated hospital a block away from our house. Seven years later, she gave birth to me, her eighth and last child, in her bedroom on St. Anthony Street. Just twelve years later, she died. So, I was never able to ask my mom why she made the choices she did, or to learn how her treatment compared in these very different institutions. But without uttering a word, her actions spoke volumes. One doesn't need psychic powers to know that neither Mobile's segregated hospital, with its white-only physicians and "colored only" wards, nor the crowded "colored" hospital, with its substandard tools, made my mother feel cared for, or safe.

Bear in mind that Mom had come of age in a place with no hospital, no doctors nearby, and truth be told, no effective treatments for most illnesses even when a doctor was summoned—and doing so was no small thing.

First of all, you had to have the money to pay the doctor. Most folks did not. Second, you had to get in your horse-drawn buggy (remember, this was the 1920s in rural Alabama—very few people owned cars) and travel miles to go get him (it was always a "him" in those days). Just imagine if nearly every time a doctor was summoned, someone was grievously ill and quite possibly near death. And so you were rarely sure whether the doctor had actually helped or hurt. Would you be quick to seek medical help? Exactly.

And let's not forget that in my parents' day, these doctors were practicing medicine before antibiotics or insulin, before high blood pressure medicine, and in many cases, without anesthesia. There really wasn't much in that old black bag except maybe a stethoscope, some bandages, a tourniquet, catgut sutures, and a bone saw. Doctors were associated with trauma, some of which they caused. Given that, even house calls must have been a terrifying experience. Imagine the agony that was witnessed; imagine how it felt to be sick and in a doctor's so-called "care." These deeply disturbing associations were cemented in the minds of generations of people, my mother's included.

Mom believed in hard work, education, and the power of God—not necessarily in that order. She insisted on a clean house and did virtually no socializing outside of her church and family. And she was deeply suspicious of white people, especially of white doctors and their versions of care. With this history, is it any wonder that when my proud, self-contained mother got sick in her mid-50s, she didn't seek help until she was so ill that there was no viable option for treatment?

And is it any surprise that, for better or worse, her orientation toward doctors (and what little we experienced of their orientation toward her) shaped her children's suboptimal approach to medical care? Even mine.

My siblings and I had no model for interacting with doctors on anything but an urgent basis. We knew medical treatment was expensive and hard to access. Even when it helped you, there was little to recommend it or make you want to repeat the experience.

Sadly, despite the amazing medical advances available today, that general point of view still stands, especially if you're poor, or a person of color, or elderly, or female, or a resident of a remote area, or—God forbid—any combination of these. Geographic and economic inaccessibility, lack of representation, lack of adequate facilities, lack of information (both within patient communities *and* within the medical community), and lack of trust: These are not the cornerstones of progress or positive outcomes. So, you're just not sure. But here's the good news: You can be.

In the Changing Medical Landscape, It's Every Woman for Herself

No one is coming to save us [♪ "Wake Up Everybody"]. I mean this in every way possible and I mean for it to motivate, not discourage, you. You must take full charge of your health, and your healthcare.

While the underlying disparities in healthcare remain stubbornly entrenched, the practice of medicine has changed dramatically in the past twenty years. So, you have to shift too. That's just common sense.

Chances are, no one informed you of these changes or how they would impact your life. For the record, no one really informed us doctors either. But we all must adapt—and that begins with understanding the emerging landscape, and then embracing it at least enough to learn how to effectively negotiate its inefficiencies.

We have overlapping trends converging and most are centered not on the individual patient, but on innovative and costly technologies and economies of scale that have all led to the systemic corporatization of medicine. Doesn't exactly give you the warm fuzzies, does it?

Regardless of your race or the deepness of your pockets, for most people, the days of Marcus Welby, M.D., are gone forever (and if you don't know who Marcus Welby is, google him—my God, I'm older than I thought). But, of course, you already knew that. What you may not have realized is how drastically different the average doctor–patient interaction has become—and will continue to be.

The expectation that you will have a relationship with a doctor who is competent, caring, kind, and will be there for you in any medical situation is no longer a reality for most people. The decades-long doctor–patient relationship is history. Sole practitioners or small physician-owned group practices, where the doctors themselves are in control of their time, patients, and office staff, are becoming relics. If you're enjoying one, start looking for a replacement now, because the trends are not on your side.

In fact, you will have increased difficulty getting your doctor to return a phone call, even when you are hospitalized and at your sickest. Oh, you will see *a* doctor there, perhaps several. But you may never see *your* doctor there. Most people don't realize that, generally speaking, primary care doctors and internists no longer take care of their patients when they are hospitalized. Rather, your care will be led by a *hospitalist* (yes, that's a real word), and if you don't know what a hospitalist is, you are not alone. A hospitalist is a doctor, typically employed by a hospital, who only cares for inpatients. They are usually internists or family physicians who manage your care only while you are hospitalized. Most likely, they won't know you. They may or may not have access to your medical records (we'll discuss medical records in a bit). They may or may not inform your primary care doctor that you are in the hospital. If that sounds less than ideal, that's because it is.

How did this happen? First, there is the graying of the doctor population that was oriented toward traditional, personalized patient care. (Have you seen my picture? I'm in that number.) Juggling the demands of seeing patients in the office along with the administrative tasks of running an office while caring for sick patients in the hospital was admittedly a challenge, but no one actually *asked* doctors before moving to this new system. Hospitalists just kinda showed up in the mid-1990s, and just like that, doctors stopped caring for their patients who were admitted to the hospital. (To be clear, if you have a surgical procedure, you should expect to see that surgeon, or at least one of their colleagues, while hospitalized. But for nonsurgical admissions, chances are you will see a hospitalist.)

Hospitalists certainly relieve the stress on busy physicians, and arguably improve patient care, but at a price. From the patient's perspective, there is a decided lack of continuity of care and loss of the comfort that accompanies sheer familiarity. And, in some cases, there is a lack of context for the medical and social issues that preceded the patient's admission. Adding to that, the entire medical community is still in a state of post-pandemic restructuring that, like COVID itself, is stressing and burning out healthcare workers at every level. One recent survey reported that up to 70 percent of doctors are experiencing burnout. A combination of venture capital groups and large hospital conglomerates have bought up private practices across the country, leaving less than 30 percent of doctors in a traditional private practice setting today. And that number is declining.

As the nature of medicine is changing, the people providing regular care is changing. Physician's assistants, nurse practitioners, and traveling—or temporary—nurses are on the rise. Corporate hospital systems are creating large, standardized group practices where the pressure to fuel profits is at least as high as it is to satisfy patients' needs. Younger doctors face the added burden of an unconscionable amount of education debt that, as employees, may make them less loyal to their jobs.

This corporate takeover was made possible by the mounting inability of solo practitioners and small groups to manage the escalating rent, utilities, malpractice insurance, and personnel costs against rising patient needs and declining insurance reimbursements. Concierge medicine has stepped into the void left by the disappearing small group practices and comes at a high premium, which the average patient cannot afford.

Get What You Need When You Need It—Don't Wait!

So, where does all of this leave you?

Well, in addition to the fact that an increasing amount of your care may not be delivered by physicians, it means that the medical attention you do receive will not be as personalized or consistent. It is also just a matter of time before artificial intelligence will become an integral part of your medical care, so get ready. This is not necessarily bad; it is just the new world order, and you need to understand it. In a sense, you are more in charge than ever, so go ahead and own that power. Just know that getting what you need when you need it is going to require considerably more effort on your part. But I am confident that once you know how the system works, you can be an effective manager of your own healthcare.

You should also understand that your relationship with your doctors will have to be flexible, not merely because they are no longer likely to stay in the same job or region for a decade or more. You are less likely to as well. In previous generations, the average person stayed in the same home, or at least state, most of their life. Today, patients change addresses as often as they used to change watch batteries (back when we all still wore watches that required new batteries). Each move or job change you make could require you to pick new doctors, a process that can be more difficult emotionally than it even is practically.

Janet

Janet was a 47-year-old patient I had been treating since her college days. She had surgery for endometriosis in her 20s and she endured several rounds of fertility treatments before conceiving two beautiful babies, whom I delivered. As those babies reached college age, we talked as much about them during her annual checkups as we did about her medical issues, which were, thankfully, few.

One day, when Janet came in for her annual visit, I asked how she was doing. "Okay," she replied, but I immediately knew she wasn't. I handed her my trusty Kleenex box then asked again, and the floodgates opened.

"Oh, Dr. Malone, I'm afraid I have some bad news." Janet and her husband were getting a divorce and she was no longer able to stay on his insurance plan. Our office did not take the insurance that her job offered. Although I would have gladly seen her for less, and she could have paid out of pocket for her annual examinations, she had been putting off some much-needed surgery that she simply could not afford to cover without insurance. So, she was going to have to leave my practice.

After we both made use of the Kleenex, I referred Janet to one of my colleagues who I knew would take good care of her.

The Takeaway: Nothing can replicate a decades-long relationship with a doctor you know and who knows you, but this type of relationship is becoming a relic in today's world. You will have many changes in location and circumstances that will necessitate interruptions in your care. As you make these transitions, don't let the perfect get in the way of the good. Don't neglect your care even if you have to seek it somewhere else with someone new.

Your behaviors and expectations have got to reflect the new paradigm. I hate to say it, but while medicine was once considered a calling, today it has become more of a commodity—so you have to evaluate it the way you would any other commodity, for its value, utility, and ease of use. I know we like to think of medical care as something different, but I assure you it is not.

Suppose you need a pair of basic black pants. You can buy a pair at Walmart, or you can buy them at Neiman Marcus. Are the pants you get at Walmart functional? Yes, they are. Are they the same size and cut as the pants from Neiman's? Yes, and yes (roughly). Are the Walmart pants as good a buy as the pants you get from Neiman's? It depends. The Walmart pants cost less and are machine washable, but they may not last as long. The Neiman pants could last longer, but they'll need expensive dry cleaning. You get my drift. The overarching questions are: What is most important to you, and What pants can you afford? There is no right choice, just the one that's right for you.

The same is true for your medical care. Affordable is not synonymous with low-quality, and expensive doesn't always translate to utility. That is why you need to know what's important—to you. Only then can you effectively evaluate your primary care options.

Start Where You Are

Until our larger societal issues are worked out (a puzzle whose solution is beyond my pay grade and yours), I want you to heed the late tennis star Arthur Ashe, who wisely said: "Start where you are. Use what you have. Do what you can."

It is critical that you establish a dependable medical home. But your first goal should be to make yourself as *well* a patient as you can possibly be. In other words, before we focus on choosing the best doctors for your needs, let's focus on *you* and understanding what your needs actually are.

A lot of what we encounter in medicine is debatable, but the basic building blocks of good health don't change. So, right here, right now, recommit to the six top healthy habits that I promise will slow your aging and improve your life:

- Eat a balanced diet of nutritious whole, unprocessed foods

- Get a good night's sleep

- Move and stretch your body and mind, regularly

- Minimize your stress

- Limit your alcohol intake

- Don't smoke

Notice what's not on this list—losing weight. And yes, that's important. But as we'll see later, if you do these six things, it will be easier to control your weight. In fact, each of these factors contributes to weight gain when not managed properly. We're going to talk more about weight later.

Together, these habits form the North Star of good health. Preventative care is the Holy Grail. Our goal as we age is not just to live longer, but to live a healthier, more functional life. Who wants to live the last decade of their lives housebound? Answer: no one. How you treat yourself in the years approaching midlife will determine how well you live out your last years. Remember when I told you to get familiar with the term *health span*? Our goal is not just to increase your lifespan but your health span as well. Let's face it, wouldn't you rather spend your retirement money on vacations than on medication? Well, to do so requires investing in illness prevention, or as my mother would say, "A stitch in time saves nine." In today's world, many of us don't even know how to sew. Well, I'm going to teach you.

What's on Your Wellness Wish List?

Before you can get what you need, you have to know what you need—and maybe need to change. Start by making an objective list of your most consistent healthcare habits (check them against the list in the previous section). Then ask yourself:

- What are the values that drive (or prevent) your self-care?

- What are your areas of greatest confidence related to seeking healthcare?

- What are your fears about health and aging—and how do they get in your way?

- Who are your healthcare role models and how do they impact your behaviors?

- Who are your healthcare advisors or advocates (this can include your healthcare providers as well as individuals you'd turn to in a crisis), and how do they help or hinder your efforts to manage your medical needs?

The point of this exercise is not to beat yourself up or pat yourself on the back. It's certainly not meant to provoke a pity party—*nobody's* got time for that. The goal is to help you see where you're good and where you can course-correct.

Maybe it's time to get a new internist because yours intimidates you, so you don't speak up in appointments. Maybe this is the week you'll quit smoking or schedule a memory test, even though you're afraid of what it might show. Maybe Aunt Edna, fly as she is at 73, shouldn't be who you model yourself after, since her key to staying trim is a liquid diet—that liquid being gin. It's always high time to do better, wherever you can. As Maya Angelou put it, "When you know better, do better."

To the fatalists who subscribe to the do-nothing/we're-all-gonna-die-anyway approach, you're not completely wrong. You can be minding your own business and every law of the road and still get hit by an eighteen-wheeler. But that's no reason not to get the brakes fixed on your car.

How to Choose a Doctor

In most doctors' offices today, nobody's talking, everybody's typing. No one recognizes your face, knows your name, or asks about your kids. Of course, you'll be seen by a physician, physician's assistant, or nurse practitioner, as well as a nurse or medical assistant. And let's not even discuss artificial intelligence, Yet don't be surprised if in the not-too-distant future you're interacting with Dr. Chatbox. And how often, once you leave, will you really feel like you've been more than just Patient X in Exam Room D on Day 3 of another doctor's dispassionate week on their J-O-B?

The answer to this question depends on how carefully you choose your medical home. Start with your insurance provider and choose a primary care doctor (internist or family practitioner) within that network. If you don't, you'll leave money on the table, and you won't necessarily get any better care.

Run your provider's list by friends and family to see if there's any overlap with doctors they know or can recommend. Also pay attention to:

- **Location:** Annual appointments an hour away might work, but what if you require frequent visits? Or if you are in pain and travel is uncomfortable? Suppose you have mobility issues and walk with a cane or walker—is there ample parking nearby? Is the office easily accessible by public transportation? Convenience matters. A lot.

- **Hospital Affiliation:** Make sure you're comfortable with the ratings and rankings for the hospital your doctor is affiliated with (readily available through several sources online), as well as its proximity to you. You will ultimately want to keep your doctors aligned with the same hospital, if possible.

Once you've identified an option or two, do some sleuthing. Google is not where you should seek a diagnosis (ever!), but it's great for getting intel on some of the following details:

- **Board Certification:** You might be surprised by how many practicing doctors are not board-certified, and ideally you want doctors who are. Although board certification is not a guarantee of good care, it is a helpful data point. This information is available online (I recommend certificationmatters.org).

- **Licensing and Disciplinary Action:** Local and state medical boards maintain databases related to the licensing and disciplining of doctors. These feed into the Federation of State Medical Boards Physician Data Center, a comprehensive repository of the nation's more than 2 million licensed doctors, which includes disciplinary actions and malpractice cases dating back to the early 1960s.

- **Training:** You shouldn't base your decision solely on where a doctor went to school or where they did their residency, but it's still good to know.

- **Online Ratings:** Occasionally worthwhile, but be warned: They're always going to skew negative because happy patients rarely bother to post reviews. The worst online evaluation I ever got was from a man I never met who was mad because I prescribed his 16-year-old sexually active daughter birth control pills. He gave me a "1," but I'm sure his daughter would have given me a "5." And if your doctor has 100 percent 5-star ratings, they may actually be great, but know that there are quite a few ways to juke the stats. Think about it: Was your last Uber ride really a 5-star?

- **Top Doctors Lists:** Media-generated lists of "top" or "best" doctors can help (full disclosure: I've been on a few) but this comes with a giant caveat. They tend to be popularity contests, and often don't surface the most diverse candidates. Also, once you're on them, they're loath to take you off. So, use them to source names, but then do your own sleuthing to learn more.

After you've identified a primary care prospect, call the office and talk to the administrator—an actual human being. They will not be trying to have a long conversation with you, so come prepared and be persistent. Tell them you'd like to become a new patient and want to make an appointment, but you have a few questions first. They should be willing and able to help. If they're not, that's a red flag worth jotting down in a place you reserve for keeping track of your healthcare journey. There are several versions of mass-produced healthcare organizers and journals available online. Whether you prefer one of those or a blank journal, a binder, or a spreadsheet of your own making, create a system you'll depend on long-term. Now is no time to rely on your memory. So, keep scribbling, as you ask:

- What's the average wait time to make an appointment?

- What's the average wait time once I arrive for an appointment?

- How will test results be communicated? (Patient portal? Text?)

- Will I be seeing a doctor most often or a nurse practitioner or physician's assistant?

- Is it okay for me to bring a friend or relative to my appointments?

- Does the office have evening or weekend hours?

- How do you handle emergencies and acute care?

This last one is important because, as a rule, the emergency room should not be your Plan B for nonemergency care (see Chapter 3 for more).

Josephine

Josephine is a 52-year-old woman who has always been in great health. She exercises regularly, sees her primary care doctor annually, and only takes one medication. Just before bedtime one night, she experiences severe pain in the middle of her chest. She feels hot and sweaty and starts to have palpitations, which only make her more anxious.

Concerned that she might be having a heart attack, she calls her primary care doctor's office and gets the answering service. The message starts with, "If you are experiencing a medical emergency, hang up and dial 911." Not sure if this is a real emergency, Josephine leaves a message for her doctor to call her back. She waits . . . and she waits. Thirty minutes go by. Then an hour with no return call.

Now she's really anxious and thinks, *What if I am having a heart attack?* When the pain doesn't go away, she decides to heed the recording on her doctor's after-hours message and she calls 911.

She's taken by ambulance to the emergency room at the nearest hospital (when you call 911, you don't get to choose). Since she's a "rule out MI" (that's medical-speak for possible heart attack), Josephine is seen quickly. She gets an EKG, and her vital signs are taken, all of which are normal.

The ER doctors sense no immediate danger, but to be sure, they draw Josephine's blood and put her gurney in the hallway while they wait for her lab results. Hours go by. The pain in her chest is long gone, but she's too worried to leave. She's also exhausted, hungry, and annoyed at being left in the hallway, where she ends up spending the night.

At 6 A.M., after her bloodwork comes back normal, Josephine is discharged with a standard preprinted chest pain sheet and told to follow up with her doctor in 2–3 days. She is too tired to go to work, but she does schedule the needed follow-up with her doctor. Given his schedule, this is no easy feat, but thanks to Josephine's ER directives, the administrator fits her in two days later.

She arrives at her appointment on time. After a 45-minute wait and another missed day of work, she finally sees her doctor, who asks, "What seems to be the problem?"

Josephine thinks her head is going to explode. "The problem is that I spent the night in the emergency room two days ago. Don't you have my records?"

Okay, I'm going to stop this story right here. You need to know that this is not a unique situation or exaggerated for effect. This happens every day. I don't know when we started adding that sentence, "If you think you are experiencing a medical emergency, hang up and dial 911," to doctors' voicemail greetings, but it changed medical care forever. Just like with the appearance of hospitalists, we didn't discuss it. It just took hold and metastasized. It's as if the entire medical community in America decided that we either could not or would not call our patients back in a timely manner. And if something bad happened, the fallback would be, "Well, I told you to go to the emergency room." Don't get it twisted. That message is not there out of concern for your health. It's about medical liability. It's what we in medicine call a CYA move—as in "cover your ass."

I know. That's terrible, right? We put that "go to the emergency room" thought in your head, and we, the medical profession, have to own it. The problem is, the ER—even if there's one within walking distance of your home—is not a viable substitute for having an established medical home and an accessible doctor to advise you in times of uncertainty.

If Josephine had gotten a timely call back from her doctor, he might have been able to reassure her that she likely was not having a heart attack. A few standard questions could have elicited the fact that she'd just eaten a fast-food burrito, and that she had forgotten to fill the prescription for acid reflux medication he gave her at her last appointment. With that, she may have gotten a little more guidance about when it might be appropriate to go to the emergency room and which ER she should go to, if necessary.

Here is some news you can use: When you show up in an emergency room, they don't know you, and they probably don't know your doctor either. An ER physician will evaluate you and a hospitalist will admit you if you are deemed sick enough to stay in the hospital. If hospitalization is not warranted, you will be sent home with an instruction sheet and told to follow up with your own doctor. And let's be clear, emergency rooms are great for some things and not so great for many others. Trying to figure out what is and is not an emergency is what most patients need help deciding (more on this in Chapter 3). What you should be aware of is the fact that if you do not notify your doctor that you are in the emergency room, the chance that someone in the emergency room will let your doctor know *and* forward your records to their office is not zero, but it's pretty darn close. Bet you didn't know that it is your responsibility to arrange for your records to be sent by any hospital that is not within the same system as your doctor. This is why it is extremely helpful to have doctors and hospitals within the same network. Even if your doctor was not made aware that you went to the hospital, they will at least be able to see the doctor's notes and test results from your visit.

If you are unsure whether your doctor and hospital are in the same network, rather than guess, to be safe, create an online portal account in that hospital system. The nurse or clerk can instruct you on how to sign up. This will allow you to access all records and test results from your recent visit, which can then be printed out and taken to your doctor when you go for your follow-up appointment. It surely would've helped Josephine to know this before showing up at her doctor's office empty-handed, forcing her to wait another ninety minutes for the ER to fax (yes, people, even in 2024, doctors still fax) her records over.

This is one of those moments to confront without flinching. Once more in case you missed it: The system is broken. It is inefficient. And biased and bureaucratic. It often defies logic and reason, and on a bad day, it can actually exacerbate whatever is ailing you by sending your stress levels soaring. Speaking of which, when Josephine got her bill, she discovered that her insurance covered only 80 percent of her ER visit and 0 percent of her ambulance ride. Her total cost for indigestion? More than $2,000.

Congratulations! You Got a New Doctor

You've finally chosen a doctor and made an appointment—preferably a wellness appointment, or routine checkup. (If you've been someone who only goes to the doctor when you're sick, you're done with that!) Show up on high alert because the most important part of your assessment phase begins now.

First impressions matter big-time. Trust your gut. If the office were a restaurant, would you eat there? Order and cleanliness matter. Courteousness and efficiency matter. Plush seating and big-screen TVs in the waiting room? Not so much.

Trust how people make you feel. And here again, heed the wisdom of Maya Angelou, who said: "When someone shows you who they are, believe them the first time." Does your doctor communicate well? How about the support staff? Is everyone on the team receptive to your questions and concerns, or noticeably irked by them? Do they show you *and other patients* respect [♪ "Respect"]? Do they complain or share inappropriate information with you? Are they generally thoughtful and present or do they seem harried, disgruntled, or distracted? If the people who work there seem like they'd rather be anywhere else, you probably should be too.

Need a second set of eyes and ears to help you gauge the quality of your initial visit? Bring a trusted family member or friend to be a fly on the wall, particularly if you will be discussing complicated issues or upcoming surgery. Get their impressions afterward, but remember, this is *your* life, *your* health, *your* doctor, and *your* decision to make.

Keep in mind that nobody's perfect. I know brilliant doctors who I'd never want to party with, and charming doctors who I'd never want to treat me. Bottom line, your doctor should make you feel:

- Confident in their intellect and abilities

- Safe in their presence

- Respected

- Seen and heard

Don't settle. With a shout-out to one of my favorite showrunners, Shonda Rhimes, and all you *Grey's Anatomy* fans: Forget Dr. McDreamy and Dr. McSteamy [♪ **"No Scrubs"**], you need Dr. McSeeMe—literally and figuratively. Like the United Negro College Fund says about a mind, a doctor's visit is a terrible thing to waste. Especially when they can be so hard to get! So, find a practice that values you and your time—and theirs. Make a list of your questions and concerns and get them addressed before making a final decision. Then once you've established that relationship, let your primary care doctor refer you to specialists that you might need. You will get better referrals and better responsiveness if you work with doctors who routinely work with one another.

Concierge Doctors:
Primary Care with a Premium Price Tag

Remember when I told you about those Walmart pants and Neiman pants? Well, think of a concierge doctor as a personal stylist. If you're the type who not only requires designer pants, but also wants someone else to pick them out for you, along with a Chanel blouse and a pair of

Christian Louboutin (hello, red bottoms!) shoes to match, you might consider concierge medicine—but only if you have deep pockets in those pants, because it's going to cost you. A lot.

Concierge medicine is made up of boutique practices that limit the number of patients they take on. Most concierge doctors boast 24/7 availability. They will return your phone calls, make referrals and secondary appointments for you, and send you personalized notes. They often let you take all the time you need, in person or virtually, to get your questions answered. Did I mention that office wait-times are notoriously short? And that some of these doctors even make house calls and have private ERs?

It's the country club of medicine, and like any exclusive club, the price of entry is steep and gaining entry can be competitive. In addition to the costs for care (which may or may not be covered by insurance), concierge practices charge fees ranging from thousands to tens of thousands a year, just for the privilege of membership. That's whether you ever see a doctor during that year or not, and insurance will *not* cover that retainer. Some practices set their fees on a sliding scale based on age, where the older you are, the higher your annual retainer (because they assume older patients will require their services more).

While the heightened accessibility of concierge doctors may make you feel like a VIP, most simply do what regular doctors used to do—just faster. Those Walmart pants aren't looking so bad now, are they?

You Need More Than a Doctor to Ensure You Get Good Care

Checking your primary care doctor box is *huge*. But let's circle back to your primary caregiver: *you*.

What if you suffer an accident at work—who would your employer call? What if you're brought into the hospital by ambulance, too ill to process what's happening or even fill out the intake forms? What if you're unconscious or unable to speak?

While it can be hard to imagine yourself in crisis, you need to prepare for every potential medical interaction—including those where
you can't advocate for yourself. Bottom line: You need backup in the
form of an emergency contact and a health proxy, or medical decision-
maker. These should be trusted, capable people who are also reliable,
reachable, and prepared to make your medical decisions when you
cannot. Ideally, they are also local and physically available, but they
needn't be to be effective.

A recent study conducted at Henry Ford Hospital in Detroit found
that 95 percent of patients admitted to the ER believed that their
emergency contact was the same as their medical decision-maker, even
for end-of-life care. While that may sound logical, it's just not true—
unless you make it true. They can be one and the same, but these roles
are distinctive and equally critical components of your primary care.
With luck, you may never use either, but you absolutely need both.

Emergency Contact: The person who is notified when you are in
an emergency. That's it. They may or may not be able to show up for
you in person, but they need to be reachable and ever-ready with your
information. While they are not empowered to make medical decisions for you, your emergency contact should know your medical history (or where to find it), including any chronic conditions, allergies,
and medications. This can be lifesaving in a crisis. They should be
equipped with up-to-date contact information for your primary care
doctor as well as any additional people you want notified. They should
also be aware of any privacy concerns you have, and you should be
confident that they will respect your wishes.

Healthcare Proxy (or Healthcare Power of Attorney): This person
has the legal authority to make medical decisions on your behalf when
you are unable to do so, even if they are not physically with you. This
requires written documentation, and since this is a legal document,
make sure you know what the requirements are in your state, as they
do vary.

You should fully discuss with the person (or people) you choose for
these roles what each responsibility includes. Press, like flight atten-

dants do if you're sitting in the exit row, for their articulated consent. They should be clear on your thoughts about life support and end-of-life options and be committed to advocating for *your wishes,* even if yours differ drastically from their own. And keep in mind that, as with your primary care physician, changes in your life or theirs may necessitate changes in who fulfills these key roles.

DR. SHARON'S RX FOR

Getting and Managing Good Primary Medical Care

1. Pick a primary care doctor within your insurance network who is affiliated with the hospital system you wish to be admitted to if something happens.

2. Ask that doctor for specialists within the same provider network. It is always better to have doctors within the same network. They may know one another and will have access to your electronic medical record across specialties without you having to provide it.

3. Check your insurance coverage so you know exactly what is and is not covered. Find out ahead of time where you should go for lab work, mammograms, X-rays, etc. Going out of your insurance network can be costly but is sometimes necessary. If so, make sure you understand your out-of-network provider's costs, and shop around, if possible.

4. Always sign up for your practice's patient portal. Not only does this facilitate communication and making appointments (so you can avoid Automated Phone System Hell), but your medical records and test results can be accessible there.

5. If you choose to see a doctor outside of your network, know that you are responsible for providing your medical records. Technology has revolutionized medicine, but it still has its limits, and they will sometimes surprise you. Electronic medical records from different offices or hospital systems do not talk to one another. Never assume that your doctor has sent *anything* to another doctor, even if they referred you to them.

6. Have a good reason for why you might want to see a doctor out of network. Common things happen commonly, but occasionally you might become something you only want to be at a dinner party—interesting. If you have a problem that is not easily diagnosed or if you need a procedure that your doctor has rarely done, then by all means seek a more experienced opinion. It is quite acceptable to ask your doctor questions like "Have you ever treated this before?" or "When was the last time you did a surgery like this?" No doctor worth his or her salt should be offended by a second or expert opinion.

7. Keep a list of all your medications and doses handy (birth control pills, supplements, and stool softeners count), as well as your known allergies and emergency contacts. Your phone and wallet are good places to start. And your health proxy should be kept up-to-date on this info too. (See Chapter 12 for more.)

8. Do not call an ambulance unless necessary. Ambulances will take you to the nearest hospital, which may not be where your doctors are affiliated. They are costly and not always covered by insurance.

CHAPTER 2

Family Affair♪

Knowing Your History Helps You Build a Brighter Future

Dear Sis,

Health, like wealth, is not something we discuss enough, even within our families.

We will hold court and spill the tea on all manner of personal triumph and mess, yet we've been raised to believe our health is our private business and our own cross to bear. As a result, not only are we rarely clear about our health histories, we also haven't been taught how vitally important they are.

Add to that, in Black families there's a tradition of plowing forward and not looking back. Generations of trauma will do that to you. Intimidated by tight-lipped elders' and our own fear of the unknown, we don't ask the questions that keep us up at night. We just keep losing sleep.

That—*all* of that—has to change.

No matter how complicated or murky your family tree is (and trust me, I know how tangled and frustrating family ties can be), it's time to get all the answers you can about your genetic health. Ignorance is not bliss when it comes to your medical history. The old adage "What you don't know can't hurt you" is a lie. What you don't know can kill you, unnecessarily and too soon. Moreover, what you *do* know might just save your life. And remember, I got you!

xo, Dr. Sharon

Bertha Davis Malone was born in 1914 in a speck on the map of Alabama affectionately known as "up the country." My mother never spoke of her childhood. She shared no stories that began "when I was a little girl" or "my mother used to . . ." And she certainly didn't talk about the things I would have been the most curious about, like sex. Church lady that she was, no doubt her advice would've been a simple, "Don't, until you're married."

On countless other subjects, I will never know where she stood [♪ "A Song for Mama"]. And lest I think that by the time I came along my mother had simply exhausted her storytelling days, I confirmed with my older brothers and sisters that they heard no stories either, even about seemingly obvious things. My mother had a crescent-shaped scar about the size of a half-dollar just to the left of her mouth, and to this day, neither I nor any of my siblings has any idea how she got it. She never talked about it and we never asked. How crazy is that?

My mom worked hard, sang in the choir, loved her family, and kept her own counsel to the very end—an end that came too soon.

Her premature death changed everything for me and the rest of our family. The magnitude of losing her when she and I were both so young haunts me to this day. But my feelings about her death were compounded years later when I learned that it wasn't an isolated tragedy in our family. It seems that I come from a long line of women who didn't live long enough to impart the wisdom that only comes with time. Neither of my grandmothers lived to see 50.

My mom was 14 when her mother, Edna Davis, died. Edna was only 44. Out of necessity, Mom and her 16-year-old sister became the women of the house, cooking, cleaning, and caring for their three younger siblings and each other. No longer able to attend school, they had to learn how to mend things and manage the many illnesses, cuts, scrapes, and bruises that children inevitably have. They did so with little in the way of resources or support. I ache to think that, like me, they hadn't had enough time for conversations with their mother about growing-up things like puberty and the changes womanhood brings. I suppose they at least had the benefit of having observed her for the decade before she died. And I'm sure there were aunties and elders to advise them and occasionally lend a hand. That's about all I know.

Bertha was the type of woman who could impart a whole life lesson with a look, and she often did. What she did not do was look back or ask why. Given how harsh life was for Black people in the segregated South, there was little good to be gained from doing either. So, I have no idea what killed her mother or Charlotte Malone, my father's mother, who also died in her 40s.

Was it childbirth? Cancer? Did Charlotte have an aneurysm or fatal allergic reaction to something she didn't know enough to avoid? Had Edna been sickly or was she suddenly struck down, leaving seven children, three under the age of 10? It's more than likely my parents didn't know either.

In those days, no one spoke of the causes of death because the knowing didn't make your loved ones any less dead. Who was going to be there to make the diagnosis anyway, when access to healthcare was so limited? But how many lives in my family and yours would have been saved, and still could be, if we understood how important knowing our medical history is?

A couple of years after my mother died, her younger sister, my aunt Mildred, also succumbed to colon cancer. I wonder now—did she even know that her older sister died of colon cancer? Did anyone tell her? If she'd had that information, might she have gotten checked out sooner? Again, who knows? At least my siblings and I knew and have been vigilant about regular colon cancer screenings. But how might knowing more about our family's health have further helped my siblings, nearly every one of whom has had some form of cancer? And how much more vigilant might my mother have been about her health if she'd known what took her own mother from her at such a young age?

Like me and mine, you and your biological family members share genes, or DNA (short for *deoxyribonucleic acid*—so now you know why we stick with the acronym). You might also share common behaviors or diets. You might share environmental health risks because of where you live, and you might share religions or philosophies that shape your lifestyle and approach to healthcare. Any or all of these create the likelihood that you share a heightened risk for certain diseases or health conditions, as well as patterns in how you age.

A family health history is a written record of these things, and having one can greatly impact the quality and length of your years. It's not just a chronicle of your family's past health. It's a driver for living with greater intention, greater agency over your healthcare, and a greater sense of control. It's a tool for bringing family together and strengthening your bond and commitment to one another. And it's a road map to the future, marked by guideposts and red flags that can alter how you live, and think about living, in meaningful ways. Creating a record of your family's history and using it can improve not only your life and your loved ones', but the lives of family members not yet born.

As women of a certain age (and women of color, especially), one of the most stubborn barriers to our receiving quality medical care is the stunning lack of collective data available on us. There is a long history in medicine of excluding women from clinical trials, often under the guise of "protective" protocols and governmental policies. To be clear, these measures have always been purely patriarchal in nature. It was not until 1993 that the NIH mandated the inclusion of women in large clinical trials, and unfortunately, the largest clinical trial involving menopausal women was dangerously misinterpreted. To date, there have been no large-scale studies addressing the special health concerns of perimenopausal women. Additionally, women of color are still woe-fully underrepresented in most clinical trials.

This lack of attention paid to women's health as we age minimizes our status as tax-paying citizens, limits our rights and freedoms, and is baked into the system to this day, impeding the quality of our health-care at every stage of our lives. (*Do not* get me started on our reproduc-tive rights—that's a whole 'nother book.) Our voices have not been heard. And that is precisely why you must find it within yourself to raise your voice and demand solutions to the healthcare challenges that have persisted since time immemorial.

Every time you fill out a medical intake form—that long question-naire you receive whenever you see a new doctor—you have an oppor-tunity to be seen and heard in a powerful way. Do not just check boxes and regard it as routine. This is your doctor asking you who you are and what you're bringing to the table. Tell them! Scribble in the mar-gins and write notes on the back if you have to. In order to be seen, it's incumbent upon you to show up every chance you get, with every-thing you've got.

A Medical Family Tree: What's in It for Me?

Did you ever go on a diet that requires you to start each day on the scale? The reason so many weight-loss programs include this is not to torment you (although I know it can feel that way some days). It's been proven that weighing yourself every morning makes you conscious throughout the day of doing the things—eating better, exercising, drinking lots of water—that will keep you and your scale on the right track.

A well-maintained medical family tree (see the Additional Resources section on how to create one) has a similar cascading effect. It should be a living document, a trusty reference kept updated in real time. The base is your own medical history. Add the histories of your parents and grandparents, if possible, and siblings and children if you have any.

As you build it out, patterns will emerge. Questions will surface. Stories will be shared. Pathways to better health will be revealed. It may not all be pretty, but it will be incredibly empowering.

Once upon a time we kept a reliable record of births and deaths in the family Bible. Occasionally, there were brief notes beside the dates. "TB," for tuberculosis. "Nervous," implying mental illness. "Car accident." Or "Fever," which could indicate a virus or infection. Even small clues can give you a more vivid picture of the past. The dates alone, telling you how long your people lived, are like breadcrumbs you may follow to gain a clearer sense of your future.

Until recently, each generation has tended to live longer than its predecessor (sadly, COVID set us back). If you've already had a few centenarians in your family, then buckle up, you're probably in for a long ride. If you're related to several alcoholics, don't make a habit of happy hours (not that any of us should!). The bottom line is, no matter what there is to know—good, bad, or indifferent—you will likely live better, feel better, and do better by your family for knowing.

First Things First: Your Personal Health History

You've heard the phrase "garbage in, garbage out"? It's the first lesson of data science, shorthand for the idea that poor-quality input always yields faulty output. Sadly, one of the most glaring examples of this was the ill-fated Women's Health Initiative, which could have had a profoundly positive effect on our understanding of women's health. Instead, it was stopped early, and the repercussions of that abrupt halt have interrupted vital information about the effects of hormone therapy after menopause. More on that later. What you must understand is that every interaction you have with a doctor, from your regular annual physical to an emergency room crisis, will begin with your medical history. The more accurate and comprehensive the information *you* provide about your health, the higher your likelihood of getting the treatment you deserve and the outcomes you desire moving forward.

Creating a comprehensive record of your own health is much easier than trying to uncover the fate of your late, great cousin, twice removed—and far more important. Start by writing down the most obvious stuff, which you can channel by looking for guidance online (see Additional Resources) or recalling every intake form you've ever filled out on your first trip to a doctor's office:

- Age, height, and weight

- Immunizations (tetanus, diphtheria, and pertussis [collectively known as Tdap], hepatitis, HPV, COVID, and shingles vaccines)

- Allergies (including drug or food allergies)

- Chronic conditions (e.g., diabetes, high blood pressure, arthritis, lupus)

- Medicines (including herbal supplements, vitamins and minerals, oral contraceptives, and hormone supplements, with dosages), as well as the doctors who prescribed them

- Hospitalizations and surgeries

Try to get *all* the information about yourself that you can, including things that may seem minor. Most of us never know anything about our births other than we made it, but we are learning that even random details about your mother's obstetric history can have profound implications for you. So, it's worth finding out if you were born prematurely or your mother had difficulty getting pregnant. Did she have frequent miscarriages? Did she require emergency treatment during or immediately after delivery?

I only found out last year from my sister Joyce that my mother took a long time to recover after my birth. Mom was never one to take to her sickbed, so this was startling to me. Did she bleed excessively? Did she have postpartum depression (even though there was no name for it in those days)? At the age of 45, was she just exhausted at the prospect of caring for a new baby?

These details can matter long-term, if not to you then perhaps to your children when they are expecting. If you were born in a hospital or someplace that kept records, seek them out. You might be surprised by what you learn. I certainly was.

That's why it's also critical to engage family members, young and old, in this project. Send them copies of your medical family tree as it grows. Seeing in black and white where they fit or how they could help you might trigger their memory or motivate them to fill in some blanks. Allow it to spark ongoing, open multigenerational conversations. Discuss it freely with your doctors so they understand that you are knowledgeable, resourceful, and actively engaged in your care. Again, this will push them to *see you* and do better by you, which, at the end of the day, is why we go to the doctor in the first place.

At the start of every interaction with a new physician, expect to be required to list these fundamental facts in writing before you are examined. (If no one asks for this, it's a giant red flag. Make like Jordan Peele and *Get Out!*) But don't expect your doctor to draw connections or seek your opinion about which parts of it you think are most important. *Always assertively raise your voice about any information you believe your doctor should know, even if it's right there in black and white.* You would be surprised by how many doctors fail to read your chart—even when you are hospitalized.

In any emergency situation, your health history is the starting point for your receiving care, so your emergency contact should be accessible and kept up-to-date on this information, as should your medical proxy (see Chapter 1). We tend to think of health as a very private matter, but that attitude can handicap your ability to have support and effective advocacy, should you be really sick and need it.

Immunizations are a key part of your health history. While vaccines have become a source of global debate and divisiveness of late, let me state unequivocally and for the record that immunizations are one of the great public health success stories of all time. Are they completely without risk? No. But nothing is. As a child, I had measles, mumps, and chicken pox, which I would wish on no one. Perhaps you yourself have had shingles. You certainly know someone who has. The good news is, thanks to vaccines, future generations will be far less impacted by these diseases than previous generations were.

There are decades of indisputable evidence to show that adhering to the long-established guidelines for vaccinations from infancy through adulthood prevents tens of thousands of deaths; avoids millions of incidents of disease, including cancer; and saves billions of dollars per decade. It is generally presumed in the United States that anyone over 40 has received at minimum their full schedule of childhood vaccines for preventable diseases, including measles, mumps, and rubella; polio; and Hib (Haemophilus influenzae type b). There are other vaccines that you should get as an older adult, such as shingles, pneumonia, tetanus, flu, and COVID. Discuss with your doctor which ones are appropriate for you, and when you should have them. If you have not had these, make sure your doctors are aware of this.

Whatever your views on immunizations are, we all learned important lessons during the COVID pandemic about their usefulness and limitations. Medicine is rarely black and white, so you need to learn to make decisions in the grays. You will find that I frequently echo something my mother often said: "Don't let the perfect get in the way of the good." In healthcare, as in almost all things, I have found this to be unassailably wise advice.

Your Rights, Your Records, and Where to Find Them

We've all faced some tough lessons lately in the chaos that ensues when "alternative facts" take over. So, whenever possible, get medical records—and keep them organized and accessible. You know how we're supposed to keep three to seven years of tax returns on file? Take a similar approach to family medical records, especially those that are too old to be available digitally.

There are codes of privacy around health, and for good reason.

These enable *you* to be in charge of who has access to your health information and who does not. But, by law, you always have the right to obtain your own medical records, including billing information, test results, doctors' notes, and lab reports.

Doctors closing a practice are legally and ethically required to transfer their patient records to another provider and to inform their patients of where their records can be found. If your doctor is retiring from a practice that will still be operating, your records should remain on file there. If you decide to leave that practice as well, you'll have to request that your records be transferred. In any case, it can't hurt to ask for the records themselves.

The good news is that in the future, there will be no papers to lug around, but many doctors' offices are still operating in the Dark Ages. They may provide you with copies of medical records and charge you by the page! Fortunately, with electronic records, this will become a rarity.

By law, prenatal and delivery records must be maintained for a prescribed number of years that varies by state. In the District of Columbia, where I practiced, those records had to be maintained until the child reached the age of maturity, which is 21. Yes, you heard me right, you or your child has the right to sue your obstetrician until that child reaches adulthood. Now you know why our malpractice insurance is so high.

If you're lucky enough to see your doctor only once a year, know that a lot can occur in twelve months, including your doctor's unexpected death or an abrupt office closing. Private practices are being bought up by hospitals or venture capital groups at a record pace. Currently only about 30 percent of doctors own their practices and that number is dropping. In the wake of the COVID epidemic, doctors are closing practices and quitting medicine in unprecedented numbers. Hopefully, most of the information that you would need access to, such as operative reports, delivery records, and pathology reports, would have been scanned into your electronic record or be available at the hospitals where your surgeries or tests took place.

You will likely have to pay for printed copies of any medical records—and be aware that there can be dozens of useless documents on file. To avoid any unhappy surprises, you should get an estimate for printing costs beforehand. Better yet, request that your records be delivered to you digitally, so you can print only the pages you need.

What happens to your electronic records in the face of a sudden office closure? Now would be a good time to explain how electronic medical records work.

Marie

Marie is 56 and has spent most of her career in the foreign service. For much of the past thirty years, she has lived overseas. She dutifully returns home each year for her annual examination with the same doctor.

She has a complicated medical history, including multiple surgeries for precancerous conditions that put her at elevated risk. She doesn't keep close track of her test results or when she should follow up, because her doctor normally does that for her and reminds her when her next test is due.

She also has had a hysterectomy and one of her ovaries removed, she just can't remember on which side. She had genetic screening done for breast and colon cancer at her last visit but doesn't recall getting the results. Her doctor said they would be available on the practice's portal. But Marie, who stays on top of things related to her work and family but is notoriously unreliable about her own health records, never set it up.

While she was out of the country, Marie's doctor closed her practice. A notification sent via email and snail mail gave patients eight months to make arrangements to get their medical records and find new doctors. Marie, who never opened either communication, learned about the closure when she called to schedule her annual appointment and the phone number was no longer in service. She tried frantically to get in touch with someone to find out how to access her records, to no avail.

"Shouldn't someone be able to get my records for me?" she pleaded when we met.

"What's the name of the specialist who did your biopsies?" I asked her.

"I don't remember," she said, finally coming to grips with her reality.

"We might be able to track them down," I told her. "But it is going to take considerable detective work to do so."

The Takeaway: Keeping track of your medical information is your responsibility, no one else's.

You can see how this can become a problem—and not an uncommon one. I'm going to sound like a broken record here, but if your doctor has an electronic portal, you're in luck. Confirm that your records will be readily accessible there and use it! Trying to figure out one more password is a pain, I know, but it's important.

If you're old-school, be old-school-organized and keep a good old-fashioned file of pertinent paper documents. Even if you're totally tech-savvy and trying to save our trees, it's not a bad idea to print out the important stuff so it's accessible on a no-Wi-Fi day!

Bottom line: You must be able to access your medical records. So, however you handle it, *handle it.*

And again, give copies to your emergency contact (and your health proxy, if that's a different person) because if you are unconscious, good luck getting logged in to your portal or some locked file cabinet.

Requests for records may be made through your patient portal, fax, standard mail, or in person, of course. Should you call, the office administrator will still require your request in writing. Plan to follow up; never assume that just because you asked for your records to be sent, they actually were. A better bet is that they were not. If you want to expedite the process, call ahead and then go in person. Bring your ID and be prepared to sign a release.

If you've had surgeries that required implants, such as knee, breast, heart valve, or mesh, the surgical notes should include the model and brand, which could be important in the event of a recall or a problem with your implant, even years later. You may be given a card with the type and serial number of your implanted device. Hold on to it or take a snapshot with your phone and keep the original card in a safe place.

To obtain records for others over whom you don't have legal guardianship (elderly parents or other family members who may need you to advocate for them or serve as their health proxy), you'll need to produce their written, in some cases notarized, permission for every record you seek.

Start Talking

I have already lived more years than my mother. Having raised my children to adulthood, I cannot imagine the heartbreak of dying, all the while not knowing if your youngest children would remember you. As a daughter, I am filled with longing for answers to the many questions I never knew to ask my parents. As a physician, I am haunted by the medical history that our family lost when they died.

I don't want that for you. If you are fortunate enough to still have your parents (and other elders), it is your duty to find out everything you can from them before it's too late.

Cracking open a Pandora's box is never easy. The CDC promotes

Thanksgiving as National Family Health History Day to encourage families to use that time together (rarer in modern life than ever) to talk about their health and general wellness. Holidays, birthdays, or other times when your family gathers (even funerals or memorials, when health may be top of mind for everybody) offer an opportunity to introduce the idea that the family that talks about their health will individually and collectively thrive in ways that other families won't.

The CDC's tips for making these conversations productive:

- Explain why talking about health and creating a medical family tree matters. (Feel free to quote me!)

- Educate your family about common hereditary disorders.

- Celebrate and give thanks for any family health wins. This could be anything from Uncle Jimmy quitting smoking to Grammie's new hip allowing her to dance the Cha Cha Slide again.

- Share your own health concerns or habits that are benefiting you.

Being candid about your health journey may help your relatives open up about theirs. Allowing yourself to be vulnerable will encourage a mutuality of trust and caring. You can't expect others to do what you're not willing to do. And, while it can be awkward, inquire about people's health. Most people love to talk about themselves, they just need to be asked.

If, despite your best efforts, some relatives won't talk or can't remember, I understand—the struggle is real! But don't let that stop you, or even slow you down. There's just too much at stake.

Gloria

Gloria is 55, a bit overweight, and was recently diagnosed with hypertension. At her previous doctor's visit, a year ago, she was also told that she was prediabetic. She wasn't surprised by either of these diagnoses because two of her older siblings, her mother, and her father all had at least one of those conditions.

Six months after Gloria's diagnoses, her mother died suddenly of a stroke. Her mother had been the primary caregiver for her father, who is on dialysis. With the family in crisis, Gloria decides to change her life. She and her sisters vow that their parents' fate will not be theirs.

They meet three times a week for a two-mile walk, and they trade healthy versions of their traditional soul food recipes. They use the walks to talk openly about what being healthy means and their struggles with it. These are sometimes difficult conversations, but they are doing more to improve the long-term health and vitality of their family than any medication could. Oh, and by the way, Gloria has lost ten pounds and she is no longer prediabetic.

The Takeaway: Silence is never empowering. The price of silence can be a failure to thrive.

My family was like most Black families, where conversation is not the preferred medium of teaching. My theory is that there was too much hurt, trauma, and fear to articulate. It doesn't help that illness often walks hand in hand with isolation, and even shame. I can't tell you the number of patients I've treated who kept things like fibroids, infertility, and even cancer hidden because they felt embarrassed. Did they believe that their illness was their fault? Did they have a need to be seen as strong, even indestructible? I don't know, but hiding from loved ones handicaps us, and them.

I still long for the many talks my mother and I never had. But I realize that these imaginary life-changing moments are a fantasy that probably would never have been fulfilled even if my mother had lived, because like many of your mothers and grandmothers, my mom was a woman of her generation. God bless them all. They did the best they could with what they had [♪ **"Grandma's Hands"**]. But we've got to do better and equip our daughters and nieces to do better too.

We are living in another time. We have access to far more information and support, and we must leverage that to transform the silence and secrets we've inherited into something that will benefit future generations. We owe them our stories, our trials, and our truths. Without this, they are at greater risk than they need to be.

A cloud of secrets, lies, and unsolved mysteries hovers in the air around virtually every family. As women, we are especially protective of our loved ones, not wanting them to have to worry or fear for themselves, or us. We've got to get over that. No matter how good your intentions may be, your health outcomes will never be served by secrecy, vanity, or deception.

Keep It Simple, Stick to the Facts (and Make It Fun!)

Compiling and being the keeper of your family health history is not a small responsibility. But it can be a game changer. So, embrace it and don't overcomplicate it.

Remember, it includes just three generations of basic information: yours, your parents', and your grandparents'. Anything you record beyond that will be a bonus (and minor miracle), useful but not essential.

There's no need to channel your inner Alex Haley or hire a genealogy consultant. Keep it doable! And try to keep it light (health doesn't need to be heavy).

Technology makes it much easier. Start a family chat or email chain to introduce the idea. Outline what you need. As the late, great General Colin Powell once said, "Have a vision. Be demanding." But don't be a PITA (pain in the . . .).

Aim for consistency. Maybe once a month, post an article that might spark lively conversation—even debate is good! New information and inspiring health stories will benefit everyone. And funny health-related memes or jokes can't hurt. For example, "My boyfriend threatened to leave me because he couldn't handle my OCD. I told him to sweep the floor and close the door five times on his way out." Or this one: "Does an apple a day keep the doctor away? Yes, but only if you aim well."

Okay, maybe not that one. But you get the idea. Encourage and engage your family members, but don't burden or beat them over the head with endless questions and boring medical stats.

Above all, keep it factual. Don't guess or embellish or accept information that doesn't add up. Don't assume that old family lore or some story you overheard at your aunt's birthday party, *after* everybody took their turn at toasting her, is true. If you're over 40, you already know firsthand that memory is subject to mistakes—and biases. So, make every effort to compare stories and confirm critical details.

You can also search old family pictures for health clues. Who was smoking? Who was alarmingly thin? Who was confined to a wheelchair? Who was missing from the reunion because they were recovering from a surgery everybody was being sketchy about? Historically, "women's troubles" and mental health issues were banished to a black hole of denial and secrecy, and too often still are. Do what you can to shine a light on them.

Be transparent about what you're doing and why. Write down everything, even if it doesn't sound important. When in doubt, indicate what you know to be true, and what you don't. Also, don't judge the facts. Stay open to what is shared, with compassion. And look for patterns. This is serious business, but it can be fun.

What Can Testing Tell You?

Genetics are fascinating and complicated. For example, while not a determining factor in a woman's fertility, it is helpful to know whether your mother struggled to get pregnant or if she had an early menopause. It is also true that multiple births, premature births, miscarriages, gestational diabetes, and postpartum depression can run in families. So do fibroids, and some cancers. But is the main culprit nature or nurture? The answer can be unclear because families share far more than genes.

Mara and Morgan

Mara and Morgan were 14 and 16 when their dad, William, brought them to see me. They were lovely and energetic and beginning to hit their strides in high school. They were also just blossoming into their newfound womanhood.

Their mom had died of breast cancer when they were in elementary school. Their wonderful dad was devoted to raising his two beautiful daughters in the way he knew his wife would have wanted. William was also very worried.

He shared that his late wife died at 48 after a bruising battle with breast cancer, and that she had a daughter from a previous marriage who had also died from breast cancer, at just 34. When I asked about the girls' maternal grandmother, he didn't know when or how she died. She was already gone by the time he met his wife.

Right away, I told William that we had to be especially careful with these girls' breast health and that everything he could learn about their mother's family would be helpful. I knew there was a very strong genetic component, whether I could prove it or not. We agreed that we needed to be extra-vigilant about monitoring the girls for breast cancer without robbing them of the joy of their youthfulness.

We discussed genetic screening for the BRCA1/BRCA2 mutation, a gene most prevalent in high-risk populations, such as Ashkenazi Jews. To be honest, I wasn't optimistic that this would be a productive avenue, because the girls, their parents, and their half sister were all African American. As they got older, I referred them to a breast surgeon who would guide them on the appropriate time to start screening with mammograms and possibly MRIs.

The issue of genetic testing came up again, and after wrangling with the insurance company to get them covered, their blood tests were done. I was shocked when both came back positive for the BRCA1 mutation. In consultation with their breast specialist, they both opted for bilateral mastectomies with reconstructions in their mid-20s. Neither they nor their father could live with the constant sword of Damocles that hung over their heads, waiting for breast cancer to appear.

Mara and Morgan are now in their early 40s and have beautiful daughters of their own. They remain on alert, because BRCA1 carriers are at higher risk for ovarian cancer as well. Now done with childbearing, they are both preparing to have their ovaries removed. Most importantly, they are healthy and cancer-free.

The Takeaway: We shouldn't make assumptions about who is at risk for what. Genetic testing can be especially helpful for adoptees and others who may not have access to biological relatives or their health history or who, like many of us, just yearn to know more.

We live in the most diverse population in human history. Never has there been so much genetic mixing, although it is surely not new. Ever since African people arrived on these shores, being Black in America has included people with one drop of Black blood as well as the blackest people from the heart of the Sudan. We cannot look at anyone's outward appearance and make assumptions about their genetic makeup. As my auntie would say, "When you assume, you make an *ass* out of *u* and *me.*"

Whereas genetic testing used to be exorbitantly expensive and only check for one or two things, now you can get tested for over a hundred genetic mutations for less than $100. Let me add a word of caution here, though: We don't really know what nearly ninety of these mutations actually mean. So, be intentional about what it is you are looking for and realistic about what you'll learn. Also, be careful. Many commercially available genetic tests are notoriously unreliable. I recommend that any genetic results about medical conditions be confirmed by a reliable medical lab, especially when testing for conditions such as cancer or Alzheimer's genes.

Having a genetic mutation and having a disease are two completely different realities. Genetic tests can only give you probabilities, not certainties. If you don't have a family history of one of the more common mutations screened for—like hereditary breast, ovarian, or colon cancer—ask yourself, "Is this going to change what I do or is it merely going to stress me out?" Only you know the answer; let it lead you.

Personally, I resisted genetic testing for years. Back then, the test's cost (more than $3,000) was not covered by my insurance. But my calculation included two sisters, two aunts, and at least one first cousin who had survived breast cancer—on top of my mom's and aunt's early deaths from colon cancer. For years, I chose not to get tested because whether I had the gene or not, it wasn't going to change my family history or my behavior. I didn't need a test to know that my risk for breast and colon cancer was elevated. So, I chose to do everything in my power to minimize those risks. This included religiously keeping up with my annual mammograms and having colonoscopies early and often. Eventually, I did get tested, and I was negative. Does that matter? Not really, because there is clearly something going on in our family, be it nature or nurture. Am I going to relax my vigilant screening and lifestyle changes because I don't have the gene? Absolutely not!

In recent years, there's been a dramatic rise in genetic testing through companies that market their services more affordably. Whether a genetic testing company brands itself as beneficial to your health or plays on your desire to uncover your geographic or familial roots, know that the two are linked. In other words, your search for family could reveal unexpected information about your health and your search for health info could reveal more about your family than you ever wanted to know (or thought possible).

As when faced with any choice, you should do your homework and compare options. But remember, the right decision for you isn't about perfection or guarantees, and no one but you has to understand your decision. In addition to costs, examine privacy policies. Understand what these companies do with your data and what your related rights are. And don't forget, the biggest consumers of DNA testing are law enforcement agencies. As I told my children after I did genetic testing, don't commit any crimes out there, because they got you.

Genetics Are Not Destiny

I was quietly terrified the year I turned 57. Outside of trying to stay sane while raising three teenagers, I was good—healthy, busy, basically happy. But my mother died at 57, and that singular marker hung on the calendar like a noose. I had a family full of older siblings, some by twenty years. But it wasn't until I turned 58 that I exhaled.

So, let me repeat: Genetics are not destiny. Choosing to believe that you will inevitably be saddled with illness because it runs in your family is not helpful or necessarily true. It will lead you to normalize disease and disability. To wit, I say, "No ma'am!" Steer away from the foolish logic that can arrest your progress and your joy! Creating a family health history doesn't condemn you to sickness any more than creating a will (or the advent of my 57th birthday) hastens death.

To the contrary, confronting your genetic health history gives you power and offers you an *opportunity* to short-circuit generations of preventable problems and premature death, making better health not only a part of your life, but your legacy.

Just because your mother had multiple sclerosis and your father was on dialysis does not mean you're fated for both, or either. We must chip away at anything that makes you complacent about your health, thinking, *Oh well, what the hell,* rather than taking control and turning things around wherever you can.

The truth is, many of the health problems that we attribute to genetics or race have more to do with systemic racism, poverty, and inadequate medical care, as well as lifestyle factors such as poor diet, inadequate sleep, drug or alcohol abuse, or lack of exercise. Not everything is fixable, but you have more control than you think. And that begins with reorienting your notions about fate and foregone conclusions.

You might come from a long line of smokers who died of lung cancer. If you never smoke or quit today, guess what happens to your prospects?

We inherit predispositions and proclivities, not certainties. Remind anyone who dares to suggest otherwise that wealth and poverty run in families, too, but that makes neither a foregone conclusion.

Making Sure Your History Matters

1. Compile a family health history and discuss it with family members.

2. Keep your own medical history updated and make it accessible to your healthcare proxy.

3. Keep a current list of all of your medications (vitamins and supplements too) handy, including dosages and prescribing doctors.

4. Utilize the patient portal from your doctor's office.

5. Print out and keep a file of things like operative and pathology reports, recent test results, and imaging reports.

6. Always bring a copy of your medical record and recent test results to any new doctor.

7. Know whether your records are accessible to anyone outside of your doctor's office.

8. Utilize the health apps that include emergency contacts and test result tracking.

9. Consider whether genetic testing will be beneficial for you.

CHAPTER 3

In the Thick of It♪

Sick or Not-So-Sick?
Be Ready and Make the Right Call

Dear Sis,

There are no other medical doctors on my family tree, but I am a descendant of a long line of healers—women with the good sense, mother wit, and collective ancestral knowledge needed to keep themselves and their families well. I'm guessing you are, too, or we wouldn't even be here.

These women who nursed wounds, delivered babies, applied salves and poultices, concocted remedies, laid on hands, and prayed over us defied the odds and deserve their due.

What they lacked was the knowledge needed to predict and head off the things that they didn't see coming. And *that* (hello, wellness care!) is the great differentiator in long-term health. It cannot always eliminate the chances of bad outcomes, but an ounce of prevention *is* worth a pound of cure. So, I want you to focus on not just how to recognize and treat what ails you, but how to not get sick in the first place.

The truth is that your behaviors matter, and your health shouldn't be left to the luck of the draw. Knowing what we are at risk for helps us avoid health pitfalls as we age. Disease and death will eventually catch us all, but let's not give them a head start.

So, to boost your illness-o-meter (yes, I made that word up), we're going to combine a bit of WWBD (What Would Bertha Do) with a dash of WIWBK (What I Wish Bertha Knew), tossing in some medical know-how and a few best practices for good measure. And to be clear, we'll be leaving Dr. Internet out of it!

xo, Dr. Sharon

One of the most important lessons medical schools teach is one my mom mastered as a teenager left to fill her own mother's shoes: how to figure out who is really sick and needs immediate attention and who can wait (or what we in the medical field call "triage"). Nothing I learned in med school or since has contradicted what I learned at Bertha's knee.

With the exception of one of her sisters, who died as a toddler, my mother and her six remaining siblings survived the 1918 Spanish flu epidemic (the COVID of its day), as well as every childhood communicable disease known to mankind, without conventional medical care.

At the time, the practice of medicine was rudimentary—and that's putting it nicely. So, the diagnoses typically made at home were probably not that different from those of a bona fide doctor. The more serious common ailments were things like dropsy (now known as "swelling" or "edema," due to congestive heart failure); consumption (used to describe any disease that seemed to consume the body, like tuberculosis); weak hearts (for people who tired easily or had fainting spells due to congestive heart failure); and "fits" (which could apply to anything from seizures to strokes). These were terms my mother and aunties still used when I was a child, although I had no idea what they were talking about.

I had twelve years of training to become an OB/GYN and have benefited from some outstanding teachers and colleagues. But I still stand in unmatched awe of my mother's incredible gifts as a diagnostician.

Life is a hard teacher, but those paying attention actually learn—and Mom did. Unlike the isolation from our mothers and aunties that most of us live and raise our families in today, my mother and her people were never far away from one another and a trusted local healer. Leaning into that as well as her own experience and wisdom, Mom handled our healthcare at home—and Nurse Bertha did not play [♪"Superwoman"].

Armed with only the back of her hand to check our temperature, Mom nevertheless had a discerning gaze that not only functioned as a spot-on lie detector, it could also identify any subtle hint of rheuminess. A Jedi master at seeing our family through every manner of minor injury and illness, she had skills that were born of necessity. She couldn't afford to take off every time one of us had a sniffle, nor would she ever have entertained the possibility. So, if Mom decided you were just regular sick, she efficiently deployed a cure—usually some combination of St. Joseph baby aspirin, Luden's cough drops, and Vick's VapoRub. Throw in a cooling alcohol bath if you had a fever, a tablespoon of milk of magnesia if you had a tummy ache (my least favorite "medicine"), and maybe an enema (okay, that's worse), and she could see you through almost anything. Can I get a witness? (And if you don't recognize this regimen, ask your grandmother.)

As big and boisterous as our brood was, no family doctor or pediatrician ever saw our family on a regular basis. An earache, known in today's parlance as an "ear infection," was treated with sweet oil (which I have only in adulthood come to know was olive oil) on a cotton ball stuffed in your ear. I have no idea why it worked, but my siblings and I can all hear. And pediatricians are now acknowledging the overuse of antibiotics in the treatment of many childhood infections. Such treatments were commonly known, but by and large, prevention was not a thing. Sickness, like bad weather before Doppler radar, was unpredictable, unavoidable, and something to be endured.

Mom was confident about what she knew, but she also knew her limits. When my grandfather fell ill and she had done everything she could for him, to no avail, for the first time I saw fear in her eyes. Papa begged her not to, but she took him to the segregated hospital a block away from our house. He hadn't been there but a couple of hours when he had a heart attack and died. She was guilt-ridden, convinced that the overwhelming fright of being at the hospital had been more than he could bear. Maybe that's true, or maybe he was just so sick that there was nothing the doctors could do. But my mother always believed the former and it became just one more reason not to see scary doctors in inhospitable hospitals.

My first memory of ever seeing a doctor was not long after that. I had been sick with a high fever and sore throat, things that I am sure my mother had ministered to many times before. She exhausted her menu of home remedies, but nothing worked. So, after talking to my aunt Ola, who was the closest thing to a medical professional that she had (Aunt Ola was a nurse's aide in the nearby Catholic hospital), they bundled me up and took me to see Dr. Bell, a white general practitioner whose office was not far from where we lived.

We entered through the "colored" door and, after a quick exam, we were sent directly to the hospital, where I would undergo an emergency tonsillectomy. I must have been near death . . . I mean, who has an emergency tonsillectomy?

I can still smell the antiseptic in the operating room and see the nun, in her starched white habit, telling me to count backward from ten as she put me to sleep. I was terrified, and my mother was probably more so. She didn't know exactly what was wrong with me, but she knew my condition was dire.

This was how we accessed care—only on an emergent basis. A bit of history helps explain how this dysfunctional relationship between Black patients and their doctors came to exist, and why in many instances it continues to this day. Mobile's few Black doctors didn't take appointments, so they were often overwhelmed by waiting rooms full of sick patients and, as with old-school hairdressers, you could wait forever to be seen. My mother, the original "ain't nobody got time for that" woman (except she wouldn't have used *ain't,* because she insisted on proper English), was not about to take a day off from work to wait with a sick child, and no end in sight, in anything less than a dire emergency. In such a crisis, a Black doctor couldn't admit you to the hospital even if you needed to go. White doctors were a cash-only proposition and the indignity of entering through the "colored" door was not exactly a choice way to begin a great therapeutic relationship. Nothing about either of these options signaled ease for the patient or a respect for them or their time.

The world of my childhood was dramatically different from my mother's, but big-city doctors were no less intimidating or more trustworthy than up-the-country doctors. Nothing in my mother's entire lived experience ever made her a fan. As a Black woman, she had plenty of reason to stay wary.

For years after slavery was abolished, Black women were routinely subjected to degrading and substandard care. Fannie Lou Hamer is a famous example of the countless anonymous cases of involuntary sterilization routinely inflicted upon poor Black women. The procedure was so common, it was nicknamed a "Mississippi appendectomy." In one of the more horrific cases to gain notoriety (undoubtedly, many more did not), Minnie Lee and Mary Alice Relf, at the tender ages of 12 and 14, were involuntarily sterilized by doctors in Montgomery, in 1973. Yes, you heard me—in 1973! This was the only healthcare environment my mother knew, defined by one horror story after another. So, is it any wonder that, like her own mother and grandmother, my mom never even considered seeing a doctor unless she was desperately sick? Unfortunately, it is this history and lived experience that ultimately cost her, and us, her life.

You Have Choices: Choose Not to Suffer

Life comes with some unanticipated and unavoidable suffering. But why, when we're given the option to suffer or not, do so many of us choose suffering? The answer to this question is complex.

For starters, we've been raised to view suffering as an integral part of womanhood. In short, we have normalized suffering. We have incorporated the language of misery into the lexicon so effectively that we take suffering for granted. Girls suffer from menstrual cramps. Women suffer through childbirth and postpartum depression. We also suffer with migraines, suffer from heartbreak, and suffer through abusive relationships.

At one end of the reproductive life spectrum, we suffer from PMS, or premenstrual symptoms, only to then suffer on the tail end from the onslaught of symptoms that accompany The Change. In that sense, menopause is simply the finale on a continuum of suffering that starts the moment we begin puberty.

But the expectation that feeling bad is a natural part of growing up and growing older has got to go. Chronic pain, persistent discomfort, and feeling lousy are not normal. We have incorporated the perceived inevitability of suffering into our psyches so much that we cannot fully grasp the notion that *not* suffering is a viable option.

Where did this tendency come from? For Black women, it has its origins in slavery. As I mentioned earlier, the surgeon J. Marion Sims, once lauded as the Father of Gynecology, is documented as having operated on enslaved women repeatedly and without anesthesia, even after anesthesia became available. We're not talking minor procedures here.

Sims performed gruesome vaginal surgeries on these Black mothers, sisters, and mere girls, some of whom had been raped by their slave masters, to learn how to fix injuries sustained during childbirth. And trust me, he wasn't doing this for their benefit. Sims performed these surgeries in an attempt to restore these women's value as breeders.

The common misperception—still prevalent today in certain misguided corners of medicine—that Black people are capable of enduring more pain than white people, was reinforced by the circular logic of having to endure more pain. In fact, a study done in 2019 found that some white medical students and residents believed that Black patients had higher pain tolerances than white patients. It is galling and enraging that in the twenty-first century, Black people are still consistently undermedicated for surgical and post-op pain as well as for chronic medical conditions known to be excruciating, such as sickle cell crises. This occurs, in part, because of miseducation and the stubborn prevalence of these misguided beliefs. They must be eradicated.

Women's pain is all too frequently ignored or simply minimized as women being hysterical or overly dramatic. Even the word *hysteria* is most often associated with females, as it is derived from *hystera*, the Greek word for *uterus*. The linguistic implication is that being born with a uterus makes one more inclined to unfounded, uncontrollable emotional exaggeration, which is, of course, untrue. Back in 2020, more than two hundred women were not believed when they complained mightily of excruciating pain during their egg retrievals at a Yale fertility clinic. The following year, a nurse at the facility pleaded guilty to tampering with the fentanyl meant for the women's procedures, having replaced the opioid with saline. Now ask yourself why it took five months and two hundred women before anyone figured out what was going on. I did mention that this took place at Yale, right? Why do we continually doubt women or decide that their concerns are unworthy of redress?

The ongoing lack of gender and racial diversity, self-examination, and historical knowledge within the medical profession has led to a complicity in the acceptance of suffering, particularly for certain groups. We should never forget the hard lessons of the past, and we must continue to hold the medical establishment accountable for its ethical failings and broad inequities. But we mustn't allow these problems to prevent us from seeking every medical benefit available to us today. Mother wit and homeopathy have their place, but there are things that only modern medicine can do.

Our mothers and grandmothers did the best they could with what they had. Imperfect as things are today, we have more and better resources available. We just need to stay aware of what those resources are and how best to access them. We have to learn how to prevent disease and recognize its early warning signs. Today, we have more in our medical tool kits than leeches and rusty saws. To honor these women and the dreams they placed in us, we must do more, and be better at alleviating our own suffering and getting the care they could not.

Stay Ready—First: Aid

By now, you've gotten your doctors lined up, you've signed into your health portal, and you've established your basic medical history. Congratulations! You're a triple threat! (If not, circle back to Chapters 1 and 2. I'll wait.) That foundation will be key whenever you need medical help.

Yet most injuries and illnesses do not require immediate medical intervention. They might arrive unexpectedly and land us on our backs, but they usually require the medical equivalent of a selfie: sensible self-assessment followed by simple self-care. To be prepared, you need to keep a healthy stash of first-aid tools on hand.

When you have active kids around, emergency supplies can get used and replenished as often as the contents of your refrigerator. But it's just as important to stay well stocked as you age. A dried-out bunch of Band-Aids in that tiny size that never gets used and a few leftover (expired) medications from a decade or two ago do not count!

Ready-made first-aid kits are convenient and come in several sizes. But no prefab kit will contain everything you should have at home in a time of need. So, check what's in your medicine cabinet against the following lists and supplement where you see fit. Remember to keep these items easily accessible for you, but out of the reach of young children.

Standard Self-Care Supplies

- Antiseptic cleanser, Betadine, or alcohol (to clean ordinary scrapes and cuts)

- Antibacterial soap such as Hibiclens or Phisohex to clean dirty scrapes or cuts

- Thermometer (a digital oral one is easiest)

- Adhesive bandages (in multiple sizes, and they even now come in multiple skin tones)

- Butterfly bandages for clean cuts and liquid bandages (New Skin) for elbows and knees

- Ointments for abrasions and burns: antibiotic cream (Bacitracin or Neosporin), aloe vera gel for minor burns and sunburn

- Gauze bandages, medical tape, and ACE bandages

- Magnifying glass and tweezers (to remove ticks, insect stingers, and splinters)

- Ice packs (kept in the freezer)

- Heating pad

- Scissors, safety pins, cotton balls, and Q-tips (not for your ears)

Most Useful Over-the-Counter (OTC) Medications

- Anti-inflammatories: Ibuprofen (Advil, Motrin) and naproxen (Aleve, Naprosyn) are effective at pain relief and fever reduction, but can cause nausea and stomach irritation. Ibuprofen is good for muscle and joint pain, but use sparingly, especially if you have hypertension or kidney disease.

- Pain and fever relievers: Acetaminophen (Tylenol) does not irritate the stomach, so can be taken anytime, with or without food. Aspirin can cause stomach upset and interfere with blood clotting, so should not be taken if you are on blood thinners, are prone to falls, or are scheduled to have surgery in less than a week.

- Allergy meds: A basic antihistamine (Benadryl) can buy critical time, allowing you to get to the ER in the event of an acute allergic reaction.

- Itch relief: Calamine lotion, hydrocortisone, or topical antihistamines alleviate suffering from insect bites and minor rashes and skin irritations.

- Decongestants, expectorants, and cough medicines (yes, good ol' Robitussin).

- Upset-stomach relievers: Calcium carbonate (Tums, Rolaids) for heartburn; antacids (Maalox, Mylanta, Prilosec, Prevacid, Pepcid) for indigestion and acid reflux; antinausea (Pepto-Bismol, Dramamine); antidiarrheals (Kaopectate, Imodium); constipation relief (stool softeners, plant-based laxatives [Senokot], or high-fiber or osmotic products [Citrucel, Metamucil, Miralax]).

- Vaginal yeast medication (Monistat cream or suppositories). *Note: This is especially useful if you are on antibiotics (some of which can put you at risk for yeast infections) or are planning a beach vacation (just trust me on this one).

You might roll your eyes, but I'm going to say this anyway: Reread all product labels before each use, just to make sure of the appropriate dosing and any significant interactions (there are apps for this, including Drug Interaction Checker—see Additional Resources). If a product's label is lost or faded, the internet is a great resource for answers to explicit questions about OTC meds or treatment options, like when to apply heat versus ice to an injury; when to cover a wound versus not; and how to properly bandage a twisted ankle.

However, *do not use the internet to diagnose yourself.* I know it's hard to resist at 2 A.M. when you're sleepless and panicky, but Dr. Search Engine will likely make you feel worse. To be clear, I'm not suggesting it can't be helpful. But, in all likelihood, if you google the causes of a headache, the results will come back as varied as dehydration, stress, stroke, or brain tumor. And guess which one you are going to home in on (especially in the wee hours of hypochondria)? You will be better off if you take some deep breaths (slowly inhale through your nose, slowly exhale through your mouth), count sheep, read a good book, watch a movie. And wait to speak to an actual practitioner.

To supersize your first-aid skills, learn CPR in a program certified by the American Red Cross. This is a particularly good idea if you live with children or elders. In a pinch, you can learn almost anything for free on YouTube, but the time to start is not mid-crisis.

Develop Interoception: A Superpower for the Ages

The best offense is a good defense, and the first defensive step is to *know your body.* To do so, I want you to develop *interoception,* which is a little-known word for understanding how your body feels when it is functioning well. It is the conscious or unconscious perception of what does and does not feel right, what is and is not normal for you. Your stomach growls, your palms sweat, your heart races, you're light-headed. Your body sends you signals all day, every day, about what is happening inside it. These are clues that you'll need in order to become your own master diagnostician.

How many times have you just felt *off*? That is your body alerting you to an imbalance of some kind. Don't dismiss it. Learn to pay attention, heed it, and realize that everyone's normal is different. When we accept suffering, we blunt this vital sense and compromise our innate ability to distinguish health from "dis-ease."

At this stage of your life, don't allow anyone, even a loved one, to tell you how you feel or what to do about it. Remember, nobody knows *your* body better than you [♪ "Nobody Can Be You"]. Interoception is a powerful and underrated super-sense that everyone can cultivate. So, do!

Renee

Renee was a healthy 61-year-old writer and book editor who had never sustained a hip injury and whose parents had lived well into their 80s without needing any replacement parts. So, she was stumped when her left hip started aching badly.

The pain came on gradually. She first felt it during a weekly three-mile walk with her sister-in-law. When switching from cement sidewalks to dirt hiking trails didn't help, Renee thought maybe the problem was the weight she'd gained during COVID.

After a few weeks of eating more salad and less bread, she'd lost five pounds, but her hip felt worse. The simple act of rising from a chair had become so painful, it made her grind her teeth and groan. Worst of all was lying in bed. One night, Renee's pain was so excruciating, she woke her husband, Jake, and said she might need to go to the ER.

He told her she didn't need an ER; she needed more sex. When they finally stopped laughing, the pain was still there, but she was less panicked about it. Well-meaning Jake encouraged her to stretch more, sit less, change her workouts, ice it, soak it, maybe slather it with ointment—preferably odor-free. He even suggested a new mattress might help.

What Jake did not think Renee needed was a doctor. But she went to an orthopedist anyway, and her X-ray showed bone spurs on her hip, a sign of osteoarthritis. Treatment options included physical therapy or cortisone shots, which would likely offer only temporary relief, or hip replacement surgery, which after thoughtful consideration, she chose.

"I just felt so vindicated," Renee said. "My husband loves me, but he thinks I'm a baby about pain. I might be! But that doesn't mean that when I feel pain, there's nothing actually wrong." Preach!

The Takeaway: Feeling bad on occasion is inevitable. Feeling bad every day is not. Pain, discomfort, and fatigue are vital warning signs. Only you can feel them, so *you* should make the calls on how to respond when you do.

Patience *Is* a Virtue

It is the most basic tenet of wellness: Know when you are sick—and what to do about it. Sometimes that means doing almost nothing.

One trait that really good diagnosticians have in common is patience. If you have a cold or flu, or even some form of COVID, what's needed before anything else is rest and plenty of clear fluids (water, warm broth, tea). And the tincture of time. I understand that we've been trained by microwaves and smartphones to want everything in seconds, but "I want the answer and I want it now!" is the posture of a spoiled child, not a grown woman.

I'm a big proponent of managing common symptoms at home for 24–48 hours *before* seeking medical assistance. *Common* means exactly that—non-life-threatening sickness that may be contagious, inconvenient, or uncomfortable, but will resolve with rest, over-the-counter meds, and a bit of time. Generally speaking, if you treat your symptoms with care, your body will usually do the rest. That's what your immune system is for [♪ "Alright"].

Unless you're in a dire state, you need to let things play out a bit so you can recognize patterns. You will never come to understand the scope and course of common illnesses if you don't see them through. And for the record, if you race to the doctor every time you feel a tickle in your throat, you're more likely to catch something worse in the waiting room than you had walking in—and to gain a reputation for crying wolf. Nobody wants to be Chicken Little. (You youngsters, go google "Chicken Little.")

Cultivate Confidence

In becoming your own best caregiver and advocate, it's important that you learn to trust your judgment, and you can't trust what you never test [♪ "Strength, Courage & Wisdom"].

So, another benefit of waiting a day or two is the confidence you'll gain through administering self-care and seeing how your body responds.

If at the first sign of a sour stomach or sinus pain, you go to your doctor and ask for meds, you'll probably get them, but you'll never know if the meds cured you or if you had a minor bug that simply ran its course. Why does this matter? First off, antibiotics don't cure everything. So, you might be taking them unnecessarily. That's a bad idea because, over time, these bugs can develop a resistance to overused antibiotics and can become superbugs. And when you really need an antibiotic to treat a bacterial infection, you're going to want it to work (see Viruses vs. Infections and How to Treat Them).

Doctors can be every bit as guilty of impatience and quick (needless) fixes as patients. Ordering more tests, although sometimes taken as a measure of thoroughness, can also reflect a physician's lack of confidence in their own medical judgment and an intolerance for pausing a beat to see if their hypotheses are correct. So, be watchful of your doctor's practices. And speak up when you have any doubts. Whenever you are prescribed medicines, procedures, or expensive testing, make sure you understand 1) why this course of action is necessary; 2) what they are hoping to rule in or out; and 3) how your treatment plan is going to change as a result of this intervention. My rule of thumb has always been, if a test result is not going to change my treatment recommendation, why do it? So, always make sure you understand not just what, but why. I believe that an informed patient is far more likely to comply with treatment and testing when they understand the rationale behind the recommendations. This is not only how your own level of confidence is built, but also where it becomes essential and must be leveraged. And if your doctor is perturbed by your insistence on clarity, you know what to do.

Curb Your Fears

We women often downplay how we feel, even when we're ill. But excessive anxiety has become increasingly common across genders and generations, especially today when the news and faster-than-ever pace of life keeps us all on edge.

Obsessive-compulsive or hypochondriacal symptoms such as germophobia, preoccupation with potential illness, over-worrying about every cough and body ache, or stressing over every mole or pimple is not normal. Or productive. My mom would say, "You'll be running around like a chicken with its head cut off," meaning, if you worry about everything, you'll be effective at nothing [♪ "Mama Used to Say"].

As you age, it's normal to grow more anxious and more cautious about your health. At 50-something, you have good reason to be on higher alert than you were at 30-something. News flash: Anxiety is a symptom of menopause (see Chapter 10), but that doesn't mean you should let it go unchecked.

Anxiety can provoke increases in blood pressure. It can also overwhelm your common sense. None of this is healthy and it can worsen with age if you let it. So, pay attention to any significant changes in your attitude or patterns of behavior around health. Seek therapy if you can't control it. To paraphrase Ice Cube, check yourself before you wreck yourself. Better still, call that girlfriend who will always talk you off the edge [♪ "if you got a problem"].

Learn to Distinguish Between
Information and Data

Unlike my mother, today's mom tending her children can google "fever" and instantly generate a hundred possible causes—many of them terrifying—that my mother would never have considered. Nor should she have! Too much data can easily distract you from the indisputable facts right in front of you, killing your confidence, stoking your fears, and making you second-guess everything. Don't let it!

Doctors also now have at their fingertips every possible differential diagnosis and treatment, all the while defying Occam's razor—the simplest explanation is usually the correct one.

The proliferation of readily accessible data (and I do mean data, not information, because information is *useful*) has dulled our senses of observation and interoception. When we rely merely on data—test results, CT scans, and Dr. Worldwide Web's deeply flawed diagnostic algorithms—we disable one of the most powerful diagnostic tools we have: our brains.

I assess my patients and loved ones much like my mother assessed her children: How do you look? How strong is your voice? How well are you walking? And sleeping? Are you fidgety or eerily still? How do you smell (yes, sometimes sickness gives off a distinctive body odor)? Using these layers of information, you can make an intuitive judgment about who is sick, who is *really* sick, and who is not.

I often remind friends who float wild theories to me lifted from the internet that common things happen commonly. A sore throat means you probably have a virus or bacterial infection, not throat cancer. Try a lozenge and some warm honey-lemon tea. Rest your voice and give it a day or two. If it's worse after forty-eight hours, seek advice.

Data has its place. But common sense: Don't quash it.

Get to Sleeping, Beauty

Sometimes, you think you're sick but you're just tired. And sometimes, you think you're just tired but you're sick. Sleep is essential to good health at every age, and feeling well rested is a cornerstone of long-term aging. Yet, because so many of us undervalue sleep, we can fail to recognize the difference between chronic fatigue and chronic illness.

Let's play a little game of Family Feud. What are the top answers to why people are chronically fatigued?

- Lack of sleep

- Depression

- Stress

- Poor diet

- Lack of exercise

- Sleep apnea

- Obesity

- Overall poor health (cardiovascular disease, hypertension, diabetes, and medications)

Ding-ding-ding! All of the above. They're interrelated and serious. Lack of sleep contributes to poor diet choices and weight gain. Obesity can keep you from exercising. Stress can lead to depression. And so on. Your job is to break the cycle before it breaks you. And understand: You can!

Chronic sleep deprivation leads to cognitive deficiencies, elevated blood pressure, and inflammation. And, here again, perimenopausal women and Black women are at higher risk for developing sleep disturbances. According to the Study of Women Across the Nation (SWAN), the largest longitudinal epidemiological study of women in midlife, Black women in perimenopause and menopause get fewer overall hours of sleep and have more frequent nighttime awakenings than any other group. That results in feeling tired and unwell all the time, which is patently unacceptable. Chronic fatigue is not normal, so don't sleep on it (sorry, I couldn't resist). Normalizing this unhealthy baseline obscures the vital information that your body provides when there really is something wrong, like serious illnesses and anemia.

The good news is that you can fix it. Start by identifying what is keeping you awake at night. Is it hot flashes? Do you or your partner snore? Is eating before bed waking you up with indigestion? Are you watching TikTok videos into the wee hours or answering emails instead of turning off the light? Most of us have morning routines (alarm, shower, exercise, coffee) that signal our bodies to turn on. Create a wind-down routine leading to a consistent bedtime, and you might be surprised by how your nights—and days—improve. Make like Maxine Waters and reclaim your time.

Become a Good Storyteller

Deciding that you're sick enough to see a doctor is one thing. Effectively communicating your experience to that doctor is *everything*—at least when it comes to receiving an accurate diagnosis and appropriate treatment options. The bulk of doctor–patient problems lie in our mutual challenges in communicating. You can't fix your doctor's part in this, but I can help you speak your doctor's language. Just call me "Rosetta Stone."

There are four categories doctors routinely use to assess symptoms of every kind, from pain or swelling to bleeding or paralysis. They are: quality, intensity, location, and temporality. I find the acronym **QILT** helpful since quilt-makers just happen to be gifted storytellers.

Doctors will expect you to answer questions relating to each category. Being able to do so effectively will not only raise the quality of your doctor's care, it will also help you make sense of what's going on as you experience it. If possible, write your answers down before speaking with your doctor. This way you won't have to rely on your memory, which is often compromised when we're under duress.

Quality

- Sharp or dull?

- Intermittent or constant?

- Have you needed to take medication for it? Which medications? Did they help?

Intensity

- On a scale of 1 (barely noticeable) to 10 (stops you in your tracks), where are you now?

- Is it staying the same, getting worse, or getting better?

- Is there anything you do that makes it better or worse? (Lying still or moving?)

Location

- Where is it? Does it radiate?

- Is it on the right side or left side or both?

- Does it stay in one place or move around?

- Can you point to it with one finger or is it diffuse?

Temporality

- When did it start?

- Did it come on gradually or suddenly?

- How long has it been present?

- Has this happened before?

Viruses vs. Infections and How to Treat Them

While most of us know what healthy living looks like, not everyone recognizes sickness when they see it, and being able to is as key to good health as breathing.

In modern life, we tend to overcomplicate things, and although a lot has changed since my mother's time, the basic signs of common illnesses—like colds, stomach bugs, and the flu, all of which are viral infections—haven't. Antibiotics not only don't cure viruses, but as noted previously, their unscrupulous use can create superbugs and levels of resistance that render them useless when you do need them.

Well, you might ask, then what are antibiotics for? They are for bacterial infections, such as strep throat, sinus infections, some pneumonias, and urinary tract infections. These can be distinguished from viruses through throat, sputum, or urine cultures, tested in your doctor's office. Most viral infections will run their course. Bacterial infections will typically not get better on their own.

This is where a little finesse goes a long way, because bacterial and viral symptoms are often confused and differ in subtle ways. Fever can be a symptom with both; however, fevers tend to be higher with bacterial infections [♪ "Fever"]. How high, you might ask?

- High-grade fever: 102 to 104

- Low-grade fever: 100.5 to 101.5

- Normal temperature: 97 to 99

- Gray zone is 99–100.4 and trends are important—is it going up or going down?

  Red Flag: Adults rarely get fevers over 104. If you do, notify your doctor immediately or head to urgent care.

Both bacterial and viral infections can cause coughs and pneumonia, but viruses tend to produce less sputum than bacterial infections. Viral coughs are more likely to be dry or to produce sputum that looks more like normal mucus—clear or slightly yellow. Bacterial infections tend to produce copious amounts of greenish, rusty, or brown sputum. I know, right: gross. But as my mother would say, "Better out than in."

Urinary tract infections (UTIs) require antibiotics, because left untreated they can progress to kidney infections and full-fledged sepsis. Most of us have at some time had a dreaded UTI. The symptoms start with pain and burning during urination, urinary frequency and urgency. Occasionally, there's blood in the urine. UTIs are easily treated with oral antibiotics if caught early. Fever and back pain become symptoms once the bacteria have left the bladder and started to invade the kidneys. This is a red flag that should prompt immediate attention and possibly intravenous antibiotics.

If you experience pain, burning, and urinary frequency for months without additional symptoms, it may be due to local irritants, the genitourinary syndrome of menopause (see Chapter 10), or a condition called "interstitial cystitis"—none of which is likely to respond to antibiotics. You'll need to have your symptoms evaluated and treated— preferably not in an ER or urgent care setting, because guess what they are likely to give you: antibiotics!

Medicine vs. Too Much Medicine

Several studies have shown that women take medicine more often than men. This observation correlates with data that shows women have a higher rate of contact with medical professionals than men do. We also use more "natural" remedies, because "natural" sounds better. But for more than a decade, there have been rising concerns about Americans' overuse and abuse of medications—including so-called "natural remedies and supplements."

Lana

Lana is 62 years old and is only taking a women's multivitamin and medication for mild hypertension. She is active, walks regularly for exercise, and is in relatively good health. Her only complaint is occasional knee pain, which she attributes to arthritis.

She has had a couple of occasions when she felt like her knee was going to give out. Lana mentioned it to one of her girlfriends, who suggested that Lana attend a marketing party for a new supplement she was selling. Her friend raved about this proprietary miracle supplement, saying she'd been on it for more than a year. Not only did all of her aches and pains go away, but she said she felt more energetic than ever.

Lana figured she'd check it out. After all, what did she have to lose?

After a very convincing presentation, replete with slides and graphs, Lana decided to sign up for a subscription to the supplement, with the assurance that within weeks she'd be a new woman.

The answer to the question "What did she have to lose?" turned out to be $100 a month. Convinced it was working, she didn't seem to mind. It must be working, right? Otherwise, that would make her a sucker, and Lana is way too smart for that.

The Takeaway: Do not buy vitamins or supplements as part of multilevel marketing operations or just because they are endorsed by celebrities. Typically, the data on effectiveness is thin and the promises are outsized and unsubstantiated. And given what we know about the placebo effect, we also know that the more you spend, the more you believe in the benefits.

Polypharmacy is the regular intake of five or more medications and is a concern for older adults, according to the Lown Institute. Its 2022 study found that 42 percent of older adults take five or more prescription drugs a day, and almost 20 percent take ten or more. The incidence of polypharmacy has tripled in the last two decades, and the

Institute warns that if this trend continues, it could lead to 150,000 premature deaths and 4.6 million hospitalizations in the next ten years. The risk is not necessarily due to the number of drugs consumed regularly, but rather to the interactions of those drugs—which, if not well monitored, can be deadly.

Common indicators of possible overmedication are:

- Slurred speech

- Drowsiness

- Confusion

- Poor motor skills, which can put you at risk for falling

Prescription mistakes and overmedication happen, but you are at greater risk if you have doctors from different networks who don't communicate with one another, or if you offer an incomplete list of what you're taking when your doctor inquires.

All that said, many drugs that we regard as commonplace today have been game changers for patients with chronic, even life-threatening, conditions. The incidence of heart disease has risen but resulting deaths have steadily declined over the last fifteen years due, in large part, to our ability to keep people alive after a cardiac event. The lives of countless sufferers from chronic diseases such as diabetes, multiple sclerosis, lupus, HIV, and more have been improved, if not cured, by therapeutic advances.

Used properly, medicines offer relief and hope. But understand: The responsibility for their cautious and appropriate use lies primarily with you (see You Must Be the Master of Your Medication).

Every prescription today comes with a laundry list of warnings and potential side effects. So, always read the fine print (break out those readers, y'all!) and keep those documents handy for as long as you are required to take the medication. If you develop any troubling side effect, notify your doctor.

The most commonly abused drugs are opioids. Usually prescribed to offer short-term relief from postsurgical or acute pain, opioids are highly addictive. Whenever you are prescribed a drug that is known to be addictive or to carry any worrisome risks, or if you or someone in your family has a history of addiction, talk to your doctor before accepting the prescription. Sharing your questions and concerns may lead them to alter the dosage or type of medication they prescribe.

Along with the efficacy, side effects, and risks associated with any medications you take, consider the cost. I have a friend who insists on taking the name brand of all her medications and whenever I suggest that generics do the same thing, she sniffs that she doesn't want "the cheap stuff."

If you prefer Chanel makeup to Target's brands, I'm not mad (I use both) but it pays—literally—to make sure the difference in the products is worth the difference in the price. My general rule is, if you're taking a medication and it's working, don't change, not even for the "new, improved" version. If a company has enough money to run commercials on TV for a drug all day, unless it has no effective duplicate on the market, just ignore it [♪ **"Walk On By"**].

Joyce

Joyce, my 77-year-old sister, is extremely overweight, but despite this, she was in relatively good health until her mid-60s. The only medication she took was for mild blood pressure elevation. She was diagnosed with colon cancer eleven years ago, but has thankfully been free from recurrences. And since her cancer surgery, Joyce's only other hospitalization was for a pulmonary embolism, for which she was placed on a blood thinner. She also has osteoarthritis in both knees, but is ambulatory, feeling only moderate discomfort.

Joyce is normally quite sedentary, and COVID reinforced this tendency. For the first two years of the pandemic, due to her age and multiple risk factors, she didn't leave her house. In fact, since her grandchildren live with her, and they were out and about in the world, she rarely even left her room. Despite this and being fully vaccinated, she contracted a mild case of COVID.

Eight months later, when she contracted COVID a second time, her respiratory symptoms were more pronounced, but thankfully she was able to avoid hospitalization. However, after recovering, she developed marked swelling in her feet and legs. Walking became difficult and she was short of breath with minimal activity.

She saw her doctor, who diagnosed her with atrial fibrillation, a condition where the heart beats irregularly and often too fast. This was responsible for the excess fluid accumulating in her legs and feet. Joyce left her doctor's office with a diuretic to reduce her swelling, and medication to slow her heart rate. She was also scheduled for a cardioversion (an outpatient procedure to shock her heart out of atrial fibrillation and return it to a normal sinus rhythm).

The cardioversion was a success, and Joyce's cardiologist informed her that she no longer needed to take the medication to control her heart rate. However, two weeks later, she didn't feel any better. In fact, she was still chronically tired and winded. Having recently picked up her new prescriptions from the pharmacy, Joyce noted that she always felt worse after she took one of the medications. She skipped it for a day and felt better.

At this point, she called me to ask what she should do. I had her review all of her medications with me. It turned out that she was still taking the heart medication that her cardiologist had told her to stop. She hadn't checked to see what her pharmacist refilled, and the pharmacist was un-aware that her medication had been discontinued. She just took the medications she was given without checking.

Joyce informed her doctor of the mistake, stopped the medication, and found her symptoms improved immediately. Fortunately, her story ended well, but it could have been disastrous.

The Takeaway: This is *really* important. When you (or any-one in your care, such as your parents) see the doctor and doses of medications are changed or discontinued, know that the pharmacy is often not informed of these changes. They will continue to refill whatever they have on file. It is your responsibility to fully understand your new regimen and to ensure that it is followed. Have your doctor's office write down any changes for you. Even if they promise to update your pharmacy, make sure that what your doctor prescribed or changed is reflected in your new medication and the accompanying instructions when you pick up your prescription.

Vitamins, Supplements, and "Natural" Remedies

You might be wondering if vitamins and supplements count in the polypharmacy category. The answer is a qualified yes. Most are harmless. Some do nothing, including what they claim. But that doesn't mean you shouldn't be vigilant about them, especially if you're taking a half dozen (or more) a day. Some vitamins are known to interact poorly with certain prescription meds. Others, like vitamin A, can be toxic in high doses on their own. This is why *you must do your home-*

work and include all vitamins and supplements on your list of medications (see You Must Be the Master of Your Medication).

You should pay close attention to *anything* you ingest—including things that are purported to be good for you. Be aware that "natural" and "organic" are marketing terms. Do you know what else is natural and organic? Bullshit. There's a lot of it out there, so beware.

Here's a little bit of marketing sleight of hand. If your supplement says it "supports" things like bone health, brain function, memory, and collagen formation, there is a good chance there's little-to-no data to substantiate it.

In addition to potential health risks, all of this so-called "health in a bottle" can be extremely expensive. If the cost of your health regimen is preventing you from affording a tropical vacation, you might ask yourself if you wouldn't be better off getting your vitamin D lying on the beach in Jamaica. Just food for thought.

Vitamins and supplements are big business. According to the NIH, 77 percent of Americans took at least one supplement a day in 2022 (the older you are, the more supplements you are likely to take) and we spend more than $30 billion out of pocket on supplements annually. It's incredible that long-established health initiatives like vaccines and fluoridated water spark rebellion and conspiracy theories, while an entire industry that's unproven and unregulated gets a pass.

I'm not saying that all supplements are bad. I am saying most adults in this country can get all the essential vitamins and nutrients they need from a healthy diet. That is the gold standard. If you don't always eat right, a multivitamin might help. But as a general rule, since most vitamins are water soluble, you are just going to pee them out and flush them down the toilet. That goes for calcium pills too. Calcium derived from dietary sources is more soluble and easier to digest than calcium from a pill. But if you are lactose intolerant or do not get the required daily dose of calcium, a supplement might be in order. Remember, supplements are meant to *supplement* a healthy diet, not to substitute for it.

It pays to be aware that the science behind supplements is always changing. For years, we—and I include myself in this number—hammered home the belief that women need higher doses of calcium and vitamin D to prevent osteoporosis as we age. Even though we all need calcium and vitamin D in our diets, we later found that they do nothing to prevent or treat osteoporosis after menopause. In fact, some studies found that too much calcium, particularly taken as supplements, can contribute to kidney stones, constipation, and cardiovascular plaques. Oops! And confusing, right? Here's the bottom line: Taking the recommended daily dose of any supplement *for your age* is all you should take. More is not always better. Calcium and vitamin D do not replace bone that is already lost. So, to prevent osteoporosis, the best time to have a calcium-rich diet is when you're young and still growing and making new bone.

Medicine and science are always evolving, and we're not good at admitting what we don't know. But what we know for sure is that there is no substitute for a healthy diet. Unprocessed whole food is medicine. My mother knew that. Your grandmother knew that. Many of our pharmaceutical drugs were also derived from nature—aspirin comes from the bark of a tree. So, I do not pooh-pooh all natural or herbal remedies. All I ask is that you be aware of what you are taking and how it may interact with other medications you are on. At the end of the day, if it makes you feel better, doesn't break the bank, and doesn't harm you, I have no objection. It's your call.

You Must Be the Master of Your Medication!

Tracking your medications sounds simple, but for whatever reason, it is hard for people to do. To start, keep a list of:

- Every medication you regularly take

- Product names, dosages, and prescribing doctors

- Any and all changes in your dose (discard or remove medications that have been discontinued)

- All OTC medications, vitamins, nutraceuticals, herbs, and holistic remedies you take regularly

There are several mobile apps designed to store this information in your phone. There are also plenty of products (binders, folders, pockets, organizers, even refrigerator magnets) available to help you store medical information in visible and readily accessible places, including your wallet, medicine cabinet, glove compartment (where emergency responders can easily access them), and near your landline if you have one.

Be aware that your emergency contact should have their own copy of this list, which you must update as needed.

In managing your medications:

- **Keep track of all product and prescription expiration dates.** And note: This is the last date at which the manufacturer can guarantee the full potency of the treatment, not the last day they are safe to use.

- **Put a reminder in your phone** for two weeks *before* any prescription runs out. Trust me, Saturday night is not the time to realize you need a medication refill.

- **In emergencies, some pharmacies will give you a limited prescription** until you can get in touch with your doctor during regular business hours. In a pinch, ask!

- **Never ingest anything (medication or otherwise) that seems off.** When the texture, color, taste, or smell is in doubt, throw (or spit!) it out.

- **Honor product warnings and adhere to prescribed dosages** unless your doctor indicates otherwise. There are risks worth taking in life, but playing fast and loose with medication is not one of them.

Is It an Emergency?
How to Know and Where to Go

ERs are open 24/7 and are required by law to treat everyone who comes in, regardless of their affliction or ability to pay. This has made them a magnet for all manner of healthcare needs, including those that don't in any way resemble an emergency. The many downsides of that are both obvious and not.

In today's overburdened ERs, crowding alone presents a critical safety issue, the consequences of which can be severe for patients and providers alike. ER docs are trained to handle acute, traumatic health crises, and that's what they do best. As for the rest, they know a little about a lot of things. So, if you are not in the midst of an emergency, an ER doc is not likely to be your best option for diagnosis and treatment.

Let's put aside the impractical aspect of calling 911 or even driving yourself to an ER because you feel lousy at 7 A.M. on a Sunday. If two Tylenol didn't cure you and you don't want to wait until Monday to see your doctor, you're not necessarily doing yourself any favors. You will likely walk out of there still not knowing what's wrong with you, having spent a day or more in a room full of sick people who could give you something you didn't already have.

The kicker? You will be told to go see your own doctor or a specialist, anyway, and you'll be financially poorer for the experience. ER care is exceedingly expensive and is covered at the sole discretion of your insurer—if you have one. In fact, several insurance companies reserve the right to deny coverage for ER visits that fall short of their definitions of a true emergency. And their definitions may not match up with yours.

Bottom line: Emergency rooms were created to handle life-and-limb-threatening situations. If you're not confronting one of these, think twice before heading to an ER. But if you do experience any of the following symptoms, get to an ER—quick, fast, and in a hurry!

- Chest pain

- Shortness of breath

- Facial drooping, arm weakness, speech difficulties (Think *FAST* for a suspected stroke. The *T* is for "Time is critical!")

- Severe head, neck, or spine trauma

- Severe allergic reaction

- Loss of consciousness for >30 seconds

- New/undiagnosed seizure

- Heavy, unstoppable bleeding

- Electric shock

- Exposure to fire, smoke, or toxic fumes (even if not burned)

- Badly broken bone

- Suspected poisoning or drug overdose

- Suicidal thoughts

Where to Get Nonemergency Care

The COVID pandemic exposed and exacerbated the strain our health-care system faces daily in its quest to deliver effective care. As a consumer of that care, you have an important role to play by understanding where to go when you're in need of it.

For non-life-threatening situations that warrant medical help, there are several options, the best of which is always going to be the office of your primary care doctor. By now you should know that you are always going to be best served by a doctor who knows you (or at least your medical history) rather than a total stranger.

Barring that (if, let's say, you're out of town or can't get an appointment in a reasonable amount of time—which happens), assessing which alternative makes the most sense depends on the complexity of the issue you're facing as well as your own subjective preferences and needs. To choose wisely, consider the following:

Walk-in Clinics: The pandemic also prompted a dramatic rise in so-called "minute clinics," which don't require appointments, are usually covered by insurance (with low copays), and often have late evening and weekend hours. Big players in this space include CVS, Walgreens, Target, and Walmart.

Staffed mainly by nurse practitioners, they are a convenient and inexpensive source for vaccinations and screening for chronic problems, like high blood pressure and diabetes, making walk-in clinics a good alternative for quick check-ins. They can also diagnose and provide prescriptions (conveniently fillable on-site) for common problems such as bronchitis, ear infections, sore throats, UTIs, minor injuries, and cuts that don't require stitches. Anything more complex warrants a trip to see a doctor.

Urgent Care: Urgent care centers offer everything minute clinics do, including widespread access (especially in cities), ease of use (walk-in services as well as evening and weekend appointments), and proactive as well as responsive care options. They are typically staffed by doctors as well as nurse practitioners, physician's assistants, and registered nurses. Occasionally, they also have in-house specialists. So, they can treat urgent problems (but not true medical emergencies—that's why it's called "urgent" care), such as a mild asthma attack or a minor wound requiring stitches. And since you are likely to be seen quicker in urgent care than in an emergency room, this can save you time and money. When necessary, or if the care is not appropriate for urgent care, the doctor can give you guidance and refer you to an emergency room. Further, urgent cares usually provide standard X-ray and lab services, such as blood tests, and some can dispense medications on-site.

The out-of-pocket costs tend to be higher than those of a walk-in clinic, but lower than a private physician or specialist, and most are covered by insurance.

Telehealth Care: The COVID pandemic prompted a boom in telehealth, a fast-growing option that usually combines video, telephonic, or texting conversations between patients and healthcare providers. Telehealth can use remote monitoring devices that measure and upload key information such as temperature, blood pressure, heart rate and rhythm, and blood sugar levels.

One Mayo Clinic study reported that 22 percent of patients and 80 percent of doctors participated in video health encounters in 2020. That's three times more than in the previous year. Clearly, teleconferencing is more convenient than in-person doctor visits, but is it effective? Research has shown that it is—especially for patients with chronic conditions that need regular monitoring, such as heart disease, lung disease, diabetes, or psychological issues.

It has unsurprising limits (any diagnosis requiring bloodwork, X-rays, or other tests is better served in person), not the least of which is a patient's proficiency with the technologies themselves. This puts much older patients at a deficit. But the same 2020 Mayo Clinic study found that telehealth and in-person diagnoses matched up more than 85 percent of the time.

DR. SHARON'S RX FOR

Handling Yourself, in Sickness and in Health

1. Keep your first-aid tool kit and over-the-counter medications at the ready.

2. Maintain and keep available a written medical history and list of your regular medications with dosages available—and make sure your emergency contact has this information too.

3. When your doctor changes the dosage or discontinues a medication, make sure that the pharmacy is made aware of those changes, to avoid overdosing or duplicating. Fill all your prescriptions at one pharmacy to help ensure that drug interactions are adequately checked.

4. Take a deep breath and give yourself 24–48 hours in nonurgent situations before seeking care.

5. Call your doctor first (unless it's a red flag event) for instructions on how to proceed before showing up at urgent care or the emergency room.

6. Be clear about what you are experiencing and be able to communicate it effectively to your doctor.

7. Keep your vaccinations up-to-date.

8. Get more sleep. We are just waking up to the importance of sleep. It is one of the cornerstones of good health.

CHAPTER 4

Brave and Strong♪

What You Need to Know (and Do) About Cancer

Dear Sis,

Alice Walker said, "The most common way people give up their power is by thinking they don't have any." My patients have shown me that at every moment of your life, well or sick, you are more powerful than you know. What fuels that power? Information! This holds true, even when it comes to The Big C—cancer.

I don't know one woman whose life hasn't been touched by some form of cancer, either directly or through a loved one. In my family alone, we've waged more than our share of cancer battles, some lost and others won.

Cancer is a bitch. But it's important for me to tell you that we have come a mighty long way in reducing the mortality rates of gynecologic and breast cancers, including some of the types that we most fear. What should you take from that? Vow to be vigilant in your early detection efforts. Even better, aim to prevent cancer in every way that you can.

You're probably wondering what preventative cancer care even looks like, right? It's about your lifestyle: not smoking, not drinking too much alcohol, eating a healthy diet, exercising regularly, and getting ample sleep. Sounds basic and sooo boring (and I know I'm already starting to sound less like a deejay and more like a broken record with this list), but these simple things will make your life better and longer, whether you ever confront cancer or not.

It's about knowing your medical history and where the trouble spots might lie. It's taking care to not miss your annual physicals and making sure they include screenings for rectal, skin, and breast cancer as well as a pap test. It's about breast self-exams and mammograms—for the rest of your life. And, by the way, your dentist should be performing an oral cancer screening as part of your regular checkups. If you're not sure if this is happening, ask about it.

Cancer prevention is also about ancillary things like stress management, weight control, mindfulness, and knowing your body well enough (hello, interoception!) that when it signals trouble you heed it and get help.

"The Big C" isn't just for *Cancer,* it's for the *Choices,* big and small, that we make every day. It's for *Common Sense, self-Care, Context,* and *Control.* So, come on, let's get you some!

xo, Dr. Sharon

Three of the most dreaded words in the English language are: "You have cancer." I know. It scares us half to death. Especially when it cuts close to home, and I should know, because I come from a family rife with cancer.

Six of my eight siblings have been diagnosed with a total of eight cancers. Hang in there with me, because it gets a bit complicated. But this is important.

My three brothers all have had prostate cancer. Thankfully, due to early diagnosis, two—Clint and Elvin—are alive and well at 86 and 88, respectively. My brother Charles, who died at 77, did not succumb to cancer but to end-stage kidney failure. (Charles had, let's just say, a less-than-healthy lifestyle and he was not at all fond of doctors—present company excluded.) My sisters Vivian and Gwen had breast cancer, and Joyce, as I mentioned earlier, survived colon cancer. If you're wondering how that adds up to eight, Charles was also diagnosed with multiple myeloma and Vivian had myelodysplastic syndrome—both are cancers originating in the blood.

I know: whew! It sounds like a lot because it is. We are not just a big family; it became clear to us pretty early that we are a big cancer family. And that's just my generation.

As I previously mentioned, my mother died of colon cancer at 57. Her sister, Aunt Mildred, died of colon cancer at 61. My mother's other two sisters, Aunt Ola and Aunt Gertrude, both survived breast cancer without the benefits of the early screenings and any of the post-surgical treatments we have at our fingertips today. It was a time when many believed any cancer diagnosis was a death sentence. (Sidebar: Loved my aunties, but thank the Lord, Mom didn't believe in name-sakes.) Given all of this, one might think that a cancer diagnosis is a near certainty in my future. Yet, I am optimistic that it doesn't have to be.

Thus far, the only two of us who have not had cancer are my sister Margie, who is seven years older than me, and me. I don't think that's an accident. Margie and I have been extremely careful and intentional about altering our lifestyles, to the best of our abilities, to avoid getting cancer, or heart disease, or hypertension, or diabetes. The steps to pre-ventative health that I'm constantly drilling you with? We're all about those!

With all the cancer in my family [♪ "Cancer"], why is it worth not-ing who lived, who died, and who is still cancer-free? Because it's not intuitively obvious. My mother and her sister, who lost their lives to colon cancer, died from a lack of knowledge about its symptoms and from a lack of adequate screening. My sister Joyce, who had colon cancer decades later, knew, as we all did, to be on the lookout. Like the rest of us, she had regular colonoscopies (one a bit late) and is a thirteen-year survivor.

My aunts Ola and Gertrude lived to be 84 and 94, respectively, having both survived breast cancer. The fact that my sister Vivian's breast cancer was diagnosed when she was only 37 made her the most likely one to die from it (because typically the younger you are, the more aggressive type of cancer you have). But she did not. My sister Gwen, who by all rights should have survived her breast cancer, died at 71, because she hadn't had a mammogram in more than ten years—or maybe ever. I don't know.

The point of all this is, yes, cancer is scary. In fact, cancer strikes more fear in us than heart attacks, strokes, diabetes, and kidney failure. I believe this is partly because we associate cancer with death. Cancer is also one of the few illnesses where the treatments—chemotherapy, in particular—can strike as much fear in the patient as the diagnosis itself. The thought of losing your breast or your hair strikes at the core of most women's sense of self and femininity. I believe it is for this reason that women fear breast cancer more than lung cancer, even though lung cancer is far more deadly. But we need to take care with the stories we tell ourselves. We too often nurture narratives that are counterproductive to getting care and that only stoke our medical distrust and fear.

We've all heard folks say, "She was just fine until she went to the doctor," never mind that "she" waited months feeling off before going to the doctor. Or there's that old saw that says, "She had surgery and as soon as that air hit it, the cancer just took off spreading." Cue the instigators in the amen corner, chiming in, "See, that's why you don't let them cut on you."

We have to stop. This is not a forest fire, people. Cancer doesn't grow when the air hits it. It grows when you do nothing about it. It stems from a belief system that gets in the way of your doing what you need to do to get better. We have to break that cycle.

On the whole, my family, despite our awful cancer history, has won more battles than we have lost. And, for the record, with early screening and proper treatment, we'd have won even more, starting with my mom. Cancer scares us, but it should not immobilize us. I want you to know your family history and use it to know what to screen for and when. I cannot tell you that if you do everything right, you won't get cancer. No one can. But you can take steps to reduce your risks and a cancer diagnosis does not always equal death.

Good News You Can Use

Gynecologic cancers include:

- Cervical cancer

- Ovarian cancer

- Uterine (endometrial) cancer

- Vaginal and vulvar cancers

It may please you to know that none of these ranks among the leading causes of cancer deaths in women. Ovarian cancer does account for more deaths than any other cancer of the female reproductive system, but according to the American Cancer Society, it ranks fifth in women's cancer-related deaths. Lung cancer is still number one.

While we continue to make progress in effectively treating gynecologic cancers, much of that is linked to our advancing ability to diagnose more types of the disease in early stages. For example, the death rates for cervical cancer have plummeted due both to early intervention (pap smears) and to preventative vaccines. When it comes to cancer of almost every type, timing is not everything, but it's major. Ovarian cancer, like pancreatic cancer, poses particularly stubborn challenges, because we do not have good screening tools and, unlike endometrial cancer, it does not produce symptoms until late stage. However, having taken oral contraceptives for five years or more decreases the risk of developing ovarian cancer by as much as 50 percent.

Breast cancer is technically not a gynecologic cancer, as it impacts men as well. However, 99 percent of breast cancers occur in women and it is the second-most common cancer in women, after skin cancers. (Let's not sleep on skin cancer either! Consistent use of sunscreen may prevent it and yearly skin checks with your dermatologist will help with early detection.) The median age of breast cancer diagnosis is 62. A relatively small number of women, like my sister Vivian, are diagnosed before they are 45. In fact, less than 10 percent of breast cancers are diagnosed before age 60—except in, you guessed it, Black women, where the risk of being diagnosed at an earlier age is twice that of white women.

This should be reason enough for women to continue to see a gynecologist annually—in addition to a primary care physician—long past your reproductive years. Your gynecologist is the doctor most likely, and best equipped, to focus on your breast health.

National Cancer Institute (NCI) data put the number of people living with cancer in the United States in 2019 at 16.9 million. By 2030, that number is expected to reach 22.2 million. With a few exceptions, the death rates for most cancers have decreased over the past thirty years (by an average of 1.4 percent per year among women, from 2001 to 2017, according to the 2020 Annual Report to the Nation).

According to the CDC, the cancer mortality rate has fallen by more than 33 percent since 1991. But when it comes to the absolute numbers of deaths per year, more people die annually from cardiovascular disease than from all types of cancer combined. That's right, I said *combined*! Let that sink in for a minute. Yet we do not fear heart disease nearly as much as we do cancer.

There are as many different types of cancer as you have tissues in your body, and even within the same organ system, there are different subtypes. They can behave differently and respond differently to treatment modalities. Despite improvements in cancer treatments, the biggest wins have come from early diagnosis and preventative measures. We are much better at treating lung cancer now than we were twenty years ago. But the reality is, fewer people smoke, and this has had arguably the biggest impact on decreasing cancer deaths.

Unfortunately, the rate of lung cancer deaths has declined more slowly for women than for men (1.1 and 2.6 percent). Despite relatively few changes in cervical cancer treatment, the incidence of cervical cancer is down 65 percent in young women who have had the HPV vaccine. This is one of the best examples that we have of prevention (vaccine) and early diagnosis (pap smears) actually moving the needle.

Here is an area that doesn't get nearly the attention that it should: prevention.

Together, lung, colon, breast, and uterine cancer account for almost 50 percent of new cancers diagnosed each year. The good news is that these cancers are curable when caught early and the risk factors for developing them are fairly well established. But rather than waiting on a new medical breakthrough to cure cancer, wouldn't it make sense just to figure out how not to get cancer in the first place? And yes, we can do both. Just as we can walk and chew gum at the same time, we can innovate and prevent.

To those of you who think that just because cancer runs in your family it is inevitable, I assure you it is not. In fact, only 5–10 percent of cancers are thought to have a genetic or hereditary basis. Furthermore, it is estimated that over 50 percent of cancers could be prevented by the same things I have been harping on throughout this entire book—don't smoke, drink less alcohol, exercise regularly, maintain a healthy weight, and eat a healthy diet (oh, and use sunscreen). When you combine these healthy behaviors with regular cancer screening (pap smears, colonoscopies, and mammograms), you have done yourself a world of good.

The truth is, you *can* minimize your risk factors for getting cancer, and that should give you enormous comfort. It is also true what they say—an ounce of prevention is worth a pound of cure.

What's Age Got to Do With It?

All cancers are caused by damage to your DNA. We know that excess alcohol and cigarette smoking are directly toxic to DNA and can lead to cancer. Yet even though smoking rates have declined, lung cancer remains the leading cause of cancer deaths in women—and 16 percent of women diagnosed with lung cancer have never smoked. But let's revel in the fact that not smoking will absolutely reduce your risk of getting lung cancer, as well as a host of other cancers, and will reduce your risk of contracting a long litany of cardiovascular diseases.

According to NCI data, the median age of cancer diagnosis is 66, and if we live long enough, almost 40 percent of us will be diagnosed with cancer of some type. I know that's hard to hear, but don't shrink from it—grow, by understanding what your risks are and how you can mitigate them. And note that this is a population statistic, not an individual statistic. *Your* cancer risk is based on your health and family histories as well as on environmental and lifestyle factors.

Think of your DNA as the master cookbook that contains all the recipes on how to make a unique you. The original DNA that defines you is present only at the moment of conception. Everything from that moment forward is a copy of the master cookbook. By the time you are born, that copy has been replicated trillions of times and it will continue to be copied every time you grow an inch or need new skin cells to heal a wound.

Now let's use an analogy—because, well, I love analogies. When your master DNA is copied on a brand-new copy machine (your cells), you would expect pretty much an exact replica of the original, right? But what happens when your copy of a copy of a copy gets reproduced a million times on that same old machine—the only one you'll ever have? What if you never clean the copier screen or you spill coffee on your cookbook? Eventually, a few letters may go missing, or the period at the end of a sentence fades and now the sentence just runs on. The letters *cot* become *cut,* which changes the meaning entirely. Now instead of *cottage cheese,* it says, "cut the cheese." I think we can all agree that would make for a very different dish.

You cooks out there know a little mistake is usually not catastrophic, but imagine if over time those mistakes accumulate. Suppose instead of "add ⅛ teaspoon," the recipe eventually reads "add 8 teaspoons." Even if you've never boiled eggs, I trust you see my point.

Cancers increase with age because the damage to our DNA accumulates over time. Our immune systems, which are immensely important in protecting us from cancer, naturally weaken with age. Not to mix metaphors here, but our immune system is like our bodies' very own autocorrect—and what do we all know about autocorrect? It can be faulty.

When details in your genetic code inevitably get erased or misread over time, it changes your recipes, and usually not for the better. This is how most cancers start—with an accumulation of small genetic mistakes that, left uncorrected, can lead to more catastrophic mistakes over time. Understanding that you can't totally control the process is not meant to immobilize you, it's meant to motivate you. Aging happens, but how you age depends largely on you and the choices you make along the way. You need to keep your copier clean and get it serviced regularly, because how we fare after a cancer diagnosis is highly dependent upon how we've treated ourselves years before that diagnosis. You typically have multiple opportunities to intervene before the damage is too great—and every improvement counts.

Breast Cancer

The good news about breast cancer (yes, there is some good news) is that you are more likely to survive a breast cancer diagnosis today than at any time in history. Even though breast cancer is still the second-most prevalent cancer in women, it is not the deadliest. In fact, the number of breast cancer deaths decreased by 40 percent from 1989 to 2017, and 90 percent of women who are diagnosed with early-stage breast cancer today will be long-term survivors. The improved survivorship is due to a combination of education, better screening methods leading to earlier diagnosis, and more effective treatments targeted to specific breast cancer types. In fact, more breast cancer survivors die of cardiovascular disease than from a recurrence of their breast cancer.

We also have a better understanding of the factors that contribute to breast cancer—many of which you can modify to decrease your personal risk. For example, having your first baby before the age of 30 decreases your breast cancer risk. I don't recommend it as a mitigation strategy (and I assume this ship has already sailed for you), but it's still worth knowing. Breastfeeding your baby, regardless of your age at the time, also reduces your breast cancer risk. And now that prior broadly held beliefs have been debunked, it's important to note that having taken birth control pills in the past, or taking hormone therapy for menopausal symptom relief, does not significantly increase your risk for breast cancer.

Joanne

Joanne is 67 years old. She had her last period fifteen years ago, and although very symptomatic, she opted not to take menopausal hormone therapy because she was afraid of getting breast cancer. Her hot flashes stopped years ago, but she still has trouble sleeping.

She is in relatively good health despite being about twenty-five pounds overweight. She has no cardiovascular issues and no family history of breast cancer. She sees her internist and gynecologist annually.

As part of her annual physical, she had a mammogram, and for the first time ever, she got a callback. Given her family history, she was not overly concerned. The callback led to a biopsy, which confirmed the diagnosis of breast cancer. Her next step was to see a surgeon. Because the area of concern was so small, she had a lumpectomy followed by six weeks of radiation.

The Takeaway: The overwhelming majority of women who get breast cancer neither have a family history nor take hormones. So, don't be complacent if you don't either. Your biggest risk factor for being diagnosed with breast cancer is living long enough to get it. Get those annual mammograms. Early diagnosis leads to less extensive surgery and a higher probability of cure.

Some breast cancer risk factors, like your age, cannot be modified. Others can be—the choice is yours.

Modifiable Risk Factors	Unmodifiable Risk Factors
Obesity	Age
Smoking	Gender
Alcohol >1 drink/day (5 oz. wine or 1.5 oz. liquor)	First birth after age 30 (wouldn't recommend having a baby to decrease risk)
Stress	Radiation to the chest
Breastfeeding (women who breastfeed have a lower risk)	Genetic mutations (BRCA1/2) Family history: 2 or more first-degree relatives*
Physical inactivity	Dense breasts
Diet	

*Depends on the age of the relatives—premenopausal first-degree relatives are more significant than postmenopausal relatives.

There are now questionnaire-based breast cancer risk calculators that use information on your medical, reproductive, and family history to estimate your chance of developing breast cancer over the next five to ten years. The most commonly used calculator is the Tyrer-Cuzick risk assessment tool. The first such tool designed specifically for women of color—the Black Women's Health Study Breast Cancer Risk Calculator—was introduced in 2021. Be aware that risk calculators only assess probabilities, not certainties. They can be helpful if knowing your risk motivates you to institute risk-mitigating lifestyle changes or if they help modify your screening protocols.

As noted earlier, the biggest risk factor for developing breast cancer is living long enough to get it. The lifetime risk of getting breast cancer in the entire U.S. population of women is 1 in 8, or 12.5 percent. We doctors quote this figure regularly. That number seems high and should rightfully be a cause for concern. But we need to unpack this, and I need you to stay with me for a minute. There will be math, but just addition—nothing complicated.

The National Cancer Institute estimates the risk of being diagnosed with breast cancer within the next ten years by age group as follows:

- 30–40: 0.49 percent (1 in 204)

- 40–50: 1.55 percent (1 in 65)

- 50–60: 2.40 percent (1 in 42)

- 60–70: 3.54 percent (1 in 28)

- 70–80: 4.09 percent (1 in 24)

So, where does the 1 in 8, or 12.8 percent, *lifetime risk* number come from? This is where the addition comes in. When you add 0.49 + 1.55 + 2.40 + 3.54 + 4.09, guess what the total is? You guessed it: about 12 percent. But obviously, no one person gets breast cancer in every decade of life, so that figure is not untrue, but it's misleading. The 12 percent is the lifetime risk for the entire population, not any individual woman. See what you can do with statistics?

Even if you live to be 80, your risk of getting breast cancer is only

4 percent. Four percent is not nothing, but it is a whole lot less scary than 12 percent.

Triple-Negative Breast Cancer

We now know that there are different types of breast cancer that originate in different areas of the breast, with different receptors. We have never had more targeted treatment options or better outcomes, because we can now treat based on the individual characteristics of the cancer. But there is still much to learn about why certain cancers are more prevalent in different populations and how to treat them.

The overall incidence of breast cancer is comparable in Black and white women; however, the mortality rate for Black women is 41 percent higher. One of the reasons for this disparity is that Black women have a higher percentage of the more aggressive triple-negative breast cancers, but it's not the only reason. The other factors that contribute to this disparity are what we know as the social determinants of health, which include access to early diagnosis, exposure to environmental carcinogens, and lack of quality healthcare facilities, as well as ingrained systemic biases and racism within the medical community itself.

Breast cancers are typically categorized by the presence or absence of receptors for estrogen, progestin, and a protein called "human epidermal growth factor" (HER2). Tumors that lack all three of these receptors (or test negative for them, thus the name *triple-negative*) are typically more aggressive, and there are fewer treatment options if they recur.

While the higher incidence of triple-negative breast tumors in Black women contributes to the racial disparity in the overall breast cancer mortality rate, research published in the journal *JAMA Oncology*, in July 2021, indicated that Black women are 28 percent more likely to die than white women with the same stage diagnosis and tumor type. Black women are more likely to be diagnosed at a later stage than white women. Black women experience longer wait times for an initial biopsy and surgery. And Black women are less likely to have access to comprehensive cancer centers for treatment. This is a travesty. There is nothing about the biology of the cancer that explains this.

Black women are more likely to be uninsured or underinsured than their white counterparts. Simple logistics are often overlooked but are no less influential on a woman's prognosis. The ability to comply with follow-up treatments and/or medications can be dependent on whether a patient owns a car, has someone to babysit her children, or can take time (paid or not) off from work. These challenges and more place hourly and essential workers and many single mothers at an automatic disadvantage that is rarely acknowledged and often left unaddressed.

Endometrial (Uterine) Cancer

Uterine cancer is the most common gynecologic cancer in the United States, accounting for 7 percent of all new cancers diagnosed in females annually. Uterine cancer includes both the cancer of the lining of the uterus (endometrial) and cancers that arise in the body of the uterus. Our discussion is going to focus on endometrial cancers because they are by far the most common, as well as the most preventable and treatable if diagnosed early.

According to a 2019 article in the *Journal of Clinical Oncology*, the rates of endometrial cancer have been on the rise for the past twenty years. Although older studies have reported a lower incidence of uterine cancer for Black women, they underestimated the true incidence because of the higher rate of hysterectomies in Black women. As such, Black women had lower rates of uterine cancer because they had *fewer uteruses to get cancer in.* When this correction is taken into account, the rate of uterine cancer is roughly equivalent to the rate of uterine cancer in white women. Hispanic and Asian/Pacific Islanders have lower rates of uterine cancer.

There were several articles that made their way around the internet in 2022 trumpeting the dramatic rise in uterine cancer for Black women. There was even an article that implied the use of chemical hair straighteners was responsible for this dramatic rise in Black women's cancer. While articles such as these make for excellent clickbait, they are not helpful. And while the statistic regarding Black women is true, most articles failed to report that the rate of uterine cancer has increased for all women.

There are many complicated and nuanced reasons for the rise in uterine cancer, but perming your hair is probably not one of them. It's important to understand what the purpose of these incendiary stories is—mostly it's feeding fear and increasing viewership. Nothing draws attention like a sensational headline. It's also a prime example of victim blaming. Both the medical profession and the media have demonstrated a longtime habit of implying that if something bad is happening to women, and particularly women of color, it must be their fault.

Grammie

My mother-in-law, Miriam, affectionately known as "Grammie," died peacefully at 86 after having survived so many health scares that I could have included her in every chapter. It's hard to believe, but when I met her, she was just about my age today, and I thought of her as a very jazzy older lady. Ouch!

She saw her nice West Indian doctor in Queens, New York, twice a year. I suspect most of those visits were social ones with a perfunctory medication refill and blood pressure check, because Miriam was a minimizer. She never complained, never wanted to make a fuss. And she was in pretty good health . . . until she wasn't.

In her mid-70s, while home alone one day, she didn't feel well. Rather than bother anyone, she drove herself to the emergency room, where she was admitted after being diagnosed with a mild heart attack.

Once she was stable, we brought her to D.C., where she could have what we thought would be a routine cardiac catheterization in the hospital where I worked. (See, not all daughters-in-law are bad.) Midway through the procedure, some worrisome changes on the cardiac monitor occurred, which led to her being airlifted to another hospital for an emergency quadruple bypass. My guess is that she had some warning signs well before her heart attack, but who knows?

Grammie recovered nicely. Then, about two years later, she came to our home for an extended visit. One evening, while emptying the trash in my mother-in-law's bathroom, I saw something very odd—a mini pad wrapped in tissue. My girls were way too young for their periods, so let's just say I was concerned. My 75-year-old mother-in-law was using mini pads because she was *bleeding*? And she'd never said a word? Did I mention that I'm a gynecologist?

"Grammie, have you been bleeding?" I asked.

"Yes, just a little bit," she answered, downplaying, as usual. But when I asked her when was the last time she'd had a pelvic exam or even seen her gynecologist, it became clear that for years she had not. My babysitter then told me that my mother-in-law had been sending her to the drugstore for pads for months.

I immediately made an appointment for Grammie to see a gynecologic oncologist, who confirmed a diagnosis of endometrial cancer. In the process of confirming that diagnosis, he discovered that she also had breast cancer. A hysterectomy and lymph node dissection confirmed stage 3 endometrial cancer. She got six weeks of radiation after surgery and lived another ten years. But save for my emptying the trash that day, I never would have known, and this story would have had a very different ending.

The Takeaway: Illness is not weakness, and when it comes to your health, silence is not golden. Ever. Speak up. See a doctor. And with all things cancer-related, the sooner the better.

Women are often encouraged to believe that stoicism is strength, that sucking it up—whatever "it" is—makes us somehow superior. We are taught to endure, to shoulder the weights of loved ones—our children, partners, elders—and resist burdening others, even when we're in need. We also let fear of the unknown drive us. Sticking your head in the sand is never a good healthcare strategy. So don't!

Endometrial cancer behaves very much like breast cancer and encompasses many of the same risk factors. Advancing age, prolonged (unopposed) estrogen exposure, obesity, lack of physical activity, and smoking are known risk factors. There is also evidence that *not* having taken birth control pills is a risk factor for getting endometrial cancer. You heard me right. Birth control pills not only reduce your risk of ovarian cancer but of endometrial cancer as well. Some researchers even speculate that the decrease in the use of hormone replacement therapy (HRT) might be contributing to the rise in uterine cancer.

Ninety percent of uterine cancers arise in the lining of the uterus, or the endometrium. There are two major subtypes of endometrial cancer: Type 1, endometrioid; and Type 2, non-endometrioid, with the latter being more aggressive and—you guessed it—disproportionately diagnosed in Black women, much like triple-negative breast cancer. On the upside, the majority of endometrial cancer is the endometrioid type, even for Black women. This is important because when diagnosed early, endometrial cancer, like breast cancer, is curable, with five-year survival rates over 90 percent. But, for reasons that we don't yet understand, the risk for non-endometrioid, or the more aggressive type, is going up for all women—Black, white, Hispanic, and Asian/Pacific Islander—with the rates of increase being higher for women of color.

Most of these statistics are upsetting—and not new. We've been aware of the racial disparity in endometrial cancer for more than twenty-five years and it cannot be explained away just by Black women's higher incidence of the more aggressive type. In fact, the disparity in mortality for Black women diagnosed with endometrial cancer was so alarming that the CDC and the American College of Obstetricians and Gynecologists convened an expert panel to address these issues. Black women are twice as likely to die from uterine cancer as white women. Black women are diagnosed with later-stage disease and are less likely to receive standard treatment for endometrial cancer even when correcting for cancer type, stage at diagnosis, socioeconomic status, or insurance. Sound familiar? It should. To date, there has not been one study aimed at the interventions that might improve this disparity. You heard me right: not one.

So, what can you do? First of all, it is vitally important to understand what the early warning signs are and who is at risk. Endometrial cancer is more common after menopause, with the median age at diagnosis being 63. About 70 percent of uterine cancer cases are associated with obesity. Endometrioid (the less aggressive type) cancer usually produces early warning signs. The most common sign is postmenopausal bleeding (bleeding or spotting more than a year after your last period), which should never be ignored. Although most cases of such bleeding are benign, let your gynecologist tell you that after a thorough evaluation. To minimize the chances of getting endometrial cancer, review the aforementioned risk factors. Your weight and physical activity are important ones that you can address now.

The evaluation for bleeding after menopause can be simple, and so is the test to figure it out—a transvaginal ultrasound. A simple, relatively painless sonogram to measure the lining of the uterus (<4mm) rules out endometrial cancer in 90 percent of cases. Only if bleeding or spotting persists would a more invasive procedure—like an in-office endometrial biopsy (not entirely painless, but mercifully quick) or a dilatation and curettage (D&C) with hysteroscopy—be necessary.

This brings me to another important reminder (is there an echo in here?). Even if you are menopausal, not sexually active, and otherwise symptom-free, you should still see your gynecologist annually before age 65 and at least once every two years after age 65. Remember, Grammie saw her primary care doctor regularly but hadn't had a breast or pelvic examination or even a conversation about gynecologic issues for years. Neither she nor her primary doctor prioritized that once she was a senior. They should have. And you must!

Colon Cancer

Laila

Laila was one of my longtime patients. She married at 42 and tried to get pregnant without success, even after multiple rounds of in vitro fertilization (IVF). Many of our visits focused on her disappointment about not being able to conceive. Eventually, she made peace with this, and she and her husband decided to adopt a beautiful baby boy.

By 45, she was busy raising a toddler when she came in for her annual checkup. Given her age, I informed her that, in addition to her breast and pelvic examinations, I would be doing a rectal exam.

While performing the rectal exam, I obtained a small stool specimen, which was then checked for microscopic blood. When Laila's test came back positive, I wasn't terribly concerned because there can be many benign reasons for this—internal hemorrhoids, anal fissures, even recent aspirin use. But in an abundance of caution, I called Laila and advised her to get a colonoscopy.

Imagine my surprise when she called three weeks later to tell me that she had stage 2 colon cancer. She was able to have her surgery done laparoscopically (through a few small incisions) rather than through a large abdominal incision, making her recovery time far shorter. At this writing, it's been about seven years since her initial diagnosis, and she and her son are both well.

The Takeaway: Everyone should initiate colonoscopy screening at 45. The recommendations have changed due to an increased incidence of colon cancer in younger adults.

By now you know that colon cancer counseling and screening are never far from my mind—not only because of my mother, but also because my sister Joyce was diagnosed with colon cancer at 65. Fortunately, Joyce's and Laila's cancer stories had happy endings, thanks to screening and colonoscopies.

Colon cancer symptoms can include bloody stool, a change in bowel habits that persists, unexplained abdominal pain or cramping, a persistent urge to defecate, fatigue, unintended weight loss, and anemia. But because colorectal cancers rarely show themselves before the disease is at an advanced stage, regular screenings are imperative. And screenings not only pick up colon cancers but also precancerous polyps that, left undiagnosed, could lead to cancer.

It has always been my practice to start rectal examinations at 45—even before that became the standard recommended protocol. Imagine how different Laila's outcome would have been had she not had a simple rectal exam. I know rectal examinations are a literal pain in the ass, and to be honest, they're not one of the favorite aspects of my job, but they are important. At the time of Laila's diagnosis, the recommended age for screening colonoscopy was 50. I shudder to think what her prognosis might have been by then. The recommended interval between colonoscopies is now ten years. A lot can happen in ten years. That is why asking your doctor to add a rectal examination to your general physical is never a bad thing.

In medicine, as we learn more, recommendations change, and your doctor needs to keep current. But so do you. If your doctor does not suggest that you get a colonoscopy at 45, ask them to review the new guidelines and then press for a referral for the exam. If a doctor is mad because you've done your research or have an opinion, you probably need to go find another doctor. Also, if you have a family member who has been diagnosed with colon cancer, you should start screening ten years younger than the age at which they were diagnosed.

Now, here is a bit of art over science. Once you've had a negative colonoscopy, the recommended time before your next one is ten years, but I believe that high-risk populations—if you are African American or have a family history—should rescreen at a minimum of five- to seven-year intervals. After multiple negative screens every five years, my sister Joyce waited ten years before her next colonoscopy. By then she had stage 3 colon cancer. Again, cancer and timing are inseparable [♪ "Inseparable"].

Cervical Cancer

There is much that we do not know about what causes most cancers, so usually the best we can hope for is a good screening test that identifies the early stages. Yet with cervical cancer we hit the trifecta. We not only have a good screening test (pap smear), we also have a strong understanding of how cervical cancer behaves and what causes it. Plus, taking it one giant step further, we have a vaccine that has led to a dramatic decrease in the incidence of cervical cancer and its related mortality.

Human papillomavirus (HPV) is the most important risk factor in cervical cancer. HPV refers to a *group* of more than 150 related viruses that are sexually transmitted. Most of these viruses are low-risk and resolve spontaneously, thanks to a healthy immune system. However, high-risk subtypes of HPV are strongly linked to cervical cancer as well as cancers of the vulva, vagina, mouth, throat, and anus. It is important to note that HPV is completely asymptomatic in both women and men. In women, it is only detected with a routine pap smear or through HPV testing.

The pap smear gives us an opportunity to intervene in the "precancerous" stages of cervical cancer, much like removing polyps during colonoscopies. The HPV vaccine has also altered our approach to screenings. After decades of telling you that you need a pap smear every year, now we're telling you that you can have a pap every three years. *What?* Remember, there was a time in medicine when we thought leeches and bloodletting were good ideas. We learn constantly, thank goodness, and we adapt our practices to reflect new knowledge.

So, here's the deal: After age 30, you have two options. You can continue to screen every three years (old-school pap) or you can co-test, which means that along with your pap smear, you can simultaneously screen for high-risk HPV subtypes. If the pap and HPV screens are negative, you can wait five years before you test again; or you can test for HPV only, without the pap, and repeat that every five years if negative. Still with me? Honestly, in real life, I don't know many patients or doctors who feel comfortable with testing every five years. There is always a caveat. People with multiple new partners, or who have partners who have multiple partners, should stick to more frequent screening options.

Most of our daughters, and hopefully our sons, have already been vaccinated against HPV, so cervical cancer will become a thing of the past. That would make one down, with thirty more cancers to go—maybe not cause for a party, but at least a happy dance [♪ "Happy"].

Elizabeth

Elizabeth is a vibrant 44-year-old woman. She is healthy, has two children in college, and recently started a new career. In leaving behind her old job, she left just about everything else from her old life. Her marriage of twenty years has ended, and she is facing the prospect of dating someone new for the first time in twenty-five years.

In addition to trying to figure out how to navigate the brave new world of online dating, she wants to know what she should do to protect herself when she enters a new sexual relationship. She has had only two sexual partners and has never had an abnormal pap smear.

Allow me to interject: It should go without saying that condoms are always the right answer, particularly with new partners, at least until STI testing has been done by both partners *and* you are reasonably certain that the relationship is monogamous. Another quick aside here: The majority of women infected by HIV get it through heterosexual contact. Black women, although only 14 percent of the population, make up 61 percent of new HIV infections annually. I know, right? It can be downright depressing, but—once more—knowledge is power. Use yours. In the words of the late, great Biggie Smalls, "If you don't know, now you know."

Back to Elizabeth. Should she get the HPV vaccine? The answer is probably yes. If you're thinking she's too old, think again. Although the HPV vaccine was originally approved for girls and women aged 9–26, there have been several adjustments to this recommendation. The first extended the HPV vaccine to boys, because HPV is transmitted through sexual contact. Duh! Why vaccinate just half the susceptible population? But the most recent change has been extending the limit of eligibility for the vaccine to age 45, in recognition of the fact that older women might still have new sexual partners. And remember, with HPV as with HIV, it doesn't matter how many sexual partners you personally have had. You are taking on the cumulative exposures of your partner and your partner's partners.

The Takeaway: There are very few cancers where the precise cause is known. So, leverage that advantage here, and if you are entering a new relationship or anticipate doing so, talk to your doctor about whether the HPV vaccine would make sense for you.

Racial Disparities in Cancer: Who's to Blame and What Can Be Done?

There seems to be a cottage industry designed to scare women, and it appears that there is a full-scale industrial complex out there to frighten Black women. We are continuously bombarded with headlines that decry the worsening prognosis for Black women for just about everything health-related. This begets a tendency to blame the victim and ask: What is the problem with Black women? What are Black women doing wrong? Why can't Black women fix themselves?

Along with everyone else, Black women become desensitized to these issues as they become ill and chronic diseases become normalized. Instead of feeling a sense of outrage that fuels our demand for solutions, Black women begin to buy into the myth that our poor health and poor outcomes are inevitable. They are not.

I want you to vehemently reject any narrative that suggests simply being Black is the issue. The color of your skin does not mean that you are predisposed to illness, weaker, genetically inferior, not rich enough, not smart enough, not creative, or not well-connected enough to improve your odds and outcomes. These erroneous and offensive notions not only pose a threat to your health, your power, and your peace, but buying into them can make you become complacent and, ultimately, complicit in your own decline. Dr. Linda Goler Blount, president of the Black Women's Health Imperative, put it succinctly—"Race is not a risk factor. Racism is." Push back with all your might!

No matter what your current health status or health history may be, there is always something you can do to improve your future health, and it begins with believing in your own agency—then getting to work. This is as true with cancer as with any aspect of your life.

Black women actually have a lower overall incidence of cancer than white women do (408/100,000 for Black women and 450/100,000 for white women in 2020; Hispanic and Asian women have the lowest rates). Yet it is widely reported that Black women are overly represented in the number of cancer deaths. Has anyone really attempted to address the root cause of these disparities? And worse yet, even when the causes are known, have there been any large-scale efforts to address them?

This is critical data, more than worthy of alarm. It's a cop-out to tell you that it's your hair dye, your chemical perm, or your lipstick that is making you sick, rather than to talk about systemic racism and how Black women are underserved, under-researched, underestimated, and all but ignored by the medical establishment.

There may well be a connection between some chemicals we routinely expose ourselves to and cancer or other diseases. But the state of your health is at least equally determined by the healthcare, or lack thereof, that you have access to. It is about the lack of fresh, nutritious food options in your neighborhood. It is about the lack of safe outdoor spaces where you and your family can seek refuge and joy, and it is about the aggressions, small and large, that keep you up at night and disturb your peace, daily. It is about not being offered the same treatment options as others. It is about not knowing how to advocate for yourself within a healthcare system that was not built for you and all too often doesn't see you. It is about the compounding systemic stresses of being a Black woman in America. All of that.

Are Black women getting equal access to education about prevention? Are Black women receiving the same quality of care and range of treatment options as white women? What is it about Black women's lived experience that puts them at greater risk for death from disease? These are big, important questions, and more activism is needed around the press for answers.

Whenever you read an article about cancer and its racial disparities, there are a couple of terms I want you to keep in mind. The *incidence* of cancer refers to how many people are diagnosed each year (usually reported in number of cases per 100,000 people). The *mortality rate* is how many people die from that cancer in any given year. So, incidence tells you how common a particular type of cancer is in the studied population, and mortality tells you how deadly that cancer is in a population. And for Black women in America, regardless of the incidence, the mortality figures are almost universally worse.

When these figures vary significantly from one group to another, a mere description of the disparity, or the "what," is not sufficient. Without advancing the conversation to "why" and how to fix it, we're just spinning our wheels. Worse still, we do not have answers as to how to address these disparities, or maybe we do but just lack the will to implement them. Given that as human beings, we share 99.6 percent of our DNA, the answer may not be found in our genes, but somewhere else.

So, the next time you read a headline that says, "Black Women Have a Higher Risk of [insert your least favorite health condition here]," don't just file it under "tell me something I don't know." Instead, I want you to delve a little deeper—and demand that your doctors, your insurers, and your elected officials do as well. I know that's a lot, but while we're waiting on a societal overhaul (and yes, we can do two things at one time), I want you to be an effective advocate for yourself and your family's health. Doing all you can do today to minimize your risk of developing cancer is central to that.

Will You Tri(al)?

The 2022 annual budget for medical research funded by the NIH was $45 billion. Only about 10 percent of that budget is allocated specifically to women's health. In studies involving cancer and the brain, the commitment to understanding women is even smaller.

Clinical trials set the standards for cancer treatments. Despite the known disparities in outcomes and mortality statistics, the Association of American Medical Colleges estimates that Black people represent less than 5 percent of clinical trials. As a result, cancer research is lacking in Black stories, women's stories, intersectional stories, and the critical data those stories provide. The treatment protocols that are prescribed for us are developed without us. Racial disparities in cancer mortality rates that can't fully be explained can't be addressed. To what degree do these disparities stem from biology versus the social determinants of health? My guess is that it is less of the former and more of the latter. But no one's guess is good enough. We need to know for sure. Which brings me back to our need for inclusive clinical trials. (See Additional Resources for how to participate in clinical trials.)

All women are underserved in medical research, and for Black women this problem is even more egregious. There is no solution without us. We need to participate in studies so that future generations won't be facing the same unanswered questions. It's not melodramatic to declare this a matter of life and death. Treatment protocols should be designed to take account of the real lived experiences of Black and all underserved women. Researchers need to acknowledge women's fears and understand how to effectively recruit and retain diverse populations. Dr. Linda Goler Blount's research shows that the single most cited reason for Black people's lack of participation in studies is not the Tuskegee experiment or Henrietta Lacks. It's that they are not asked. We need more researchers of color and more researchers with cultural sensitivity to investigate these issues.

We cannot simply keep describing inequities and disparities without adequately addressing them. And we—Black women especially—cannot keep making excuses for not being part of the solution.

DR. SHARON'S RX FOR

Cancer Prevention

1. Annual mammograms starting at 40; monthly breast self-exams and yearly breast exams by a doctor, forever.

2. Consider genetic screening if two or more close premenopausal relatives have been diagnosed with breast cancer—especially if they occur in different generations.

3. Annual gynecologic examinations through age 65, then biennially.

4. Pap smears either annually or every three years with HPV co-testing.

5. Up to age 45, consider getting the HPV vaccine if engaging in sex with new or multiple partners.

6. Get any postmenopausal bleeding evaluated.

7. Colon cancer screening starting at 45 (or earlier if you know you're at high risk).

8. Investigate any persistent abdominal pain or unexplained weight loss.

9. Wear sunscreen and get annual skin checks with your dermatologist after 50.

CHAPTER 5

Control♪

Chronic Stress, Weight Gain, and Diabetes: Tame Your Triple Threat

Dear Sis,

Sometimes, we have to love one another enough to have tough conversations straight, no chaser. This is one of those times.

Obesity, stress, and diabetes (particularly type 2 diabetes, the most common kind) are three of the most significant threats to your overall health, and given their strong links to cancer, heart disease, and Alzheimer's, they are among the leading causes of preventable, premature death.

They are often discussed in isolation, but I am grouping them together so that you'll come to understand how closely interrelated they are and how serious their damage to your health can be. Most importantly, though, I want you to see how incredibly powerful your choices are in containing the risk they represent.

Stress is unavoidable and its causes are often beyond our control—which is part of why it's so damn stressful! But while we can't control its causes, we can do a better job of controlling how we respond to it—because those responses can make things far worse. Stress is related to weight gain and obesity in a cyclical way: Chronic stress can trigger the unhealthy behaviors that lead to weight gain (and, sometimes, obesity), and excess weight can also cause undue stress, creating a damaging cycle that's not easy to disrupt.

Both obesity and stress have been linked with type 2 diabetes—which, in turn, places you at higher risk for diseases of the heart, brain, and joints, each of which we will address in the next few chapters. Think of them as a trio of devious cousins who are always trying to be where you are. When you run into any of them (and you will), wave and keep walking, because they mean you no good. They are killing us. Every day. And you have the power to stop them. Just by making better choices. Start today.

xo, Dr. Sharon

There are three types of diabetes:

- Type 1 diabetes is thought to be an autoimmune disease that usually presents in childhood or young adulthood. Researchers have not yet identified how to prevent it. But it is treatable with insulin.

- Type 2 diabetes, or what used to be called "adult-onset diabetes" (today, children are increasingly being diagnosed with type 2 diabetes), is the most common and can be controlled with diet, oral medication, or insulin.

- Gestational diabetes occurs during pregnancy and usually resolves after delivery. However, gestational diabetes does increase the likelihood of developing type 2 diabetes later in life.

All three types of diabetes result in high levels of blood sugar (or glucose). Your pancreas produces insulin to help your body utilize the sugar in your bloodstream released from the foods you consume. Only type 1 diabetes is due to an inability to produce insulin. The other types are due to insulin resistance, or the inability to efficiently respond to insulin. Insulin moves the sugar from your bloodstream to your cells, where it is needed for energy production. (Think of it like gas for your car, but the gas only works if it's in the tank.)

When your body doesn't make enough insulin or you become resistant to insulin's effects (seen in obesity and polycystic ovary syndrome), the sugar in your bloodstream cannot be utilized by your cells for energy consumption. When that sugar can't make it into the cells where it is needed, the sugar levels in the blood spike and the high levels of circulating sugar are damaging to your blood vessels, with the smaller vessels (for example, those that feed your eyes, kidneys, brain, and lower extremities) being at greatest risk. But to be clear, the greatest risk diabetes poses is to your cardiovascular health. According to the CDC, if you have diabetes, you're twice as likely to develop heart disease or have a stroke—and at a younger age than someone without it.

Women and men are affected by diabetes at similar rates, but the disease affects women differently. Diabetic women are at greater risk for heart disease and stroke than diabetic men; they are at higher risk for blindness and depression; and diabetic women have lower post–heart attack survival rates and poorer quality of life than their male counterparts.

Native American/Alaska Native women have the highest rate of diabetes in the United States, according to the U.S. Department of Health and Human Services. Black people are 50 percent more likely to develop type 2 diabetes than whites—and that's not even the most shocking statistic. According to the American Heart Association, Black people are:

- Twice as likely to die of diabetes or its complications

- Three times as likely to end up hospitalized because of diabetes

- More than twice as likely to have a diabetes-related amputation

- More than three times as likely to have diabetes lead to end-stage kidney disease

The good news is that type 2 diabetes is not difficult to detect and treat. Today, doctors can identify, particularly in those who are obese or at otherwise high risk for diabetes, a prediabetic condition (meaning that your blood sugar level is higher than normal but not at diabetic levels—yet). This requires two simple blood tests, a fasting blood sugar and a hemoglobin (HgA1C), which not only measures your blood sugar on any given day but also gives you an idea of what your blood sugars have averaged over the past 2–3 months.

An estimated 27 million American women have prediabetes. If faced with this predicament, this is your chance to be your own superhero, because prediabetes is completely reversible with healthy nutrition, weight loss, and exercise topping the leaderboard of tools at your ready disposal. (If you're thinking, *That again?* so be it. That. Again.)

Even if you reverse your prediabetes, stay vigilant about getting your blood sugar and HgA1C checked annually, just to make sure they remain under control. It's also worth noting that losing just 10 percent of your body weight (or going from 200 pounds to 180) can lower your risk of developing diabetes by more than half. Your goal is to be metabolically healthy, not just an arbitrary number on a scale. If you are morbidly obese, this is a more complicated equation and you should discuss with your doctor how much weight loss will result in a significant improvement, but every little bit helps.

The fact is, diabetes and obesity tend to coexist—and having one, or both, puts you at significant risk of developing heart disease. Like the connection between heart and brain health, the same behaviors that lead to obesity cause type 2 diabetes, and vice versa.

Obesity

If you have pictures of your grandparents, take a walk down memory lane (if not, just google "March on Washington" and eyeball the crowd). You know what you won't see? Lots of fat people. That's barely two generations ago.

It is not possible to have inherited new or altered genes in such a short period of time. So what happened, and why is obesity getting worse?

It's not about your character flaws or lack of willpower. It's not likely to be your thyroid. And it's not as simple as calories in and calories out or how much we eat (although our perception of what a normal-sized portion is has changed dramatically over the years). It's a lot of things, all of which converge at middle age to create the perfect storm of weight gain.

The result? America has gotten fat and Black and Hispanic women have gotten fatter faster. According to CDC statistics, from 2014 to 2018, the rate of American women who were either overweight or obese was close to 70 percent, with the rates for Black women topping out at 80 percent. Hispanic women were close behind at 79 percent. Furthermore, the percentage of Black women with Class 4 obesity (BMI greater than 40) has increased from 7 percent to 16 percent in recent years.

Not only are we fatter, but so are our children, and at younger ages. Remember when I told you that type 2 diabetes is also known as "adult-onset diabetes"? More and more children and young people are being diagnosed with type 2 diabetes, and it is directly related to the increased rate of obesity in children. We are living in a time when 1 in 3 young adults is not physically fit enough to serve in the armed services.

Given the realities of cardiovascular disease, this will have devastating effects on our long-term health individually and as a nation. And in addition to significantly increasing the odds of developing cardiovascular disease and all its attendant risks, being overweight also increases your risk for joint pain, arthritis, and cancer.

Now that I've gotten your attention, I want to explore not just the what but the why of obesity. And, of course, how to fight it. Buckle up, this is going to be a large section (with a few bumps), but it's too important to gloss over.

Apple, Meet Pear: Where Your Weight Is Matters

Whether in a doctor's office or the privacy of your own full-length mirror, the focus around weight is usually on what the scale says. But when it comes to your health, and cardiovascular disease risk in particular, where your weight is located is almost as important as your total avoirdupois. I know, unnecessary word, right? I'm just making sure you're still with me. It just means *weight*. (Put that one on your child's spelling bee list.)

Weight is a sensitive subject, even for us doctors (myself included) and especially for those who have struggled with weight for most of their lives. According to the American Heart Association, 37 percent of all Americans are overweight (note that this figure does not include those classified as obese), but if you are Black or Hispanic, these numbers are even higher, coming in at 42 percent and 40 percent, respectively.

Now, we could debate why that is, or if that is, or how the traditional tools (body mass index, or BMI) and "norms" used to measure and define obesity are skewed by race-based biases. But none of that would change the fact that most of us need to lose some weight. And no, this is not body shaming. This is about the quality and quantity of your remaining years. Everything I'm about to say is out of love, so take it as such. There's no finger-wagging here.

Start with the fact that weight gain after 40 is, for most women, a rite of passage. However, we each have our own metabolisms and make our own choices every day—and this is where we as women, and particularly women of color, must make better choices. I know I'm walking a tightrope here, but I need to say, without judgment or blame, let's collectively do better with our diets, our exercise, and most of all, our attitudes about weight, body size, and what is normal versus what is not.

Why? Because our long-term health and our lives—in other words, our *health span*—depend on it.

Thick and obese are not the same thing. No one body type is exclusively beautiful. One person's physical idea of perfection can be another's reason for medical intervention—at either end of the weight spectrum. But obesity—as in excess weight that is placing you at risk for life-threatening illness—does have some hard-and-fast parameters, and the Body Mass Index (BMI) is not the only one and inarguably is not the most accurate assessment of risk.

Is it possible to be obese and metabolically healthy? Yes, but it's harder. In fact, figures from the National Institute of Diabetes and Digestive and Kidney Diseases estimate that 38 percent of people who qualify as obese do not have what is called "the metabolic syndrome," the unholy and dangerous combination of elevated blood pressure, diabetes, and elevated lipids and triglycerides, and markers of chronic inflammation. That, of course, means that 62 percent of obese people do have the metabolic syndrome.

Conversely, can you be thin and metabolically unhealthy? Yes. Among normal or underweight individuals, about 22 percent are metabolically unhealthy. Just because you are not fat does not mean you are not at risk for cardiovascular disease. So, if a size 6 is your calling card, don't pat yourself on your back just yet. A lot depends on where your body fat is distributed. If your BMI does not classify you as overweight but most of your weight is centered around your midsection (what I call "skinny fat"—thin arms and legs and a big belly), and you also have the metabolic syndrome, then you run three times the risk of developing cardiovascular disease and dying from it than a person of similar weight who does not have it. Weight alone does not determine health or lack thereof, so just calculating your BMI can be misleading. BMI is calculated using only your height and weight. Whether or not you develop the metabolic syndrome depends not just on your weight but also on your lifestyle, your genetic risk factors, and the distribution of your body fat. BMI does not capture those key details.

The simple measurement of weight and height used to calculate the

BMI is a rather blunt instrument and does not accurately assess body fat. A quick, easy, and more telling measurement would be the waist-to-hip ratio, which for women should be no more than 0.8. For example, if your hips measure forty inches, your waist should be no more than thirty-two inches. You don't really even need a measuring tape; you can eyeball it. Is your waist circumference bigger than your hips? Have you noticed that most of the weight you gain takes up permanent residence between your neck and your waistline? If so, you are considered apple-shaped (versus the more bottom-heavy pear) and that puts you at higher risk for diabetes, regardless of your weight (although weight itself does still matter).

Causes of Weight Gain After 40

Breathing

(Otherwise known as aging.)

Menopause Transition/Low Estrogen

The SWAN study revealed that in the 5 to 10 years that it takes to transition to menopause, women will gain anywhere from 5 to 10 pounds (it's more like 10–20 in real life, IMHO. And if you don't know what that acronym means, ask a millennial). Black women, who take longer to transition during menopause, also have more disrupted sleep, which, in turn, is associated with increased weight gain and increased risk of cardiovascular disease.

Now, we can argue about whether menopause specifically is making you gain weight or whether it's just aging, but the irrefutable fact is this—whether you gain weight or not during the menopausal transition, as your estrogen levels decline you will lose muscle and gain fat. And less muscle mass makes it more difficult to lose weight.

Unfortunately, when you gain weight, you don't get to decide where that weight goes. In midlife, a big chunk of it lands right in your midsection. As noted earlier, from a cardiovascular point of view, it's the worst place to gain weight because that fat gathering around your waistline is also gathering around your internal organs. This "visceral fat" is not only more dangerous to your cardiovascular health, but it's also associated with inflammation, the development of type 2 diabetes, disruption of your gut flora (see Highly Processed Foods), and heart disease.

Disrupted Sleep/Stress

Two other factors that negatively affect your weight as you age are stress and sleep deprivation. I am discussing them together because they tend to coexist, and the effects of one actually exacerbate the other. The more stress you experience, the worse your sleep patterns are, and vice versa.

Who among us has not awakened in the middle of the night (sometimes on repeat) thinking about what needs to be done tomorrow or what wasn't done yesterday? Hot flashes and night sweats are two other ways to guarantee that most women over 40 rarely get a good night's rest. The less sleep you get, the more fatigued, less productive, and more stressed you are the next day. And if you've been told that you snore, you are at risk for sleep apnea, which can be extremely disruptive to the quality of your sleep and your health. So, go get that checked out.

It doesn't matter which came first, the stress or lack of sleep. The two together create a doomsday loop that ultimately leads to increased weight gain and a higher risk of developing cardiovascular disease. Stress triggers the release of the hormones cortisol and adrenaline, which increase blood pressure, heart rate, and blood sugar. The high blood sugars stimulate insulin release. The insulin and cortisol stimulate your appetite, which increases food intake—which, of course, makes you fat.

Stress

Workplace stress is real [♪**"Stressed Out"**]. Financial stress is real. Micro- and macro-aggressions are real, and cause stress. When I speak of toxic environments—be they at home, in your relationships, or at work—I mean it literally, not figuratively. Life's built-in hardships and toxic environments not only disturb your peace, they also damage your health. Left unchecked, they can take an irreversible toll.

Black women tend to have higher levels of stress hormones even when they do not self-report feeling stressed. (See how we have come to normalize how we feel?) The release of these hormones is helpful when you are trying to save a baby from a burning building but is decidedly harmful when you are just sitting at your desk trying to get your work done.

Chronic stress is the worst, and it can contribute to prolonged periods of addictive eating, disrupted sleep, alcoholism, unhealthy drug use, and an entire array of poor coping mechanisms that pack on weight and suppress your motivation, all of which only make things worse long-term—especially when it comes to your heart and brain health.

Highly Processed Foods

Unsure about what ultra-processed food is? Here is a quick test: If you can eat that package of cookies in your pantry three months from now and they still taste delicious, it's ultra-processed. Try eating the oatmeal cookies or loaf of bread you baked last month and see what that tastes like. After scraping the mold off and getting new dental work, you will understand that real food isn't supposed to last for months (okay, maybe with the exception of canned and frozen goods and a few rutabagas and potatoes in your root cellar).

Ultra-processed foods do not exist in nature and our bodies literally don't know what to do with them. We have trillions of bacteria, viruses, and fungi (yes, some of them are helpful) that live in our gut. This complex ecosystem makes up our gut flora. These organisms not only help us digest food, but they also play an important role in weight regulation and immune function. Their job is to keep your blood sugar stable, help balance your hormones and moods, signal when you've had enough to eat, and tamp down inflammation.

Ultra-processed foods wreak havoc on your metabolism and alter your gut flora, which triggers inflammation throughout your body. Today, most grocery store staples have unnatural combinations of high-fructose corn syrup, salt, fats, and chemicals. Don't believe me? Read the nutritional label on a box of butter crackers. Added to enhance flavor and lengthen shelf life, these chemical concoctions also hijack your brain chemistry and digestive hormones to make you feel hungry even as they fill you up with empty calories.

That we crave these dangerous concoctions is not an accident. Right now, there are scientists in laboratories whose job it is to get you addicted to their potato chips, salad dressings, and candy bars by tweaking their recipes. I mean, come on, is pizza not fatty and delicious enough in its basic form? Do we need to bake more cheese *into* the crust and add "all the toppings you can eat," including bacon and ranch dressing? When did *that* become a thing? And don't get me started on the fast-food industry's enticements to "supersize" everything. Is it any wonder that what we end up supersizing is ourselves? And our children? As long as there is a food industry incentivized to make unhealthy foods so delectable that no one can eat just one, obesity will be on the rise and more people will die because of it. How's that for saying the quiet part out loud?

A recent study of over 22,000 people, published in the British medical journal *The BMJ* showed that those with diets high in ultra-processed foods had a higher risk of cardiovascular disease and a higher rate of premature death. If we used the same standard for the food industry that is applied to cigarettes, those ultra-processed foods would come with warning labels (and in some countries, they do).

We were not built for this. A healthy gut flora requires a fiber-rich, varied diet full of fruits, vegetables, and complex carbohydrates to survive. (See Mediterranean diet in Additional Resources.) When deprived of these nutrients, we can't thrive. Somehow, my mother knew this. Now you do too.

Lack of Physical Activity

Stress, poor diet, and inactivity are interrelated. Overeating makes us gain weight. The more weight we gain, the less active we are, the worse we feel physically and emotionally, and the more we crave the sugar rush (or chips!). Satisfying these sweet and salty rushes further damages our gut microbiome, crowding out the type of bacteria that strengthens our immune system and protects our arteries. This stresses our bodies, causing a release of hormones that raises our blood sugar, which leads to more binge eating and more inflammation. Inflammation leads to sluggishness and pain, which then keep you from exercising or maybe even getting out of bed. Need I go on?

The cycle can be toxic to your DNA. And as we all now know, damaged DNA leads to—you guessed it—chronic illnesses and cancer. The cycle is also unending, unless you slam on the breaks and end it.

Start now.

Get up and take a walk or bike ride. Do some squats or jumping jacks. Go for a swim or stretch from head to toe. Crank some music and dance it out—and take your time. I'll wait right here. And to be clear, you do not need expensive gym memberships or trainers. Regular physical activity of any type (extra bonus points if you raise your heart rate while doing it) is helpful.

Losing It

It's tough to realize that if you eat the exact same number of calories per day at 50 that you consumed at 40, you will gain weight. But that doesn't mean we have to sit back and take it. I know it's hard to lose weight (and yes, it's harder than ever when we're older), and if I had an easy answer for how to do it, I would be writing this book from the deck of my new yacht. And let me just put this out there, I am not overweight. Although I certainly don't weigh what I did twenty years ago, I have managed to keep my weight in a healthy range. And no, I don't have any special skinny genes. Did I mention that six of my seven siblings at some point in time would have been classified as obese? This even though neither of my parents was overweight.

I have no unique regimen and I'm no gym rat, but I do work out regularly and watch my weight, literally. Weighing myself first thing in the morning helps me stay mindful and chart a course for the day. I've done this, quite consciously, for years because I am most certainly not in the possession of the special skinny genes that my husband appears to have.

Although my parents stayed fit, one by one, I watched as most of my older siblings went from normal-weight young adults to overweight middle-agers to obese seniors. Only Margie, the sister next to me in age, has managed to stave off the seemingly inexorable march to obesity that the rest have been on. And trust me, she works really hard at it. As the two youngest, we had the benefit of ample time to watch and learn.

I've had the extra incentive of being a physician. How could I advise my patients to do the things that I was not willing to do myself? I've always tried to adhere to the adage "Physician, heal thyself!"

Little Sharon

When I was growing up, we ate vegetables that my father grew in his garden, and my mother cooked dinner every night. On occasion, she made liver. I never asked for seconds.

Mom shopped for groceries once a week and didn't believe in store-bought snacks. She made pound cake on holidays, cookies for Christmas, and ice cream on the Fourth of July. Oh, how I longed for Breyers ice cream from the grocery store freezer.

There were no fast-food restaurants near us until I was in

fourth grade. Then came the Burger King. I tasted my first Whopper, and I was in love. But Mom surely wasn't treating me, and I didn't have the cash.

That being said, did I eat junk? Indeed, I did. But it was always on my own dime . . . and I rarely had more than that to spend. So, let's just say the acquisition costs were prohibitive.

It was a simpler time. Parents had more control over what their children ate. School lunches were hot and made on the premises by real cafeteria ladies in hairnets. No soda machines. Just milk. White. Maybe chocolate.

Trust me, if little me had access to all the Oreos, Breyers ice cream, and Whoppers my little heart desired, I would have eaten them. And you now know me well enough to know why. Because a burger and fries are waaay more delicious than liver and onions.

The Takeaway: If you are 40 or over, take my advice: It's easier to avoid gaining a pound or two a year than it is to lose ten or twenty pounds a decade from now.

I know this is easier said than done, but I'm going to say it anyway: If you know there is a tasty treat or snack that you can't resist, don't buy it. If cookies are your kryptonite, make them from scratch. Not only will you expend some calories prepping and baking them, but your time and effort will limit how often you eat them. No matter what you cook, preparing things yourself allows you to control the ingredients and portions and make healthier versions.

Do all you can to keep the scale from climbing as your age does. That alone will be a significant win.

If you're already 50, or older, and didn't get the memo until now, not to worry, the ship has not sailed. We all have the ability to take control of our weight, and that process doesn't start at the kitchen table or on the scale or as you wait in the drive-thru line at [insert your favorite fast-food eatery here]. It begins in your head—and not with obsessing about losing weight.

Believe it or not, I want you to stop thinking about how heavy you are and start thinking about how healthy you are (or aren't but can be), because fad diets *don't* work! At least, not long-term. What *will* work is changing how you think about yourself, your life, and your health, and modifying your behavior to meet your health goals, not just your weight goals. You have to crave good health more than you crave donuts or *anything* that tastes or feels good for a moment but is ultimately holding you back.

Taking a page out of my friend Michelle Obama's book *The Light We Carry*, I want you to start small. Whether you need to lose ten pounds or a hundred, you still must lose it one pound—and one day—at a time. This isn't a sprint, it's a marathon. Slow and steady truly is the key.

The diet industry is a multibillion-dollar business pitching a new plan every fifteen minutes that's guaranteed to help you lose thirty pounds in thirty days. It's an enticing offer. But it's unrealistic (and, might I add, unhealthy). And here is another essential point that I don't want you to miss (thus, I'm repeating myself from the previous chapter): Losing as little as 10 percent of your body weight will improve your blood pressure and lower your risk of diabetes. So, do it! Commit to losing that 10 percent, for starters. The goal should be to get yourself into the metabolically healthy range, not necessarily to fit into your college jeans. And if you maintain that weight loss for a year and avoid gaining the extra one to two pounds that shows up just for living, then take an extra bow. You deserve it [♪"I Got You (I Feel Good)"].

I must offer one more cautionary note about weight-loss shortcuts, given the widespread use of relatively new drugs such as Ozempic, Wegovy, and Mounjaro. Without putting you to sleep by trying to explain how these medications work (full disclosure, I don't completely understand them yet myself, and I have not prescribed any of them to anyone), I can explain who they are for and what they do. Ozempic and Wegovy are semaglutides and Mounjaro is a tirzepatide. (IKR. I've already bored you.) All of these medications are indicated for the treatment of type 2 diabetes. But here's the kicker—in addition to helping to reduce your blood sugar, use of these medications also results in significant weight loss.

Remember when I told you that simply losing weight would reduce your risk of getting type 2 diabetes? Well, these medications offer a double whammy. So, you might say, what's not to love about them?

First, there's the price tag. These medications, without insurance, can cost anywhere from $900 to $1,200 a month. Second, they are administered as weekly injections, not pills. So, ouch! And third, there are many outstanding questions about these medications that we simply don't know the answers to: How long should you take these medications? What happens when you come off them? What are the long-term health implications of taking them? Those of you who are old enough to remember fen-phen know that these are important questions worth considering. (If you're too young, look it up and take heed as you consider weight-loss options.)

These medications may be extremely helpful as a kick-starter for those with refractory and recalcitrant weight issues that accompany type 2 diabetes and increase your risk for developing the metabolic syndrome. But make no mistake, there is no pill or portion that alone will substitute for the substantial lifestyle, behavioral, and dietary changes needed to maintain the weight loss. Remember, the goal is for you to be healthy, not just thin, and the two are not always related.

Felicia

Felicia was always overweight. She weighed more than ten pounds at birth. She was a chubby child, a fat adolescent, and an obese adult. Just before she started high school, her mother sent her to weight-loss camp. She managed to lose twenty pounds over the summer, but in less than six months, she gained it all back. For the next thirty years, Felicia tried just about every diet known to womankind: Optifast, SlimFast, the cabbage soup diet, Jenny Craig, WeightWatchers, keto. You name it, she's tried it. She could lose 10–15 pounds here and there, but she was never able to keep them off.

After Felicia turned 45, she noticed that even the diets that had worked in the past were no longer working. She couldn't lose weight, even when she nearly starved herself. The kicker came when she saw her primary care doctor for her annual examination. Her blood pressure, which had been steadily creeping up, had crossed over into hypertension territory, requiring medication. To make matters worse, she was also prediabetic. Felicia had watched her parents struggle with health issues as they got older, and most of their problems were complications from diabetes and high blood pressure.

During a tearful discussion with her doctor, Felicia vowed that this would not be her fate, and said she was determined to lose weight by any means necessary. Her physician referred her to a surgeon who specialized in weight-loss surgeries. Since she had few other health issues, they decided on a gastric bypass operation, where a small pouch is created that decreases the size of the stomach. The pouch is connected to the small intestine, bypassing a considerable portion of the small bowel. The procedure not only limits the amount of food that can be consumed, but it also limits the absorption of sugar and fats.

The procedure worked like a charm. Within the first

eighteen months after her surgery, Felicia had lost more than seventy-five pounds. She no longer needed blood pressure medication, and she was no longer prediabetic. Other than some occasional nausea and diarrhea triggered by certain foods, she was doing well. She had never felt better about herself, and she was killing it with her new wardrobe.

Felicia's weight loss plateaued at the two-year mark. Over time, she gradually fell back into old habits around her diet and exercise. She noticed that she was not losing any more weight and that she had started to regain some. At first, it was just two or three pounds here and there, but once she gained it, she couldn't get back down to where she had been. Five years post-surgery, she had gained thirty-five of those hard-lost pounds back. When she hit menopause at 53, eight years after her surgery, Felicia had regained almost fifty pounds. Her blood pressure was back up and she was again prediabetic.

I know you're probably wondering how that is even possible. The reality is that even with weight-loss surgery, it is still possible to regain the weight you lost.

The Takeaway: In fact, ten years after weight-loss surgery, almost 50 percent of people have regained some or a substantial portion of the weight they lost. I know that sounds depressing, but let's look on the bright side: 50 percent of people *didn't* regain the weight. Most likely, the 50 percent who didn't regain it altered their diets and lifestyles in addition to the surgery. The point here is simply that surgery and medication can be quite effective at helping you lose weight, but the real work of keeping it off is still in your

hands. Don't ever forget that. You have the ultimate control. Not your surgeon. Not your medication. Not your favorite snack.

Beware of Chronic Stress

My dear sister Vivian had a stressful life. She was the oldest daughter
in our family and the younger sister to three rambunctious boys. Everything in her life was a fight, from surviving the constant teasing and
roughhousing with our brother Charles to being the protective older
sister to the rest of us.

But Vivian was built for her lot in life. She was smart, strong, and
confident. She never backed down. These traits served her well when
she became one of two Black students who integrated the University of
Alabama in 1963. Staring down Governor George Wallace as he stood
in the schoolhouse door hell-bent on blocking her path, my coura-
geous sister, accompanied by a clutch of armed U.S. Marshals, walked
on by, unbowed.

Every day, Vivian walked through those doors, even as the world
seemed to implode around her. The assassination of Medgar Evers in
nearby Mississippi, the bombing murders of four little girls at Bir-
mingham's 16th Street Baptist Church, and the assassination of the
President of the United States—the same president who had upheld
her right to the same education only white people had been afforded
in Alabama before her—all occurred in less than six months of her
enrollment. Tuscaloosa, Alabama, also just happened to be the home
of the Imperial Wizard of the Ku Klux Klan.

During her time at the University of Alabama, she endured a constant stream of overt and covert threats, about which she rarely spoke.
She graduated a mere two months after John Lewis was beaten and

bloodied on the Edmund Pettus Bridge in Selma, less than an hour and a half from her campus.

After graduation, she married her college sweetheart, Mack, who graduated from the nearby HBCU, Stillman College. After living in D.C. for a few years, they packed up their blue Mustang, hitched up a U-Haul containing all their earthly possessions, and moved to Atlanta. Mack had gotten accepted to medical school. Vivian had their first child, and for the next eight years she was her family's primary bread-winner while Mack finished medical school and residency.

Not long after Vivian had her second child, our mother died. At 29, working full-time and already raising two small children, she inherited me—a grieving, too-grown-for-her-own-britches, smart-mouthed 12-year-old. As always, Vivian managed. Stable, resilient, and tough, she never let anyone see her sweat. She did what generations of Black women before her had done: She simply did what she had to, never complaining, never ever showing a crack in that armor [♪"Do Whatcha Gotta Do"].

Before she reached 50, Vivian became the primary caretaker for her husband, who was plagued by poor health for the last decade of his life. She stayed tethered to Mack for his daily dialysis before his kidney transplant, and for a couple more years after his transplant failed. During that time, Vivian, who had never been seriously overweight in her life, gained more than forty pounds. After Mack died, with her children grown, for the first time in her life Vivian lived alone—and was free to do as she pleased.

Barely a year after her husband died, I got a call from my niece saying that Vivian was in the emergency room. She had passed out at home in the middle of the night. Her blessedly persistent contractors called 911 when she did not answer the door the following morning. Firefighters entered through a window and found Vivian on her bathroom floor, conscious but unable to move.

I immediately went into doctor mode. A stroke? How could that be? Her husband had had high blood pressure; she didn't. I started grilling my niece, trying to put the pieces of this puzzle together, when she asked if I wanted to talk to my sister. Relief coursed through me. *If Vivian is mentally alert and can talk,* I thought, *it's all going to be fine.*

My brief conversation with Vivian was lighthearted, and it reassured me. I teased her, saying she was the only person I knew whose contractors a) showed up on time and b) refused to leave when she didn't answer the door. We laughed. Her speech was a bit slurred, but she knew me. She had even remembered my phone number, for goodness' sake. She was going to need rehab, but people can relearn and fully recover after a stroke. I started making mental plans to take care of her the way she had always taken care of me. I would clear my schedule, get to Atlanta by the end of the week, and arrange for her discharge. Finally, I said, "I'll see you in a couple of days." Our last words to each other were "I love you."

By the next day, everything had changed, and I was rushing to get to Vivian's side. What I saw when I arrived was unfathomable. My strong, beautiful, "I got this" sister was unconscious and intubated, with a bandage encompassing her entire skull. A neurosurgeon explained that Vivian lost consciousness a few hours after we talked. She'd suffered another large intracranial bleed. They tried to stop it, but the effort to contain the bleed caused considerable damage.

Doctors hearing this kind of news are no different from anyone else. Everything went dark and fuzzy as I pushed back hard against every word I was hearing. *But I just spoke to her,* I thought. *How can this possibly be?* I struggled to ask the only two questions I had: "Do you expect her to wake up? And if so, what do you think her level of functioning will be?" The responses were grim.

I am in the habit, especially in the bleakest of times, of looking for silver linings. There were none to be had here. Except this: I was never in doubt as to what Vivian's wishes were. She and her husband had explicit advance directives. In fact, we had just had a detailed conversation about it at Mack's bedside the year before. So, as a family, we informed the doctor that a DNR (do not resuscitate) was to be placed on Vivian's chart, and given the unlikely event that she would ever awaken, we made a plan to gather at her bedside the following morning to allow everyone a chance to say goodbye.

On October 13, 2005, after a prayer by her minister, with all of us surrounding her and holding hands, my precious Vivian's respirator was disconnected. She passed away peacefully. Only we were in turmoil.

I tell this story because, as with so many women—and women of color especially—Vivian's sacrifice, her bravery, and her meaningful mark on history have not been amply recognized. I also share it because, as painful as it is to recount, it is vitally instructive in many ways.

My sister, who was in no way neglectful of her health, died at 63. (Only now that I am past 63 do I realize how truly young that is.) She did not have cardiovascular disease or hypertension of the stroke variety that in and of itself should have killed her. She had survived breast cancer at 37 with no signs of recurrence more than twenty-five years later. From a purely medical standpoint, her death just didn't make sense. It was only after her death that the cause was identified. She died of a stroke, not due to high blood pressure, but due to an aggressive leukemia-like blood cancer: myelodysplastic syndrome.

Searching for answers, I contacted her collaborator on that elusive autobiography she kept trying to write. He shared that he and Vivian had spoken at length over the years about her life, her children, her work, and her faith. But he said that whenever the subject of the University of Alabama came up, she would draw a blank. She would promise to think about it. He would give her a writing assignment. They would reconvene in another couple of months or so, and she would have nothing.

This is a woman who was otherwise never at a loss for words. She expressed herself thoughtfully, with passion and confidence. Yet she could speak about her time at the University of Alabama only intellectually, as if she were describing a scene or tableau that was happening to someone else. When she gave the university's commencement speech in 2000, they referred to her as "a singular figure of courage and grace in the history of [the] institution," and presented her with an honorary doctorate. Even then, she could not—or would not—access the emotions associated with specific events or articulate the terror or sense of loneliness and isolation she must have experienced.

"I think she suffered from PTSD," her co-writer said, oblivious to the shock that simple phrase caused me. Well, shut the front door! Surely not my happy, competent sister who never met a challenge she couldn't face and who I never saw shed a tear or wallow in self-pity! What was he talking about?

Then it hit me like a ton of bricks: The price we pay for being strong and stoic, getting it done on time and under budget, and making a way out of no way can exact a huge, unseen toll. Sometimes it costs us our lives.

I began to realize how much my sister was like my mother, adopting a better-to-ignore-it-than-give-in-to-it approach to life's harsh blows. The price they paid for survival was sublimation—a compartmentalization of sorts that took an invisible but devastating toll on their bodies.

Renowned public health researcher Dr. Arline T. Geronimus coined the term *weathering* to describe the devastating effects that systemic oppression, including racism and classism, take on the body. Her book, *Weathering: The Extraordinary Stress of Ordinary Life in an Unjust Society*, sheds a blazing light on the ways in which the chronic stresses induced by systemic injustice steadily erode the health of marginalized people, causing them to become ill and die at younger ages than their more privileged, and societally validated, counterparts.

Just like my mother, Vivian never once dealt with her own mental well-being in any fashion (unless ignoring that a problem existed counts). But she carried the scars of a very difficult life on the inside. The layers of trauma that she endured over time overwhelmed her immune defenses. Believe me when I say that chronic stress will wear you down. It erodes your physical as well as your mental health. We, as women, are socialized to absorb other people's trauma and problems, and deflect or suppress our own. This is exactly where the strong-Black-woman stereotype is derived. But we simply are not built for it.

Whether we acknowledge it or not, stress takes a visible and invisible toll on all of us.

I believe Vivian's death is an important illustration of the cumulative effects of lifelong stress. I don't think that given the chance again, she would have changed any aspect of her life. What I do wish is that she would have availed herself of help or that she had given voice to the many difficulties that she faced. Maybe then she would have found more productive ways to deal with her stress. We may not be able to avoid stress, but we need to stop simply accepting it. Stress must be managed as carefully and intentionally as you would any other threat to your health. My message to you is simply this: Deal with stress before it deals with you.

DR. SHARON'S RX FOR
Breaking the Cycle of the Triple Threat

1. Exercise: Increased muscle mass makes you stronger and more fit, and helps you maintain weight loss. (Notice I didn't say exercise helps you lose weight, because it doesn't, but it does make your weight loss easier to maintain once you've done all the other things you're supposed to do.)

2. Increase your fiber intake and add fermented foods—such as miso, kimchi, and sauerkraut—to maintain healthy gut flora and cut down on those ultra-processed foods.

3. Treat prediabetes as seriously as you would diabetes; don't wait until you have crossed the line.

4. Get a good night's sleep; sleep is vitally important in helping you minimize weight gain. Schedule a sleep study if you snore.

5. Consider menopausal hormone therapy. It decreases the risk of type 2 diabetes and improves sleep quality. MHT doesn't make you lose weight, but it does help you maintain your muscle mass and minimizes the unhealthy weight gain in your midsection.

6. Pay attention to your mental health. Depression is independently associated with increased weight gain, dementia, and heart disease.

7. Minimize the stress in your life. Try yoga, prayer, meditation, counseling, or whatever works for you. Develop coping skills that at least help you manage your stress even if you cannot eliminate it.

CHAPTER 6

Key to Your Heart♪

Guarding Against Cardiovascular Disease

Dear Sis,

You know I generally think worrying is a waste of time. Fret less and focus more on healthy habits. That's our mantra. But we do run the risk of not being concerned enough about conditions that affect the heart and blood vessels, or cardiovascular disease (CVD).

In every decade of life after 40, anywhere from two to seven times more women die of CVD than die of breast cancer. A stunning 49 percent of Black women aged 20 and over have signs of incipient CVD. Even more heartbreaking? According to the American Heart Association, only 1 in 5 Black women thinks she is even at risk for heart disease.

I know. Per usual, it's a lot. But this is one place where knowing more and doing better will absolutely improve and lengthen your life. There are some things that you can't do an awful lot about, but this is not one of them.

Our incidence of heart ailments is so high because our incidence of contributing factors—such as diabetes, obesity, and high blood pressure—are so high. Your family history plays a role—but that's more likely because of cultural and generational habits and beliefs around diet and exercise than it is genetics.

Every chapter in this book represents an "I love you" moment, but this is one of the most important. You can change your life for the better. You can change your habits in ways that will positively influence your children and grandchildren. And when you do, generations of your family will live longer and have a greater chance to prosper, because they will be healthier and stronger as a result.

With all my heart, I'm asking you to show yourself more love. One healthy choice at a time.

xo, Dr. Sharon

We're all familiar with the term *cardiovascular disease,* but there are plenty of misconceptions about what it actually is. Is it a heart attack, heart failure, a stroke? It's all of that, plus some things you may not have thought of, like peripheral artery disease, deep vein thrombosis, and pulmonary embolism.

Cardiovascular disease (CVD) is a constellation of ailments that affect not just your heart but also your entire vascular system—meaning your arteries and veins. CVD has far-ranging consequences that, when taken in aggregate, make it the number one cause of death in the United States, and in the world. To put that in context, CVD kills more people every year than all cancers combined. And for women, at each decade of life, starting at age 40, CVD kills anywhere from two to seven times more women than breast cancer does.

Somehow, despite the ubiquity of heart disease and the seriousness of its consequences, it doesn't really register with us with the same sense of urgency as cancer. Why is that? My theory is that we talk more about breast cancer, and that's not a bad thing. It's just that we don't always have the proper perspective when it comes to heart disease. Getting a mammogram every year is an easier task than making all the daily lifestyle changes that might decrease your risk of heart disease. But the good news is, if you implement the healthy habits that I keep hammering home (you know: exercise, diet, mindfulness, etc.), you will not only decrease your risk of developing CVD, but you will also decrease your cancer risk [♪ "With Each Beat of My Heart"].

Perhaps the commonplace existence of the predisposing risk factors that lead to CVD has inured us to the real dangers posed. Let's talk about a syndrome of metabolic derangement known as the "metabolic syndrome." Clever name, right [♪ "Cleva"]?

What are the components of the metabolic syndrome?

- High blood pressure (>130 systolic or >85 diastolic or taking medication for HBP)

- Diabetes (fasting blood sugar >100 mg/dl or currently taking medication for diabetes)

- Abdominal fat (waist >35 inches or a waist-to-hip ratio >0.8)

- High triglycerides (>150 mg/dl)

- Low high-density lipoprotein (HDL) cholesterol (<50 mg/dl)

If you have three or more of these risk factors, you have metabolic syndrome, and shockingly, over 90 percent of Americans have at least one of these risk factors already. The incidence of metabolic syndrome goes up with age, ranging from approximately 20 percent in people under 40 to over 50 percent in people over 60. Do not ignore these obvious warning signs and do not accept an ailing heart as an inevitable consequence of growing old. I'm here to tell you that nothing could be further from the truth. Most of the risk factors for developing CVD are known and avoidable. And here again, women of color need to be especially mindful [♪ "Un-Break My Heart"].

Black women are 60 percent more likely than white women to get hypertension and 30 percent more likely to die from heart disease. That translates into nearly fifty thousand Black women dying from heart attacks and strokes each year, and this number pales in comparison to the millions of women who live compromised lives resulting from the symptoms of chronic CVD. Our goal is to change all of that, so you can enjoy your ride through your 40-plus life and never reach any of these final destinations.

Here comes the good news: CVD is not an inevitable consequence of middle and old age, and there is *a lot* that you can do to minimize your risk. In fact, the lifestyle and diet modifications listed in my Rx at the end of the chapter will increase your odds of staying healthy longer than any medications you take after the fact. So, let's beat that prevention drum together, shall we? And yes, CVD may run in your family, but a family history only tells you what you are susceptible to. You may not get to choose the hand you're dealt, but you do get to choose how to play those cards.

CVD Risk Factors

The risk factors for CVD will sound very familiar to you by now because they are the same biomarkers that are associated not just with heart disease but with poor health generally. CVD is caused by the accumulation of damage to your blood vessels due to cholesterol plaques, blood clots, chronic inflammation, and/or high blood pressure. How, you might ask, do your blood vessels get damaged? The main culprits are poor dietary choices (those darn ultra-processed foods again), physical inactivity, smoking, and poorly controlled blood pressure and blood sugar.

Diabetes alone increases your risk of heart disease by 50 percent. With the unholy triad of obesity, hypertension, and diabetes, the risk skyrockets even more.

Once again, family history does play a role, but it is dwarfed by the aforementioned factors. And remember, being predisposed to something does not preempt your ability to prevent it. So, rather than throw your hands up in surrender (or despair—no one needs *that*), embrace knowing what your susceptibilities are and redouble your efforts to stay well. We talked in great detail about diabetes and obesity in the previous chapter, so let's talk a bit about the third potent risk factor in that unholy triad: hypertension.

High Blood Pressure (HBP)
Hypertension (HTN)

Your blood pressure rises when your heart pumps (systolic) and falls when it rests (diastolic). That combined measurement is expressed as your blood pressure (BP) ratio—systolic blood pressure over your diastolic blood pressure reading.

There's a reason why every time you go to the doctor they take your BP first. It's that important. While your BP fluctuates naturally from minute to minute, depending on your levels of exertion or stress, blood pressure readings are typically taken at rest. Pay close attention here because the definition of what constitutes high blood pressure has changed.

Prior to 2017, hypertension was defined as a blood pressure reading of more than 140/90. The newer guidelines define hypertension as readings greater than 130/80, with a goal of decreasing blood pressures to 120/80 or less. (Blood pressures between 120–130 systolic and 80–90 diastolic are deemed elevated and worth monitoring.)

It's just a number, right? What difference does it make? Just life or death—or permanent disability. But early intervention with lifestyle changes and/or medication can significantly decrease your risk of heart disease and stroke—and women are at high risk for both. Women represent nearly half of all adults with high blood pressure and almost 52 percent of hypertension-related deaths, and yet a misconception persists that HBP is a disease that affects mostly men or people with a Type A personality. Let me be clear: That's a no.

You may have had normal or even low blood pressure all your life, but your chances of developing hypertension increase as you age. And you should be on extra alert if you had pregnancy-induced hypertension or preeclampsia, a condition that affects 1 in 25 pregnancies. Pregnancy-induced hypertension is more prevalent in Black women, and even if it resolves after delivery, it places you at a higher risk of developing hypertension later in life.

Understanding your blood pressure and what you should do about it is mission critical. You're only going to see your doctor once or twice a year, so get a blood pressure cuff (available online or at your local drugstore), learn how to use it (it's not rocket science), and keep track of your pressure year-round. Note trends but try to take your blood pressure under similar circumstances—not after a vigorous workout or a double espresso. One elevated reading does not high blood pressure make. Relax, repeat it in a day or two or next week, and record your numbers. Consistently elevated blood pressure readings require a visit to your doctor. Here are some numbers to keep in mind:

- Ideal: Less than 120/80

- Elevated: 120–129 systolic and less than 80 diastolic

- Hypertension stage 1: 130–139 systolic or 80–89 diastolic

- Hypertension stage 2: 140 and higher systolic or 90 and higher diastolic

- Hypertensive crisis: 180 and higher systolic and/or 120 and higher diastolic

Most people can avoid or minimize high blood pressure through maintaining a healthy diet, doing regular exercise, minimizing stress, and managing weight (see my full Rx). Sugar doesn't cause diabetes, nor does salt cause hypertension, but a diet with too much added sugar will make you fat, and the excess weight will increase your risk of developing diabetes. Likewise, too much added salt in predisposed individuals will elevate borderline blood pressure readings and tip the scale, landing you in hypertensive territory. If you already have a diagnosis of either, too much sugar and salt in your diet will definitely make both harder to control.

If you have been diagnosed with hypertension, please take your medication [♪"Please, Please, Please"]. And not just when you feel like it, have a headache, or happen to remember. Every day that your blood pressure is elevated is another day of potential damage to your heart, your kidneys, your blood vessels, or your brain. Keep those blood pressure logs and report them to your primary care doctor at your next visit (sooner if the readings are consistently out of range). If you're on blood pressure meds, self-monitoring is the only way to ensure that the medication is working as intended. Also make sure to note any side effects or symptoms you might be experiencing. Your doctor can adjust your medications as needed.

CVD Complications

Women have been lulled into a false sense of security about heart health that the American Heart Association is trying hard to combat. Until menopause, women have about half the risk of having a heart attack as men. But within ten years of menopause, the rate of CVD and its complications equals or exceeds that of men. Women are also less likely than men to survive their first heart attack. And for the record, heart attacks (or, as we call them in doctor speak, myocardial infarctions) in women present with a slightly different symptom profile than in men. And as Dr. Jayne Morgan, a cardiologist and the executive director of Health and Community Education at Piedmont Hospital, has stated, we should stop saying that women have "atypical" symptoms. What's normal for men is not necessarily normal for women, and it is our job as physicians to educate our patients *and* ourselves about how women present with symptoms of heart attacks. Chest pain is a common symptom in both men and women, but women's chest pain can be less severe and present with flu-like symptoms and nausea. In part, because women's heart attacks may masquerade as indigestion, shortness of breath, or fatigue, they are easy to miss or to mistake for lesser illnesses. Not only do women minimize their symptoms, but many doctors do as well and are more likely to *misdiagnose* heart attacks in women than in men.

In fact, it's estimated that upwards of 50 percent of patients who show past evidence of a heart attack on an EKG or through other testing are unaware of ever having had one. Known as a "silent heart attack," this is not the chest-clutching, "I'm coming to join you, Elizabeth" variety made famous by Redd Foxx. (If you're too young to recognize this reference, God bless you. Go watch an episode of *Sanford and Son* on YouTube.) But this silent heart attack nonetheless damages the heart, rendering it more vulnerable to long-term complications like congestive heart failure.

It is important that you know what the signs and symptoms for heart attack are, particularly if you have a family history or underlying risk factors for heart disease. This is also where it's critical that you develop and maintain a strong sense of your normal (interoception, y'all!)—and fatigue and discomfort should not be your baseline. Let me repeat: Don't get used to chronic exhaustion or pain. Don't accept them. Don't normalize them. They are vital signs when something is amiss [♪ "How Can You Mend a Broken Heart"].

Stroke

While heart attacks tend to dominate our thoughts at the mention of CVD, stroke is the third-most common cause of death in women, and many stroke survivors are left with permanent physical or mental disabilities.

A stroke can occur at any age, and in an average year in the United States alone, more than 100,000 women under age 65 will suffer one of the two common types of strokes—ischemic, sometimes referred to as occlusive or embolic strokes, and hemorrhagic. The severity, location, and type of symptoms associated with a stroke vary tremendously, depending upon where in the brain the damage has occurred. When the attack occurs in a part of the brain that does not control speech or movement, it may not be detected immediately. Sometimes a stroke can present as sudden memory loss or a change in cognition, vision, or even personality.

While many of us are at least somewhat aware of stroke symptoms (see FAST: What a Stroke Looks Like), it always helps to understand what something actually is. The brain, just like the heart, needs a near-constant supply of oxygen and glucose via the blood vessels that feed it. Even though the brain only represents 2 percent of our body weight, it consumes 20 percent of our oxygen and glucose supply. So, when that supply is interrupted because of a clogged or leaking blood vessel, there is a limited amount of time before the area of the brain supplied by that blood vessel is also damaged, sometimes irreversibly. Thus, every second counts when it comes to stroke treatment. Which is why knowing stroke symptoms cold is critical (again, get real familiar with FAST: What a Stroke Looks Like).

Ischemic strokes are caused by the occlusion of blood vessels to the brain. Think of a heart attack, but in the brain. A stunning 87 percent of strokes are clot-related.

Blockages in the blood vessels that feed the brain are caused by an accumulation of debris (typically cholesterol), inflammation, and damage to vessels from diabetes or hypertension—or by blood clots that form in the heart and travel to the brain. This is why people who have persistent atrial fibrillation are frequently on blood thinners to prevent strokes.

Hemorrhagic strokes are caused by exactly what the term implies—hemorrhage or bleeding in the brain. These strokes can be catastrophic and are seen more commonly in people with uncontrolled high blood pressure. High blood pressure over time damages the small blood vessels in the brain, which can burst and bleed. This is one reason why hypertension is considered a silent killer. Hemorrhagic strokes can also be caused less commonly by aneurysms or abnormal blood vessels in the brain.

Those who survive hemorrhagic strokes often report having had the worst headache of their lives just prior to or during the bleed. In that condition, you are literally a ticking time bomb. So, in case I haven't made myself entirely clear, high blood pressure is nothing to be trifled with. If you have it, treat it. It's just that simple.

Transient ischemic attacks (TIA), usually lasting minutes to hours, are commonly known as mini strokes. TIAs resolve spontaneously without treatment, in twenty-four hours or less. Even though TIA symptoms can seem less severe, doctors sometimes refer to them as "warning strokes" because your risk of having additional strokes increases once you've had a TIA. In fact, 1 in 4 ischemic strokes happens after a prior TIA. That risk is highest in the first few hours after a TIA and remains elevated for at least a week. So, as with any stroke, receiving medical attention and a full evaluation as soon as possible is critical.

Because many ischemic strokes are due to blood clots, there are powerful "clot-busters" that when administered within three hours of symptom onset can limit and, in some cases, completely reverse the damage. Early intervention can also minimize complications such as brain swelling, permanent disability, or death.

Large brain bleeds may require the intervention of a neurosurgeon, whereas small, limited bleeds can be monitored. Either way, FAST and accurate diagnosis is key to any stroke outcome.

Gail

Gail is 48 years old. Like most women her age, she gained about fifteen pounds during perimenopause but was still able to rock that St. John suit she bought six years ago (this is why women of a certain age love them—they stretch!). She has been treated for high blood pressure since her late 20s. Her doctor has had trouble adequately controlling her blood pressure, mainly because, as Gail admits, she does not always do her part.

Her cholesterol numbers have been rising and she was recently informed that she is prediabetic. Although she always intends to exercise, most days she is just too overworked or too tired to do it. And her diet is not exactly what the doctor ordered. She rationalizes by telling herself, "Life is tough. You gotta have some joy, right?"

On a lovely Saturday afternoon, Gail was sitting at her kitchen table eating an egg salad sandwich when she saw a look of concern come over her husband's face. "Honey, are you okay?" he asked.

"Sure," she said, struggling to form the word. She jumped up and looked in the mirror, and to her horror, she saw the right corner of her mouth drooping and her right eye was half-closed. Because her mother had had a stroke five years ago, she and her husband knew what this was and what to do.

Her husband immediately took her to the emergency room and said these words: "I think my wife is having a stroke!" Fortunately, in most hospitals this will quickly get you moved to the front of the line. Since Gail got to the hospital within one hour of her symptoms' onset, she was a candidate for clot-busters, and they succeeded in dissolving the blockage responsible for her stroke.

Gail was discharged in two days. She had no residual symptoms and was given a prescription for blood thinners.

The Takeaway: Fortunately, this story has a happy ending. It nonetheless illustrates two very important points: Time is of the essence when dealing with a stroke, and take your risk factors seriously. Gail had quite a few. They now have her full attention.

FAST: What a Stroke Looks Like

A timely diagnosis is critical not only to the survivability of a stroke but also to one's degree of disability after a stroke. If there was ever a time to go to the emergency room, this is it. So, know the warning signs. Keep them in your phone, post them on your refrigerator, and make sure your friends and loved ones know them too.

FAST is the acronym used to help you respond that way should you suspect someone in your company (or you yourself) is having a stroke:

F—Facial Drooping: Ask the person to smile and note any facial paralysis or lack of symmetry.

A—Arm Weakness: Ask the person to raise each arm or squeeze your hand.

S—Speech Difficulties: Ask the person easy questions (e.g., What's your name? What day is it?) or have them repeat a simple sentence, such as "It's time to go."

T—Time: If any of these factors is a problem, call 911 if you are alone, or if someone is home, have them take you to the hospital immediately. Having someone drive you is usually quicker than calling an ambulance, and you get to choose the hospital best suited to treat strokes. (Large or academic hospitals are typically best.) Remember to note the time when the symptoms appeared—this is crucial information for the medical team. Post-stroke, every minute counts.

Peripheral Artery Disease (PAD)

Peripheral artery (or arterial) disease is the third-most common form of CVD, following heart disease and stroke. It occurs when narrowed arteries interfere with the efficient blood flow to your extremities—most often, legs. The narrowing of blood vessels is most often caused by a buildup of fatty deposits, or atherosclerosis, or by diabetes. Remember when I told you that an ischemic stroke is like a heart attack in the brain? Well, peripheral arterial disease is like a heart attack in the legs. Same causes. Same risk factors. In advanced cases, the surgeries are even the same: arterial stents and even grafts and bypass surgery to reestablish blood flow.

The classic PAD symptom is pain or cramping in the legs (or secondarily, buttock or hip) during mild activity, such as walking or climbing stairs, or persistent sores on the feet. But 4 out of 10 people diagnosed with PAD report no pain, and that is most likely due to a concomitant diagnosis of diabetes. Diabetes damages the nerve endings in the feet. Not being able to feel your feet leads to inadvertent injury, and their poor blood supply leads to poor wound healing. And if this combination of challenges occurs, Houston, we have a problem. The complications of severe peripheral arterial disease are the most common causes of amputations.

It has been well documented that more women over 40 than men have PAD. According to the National Institutes of Health, the prevalence of PAD increases with age. In the United States, PAD affects an estimated 20–30 percent of women aged 70 and older, with Black and Native American women affected more than any other group.

But existing statistics are insufficient because, as noted by the American Heart Association, PAD in women is underdiagnosed and undertreated. This is likely because women have higher rates of asymptomatic disease or *atypical* symptoms. I know, there's that word again, but we're working on understanding how diseases affect women differently. When we do understand, I promise, we're going to retire the "atypical" descriptor for women. And, as with virtually all other health conditions, the subpar recruitment of women, minorities, and older subjects for cardiovascular trials has hampered our ability to develop targeted solutions.

Quitting smoking, increasing exercise, and improving diet improve symptoms and outcomes. More severe cases could require prescribed blood thinners and/or surgical intervention. Untreated, severe PAD can lead to the loss of toes, feet, and limbs.

Deep Vein Thrombosis (DVT) and Pulmonary Embolism (PE)

A deep vein thrombosis is a clot that usually forms in your lower extremities but can potentially form in any large vein. Deep vein thromboses in the arms or legs produce pain, swelling, and redness. The diagnosis is confirmed by a noninvasive test—an ultrasound with Doppler to check for blood flow in the affected vein. DVTs should be diagnosed and treated promptly, because left untreated they can lead to a pulmonary embolism, which is much more serious and potentially life-threatening.

PEs come on suddenly and are often associated with all the risk factors for other forms of CVD, as well as prolonged inactivity, malignancy, recent surgery, long periods in confined spaces (airplane trips or car rides), dehydration, and estrogen-containing medications, such as oral contraceptives and hormone therapy.

Less common causes of DVT/PE are genetic mutations, which often run in families, that increase the risk of blood clotting. If you have more than one family member who is otherwise healthy and who has had an unprovoked blood clot, you should inform your doctor and get tested yourself. The risk of developing blood clots is markedly increased in the immediate aftermath of surgery (yet another reason why after surgery your doctor wants you up and out of bed quickly) and in patients with cancer. Post-op patients are always kept well hydrated and are often outfitted with compression socks or an intermittent pneumatic compression device (compression sleeve). These devices are now available for home use and can be helpful for people who are wheelchair-bound or confined to bed.

Always pay attention to acute sudden changes in your body. If every time you take a breath it feels like you're being stabbed, tell those around you that you're in crisis. More PE warning signs:

- Sudden shortness of breath

- Chest pain

- Cough (sometimes bloody)

- Light-headedness or dizziness

- Excessive sweating

- Clammy or discolored skin (called "cyanosis")

Simple, common preventative measures: If you know you have a long plane, bus, or car ride ahead, take one baby aspirin per day, starting 1–2 days ahead and continue only for the day of travel. Obviously, if you are already on a blood thinner for other reasons or if you have an allergy to aspirin, don't take it. Drink plenty of water before and during trips. Not only will it keep you hydrated, it will force you to keep getting up to go to the bathroom—inconvenient but potentially life-saving. *Never* normalize new onset swollen or painful legs; seek an immediate diagnosis. If you can't get in to see your doctor, this would be an appropriate use of an urgent care clinic.

Joyce

My sister Joyce was 65 years old and had been recently discharged from the hospital after extensive but successful colon cancer surgery. Despite being extremely overweight, she was relatively healthy. In fact, other than for the birth of her children, she had never been hospitalized. Her post-surgical recovery had been slow. She was still having some issues with wound healing, but she was happy to finally be able to go home.

Three weeks after being discharged, she developed some chest pain. Initially she thought it might be indigestion, but it got increasingly worse throughout the evening. Every time she took a deep breath, it felt like someone was stabbing her in the chest. She grew sweaty and short of breath. She felt worse than she did on day one after her surgery.

Fortunately, her daughter, Tanya, was there. Tanya quickly realized she had never seen her mother in so much pain. Concerned that she might be having a heart attack, Tanya drove Joyce to the nearest hospital.

Given her symptoms, Joyce was seen quickly and had bloodwork done, which ruled out an acute myocardial infarction. Once she was deemed to be in no immediate danger, her gurney was rolled into the hallway, where she sat for the next three hours. She was given some Tylenol for her pain, which did not touch it. Her shortness of breath also continued, unabated.

After another couple of hours, her ER physician told her she was free to go home but should follow up with her doctor in 3–4 days. By this time, Joyce was in tears. Tanya's response was plain: "I don't know what is wrong with my mother, but she cannot go home like this." The doctor appeared a bit annoyed, but agreed to order one more test, a CT scan, which revealed that Joyce had a large pulmonary embolus. Once she was adequately diagnosed, she was given medication to dissolve the clot, another medication to manage her pain, and oxygen to help with her shortness of breath.

Joyce was lucky. She had an advocate there to speak up for her when she couldn't do it for herself. A pulmonary embolus can often present like a heart attack, with shortness of breath and chest pain. So, the doctors were right to rule out a heart attack first. However, they hadn't ruled out a PE, even though Joyce was a textbook example of who is likely to experience one:

- She was three weeks post-surgery
- She had cancer
- She was obese
- She had been bedridden since her surgery

The Takeaway: PEs can be every bit as serious as heart attacks. There is no doubt that if Tanya had followed the doctor's orders and taken her mother home, this story could have had a devastating ending.

DR. SHARON'S RX FOR
Heart-Happy Health

The things you most need to do to keep your heart healthy aren't complicated or endless in number. They are simple, finite, and doable. But their benefits are boundless and compound over time. No one knows when you will get sick, but this I do know—whether you are recovering from an illness or surgery, if you're in strong cardiovascular health, you will recover faster. Starting today, you will be better. So, why wait?

1. Don't smoke.

2. Limit alcohol to fewer than seven drinks a week. Less is more. Turns out drinking alcohol isn't as beneficial for preventing heart disease as we thought.

3. Monitor your blood pressure at home. It's as good a habit to develop as any.

4. If you have an early menopause or have your ovaries removed before the age of 45, definitely discuss menopausal hormone therapy with your doctor.

5. See your doctor annually to monitor for signs of the metabolic syndrome.

6. Eliminate ultra-processed foods and adopt a diet high in fiber, vegetables, fruits, and lean protein. (I hate to break it to you, but bacon is processed food and, yes, the turkey kind, too, and deli meats. So, you might skip that turkey club.)

7. Mindfully manage stress.

8. Do at least thirty minutes of exercise, preferably cardio, five days a week, every week.

9. Maintain your village. Friends and community matter.

That's it. No magic. If you do these things, you will not only decrease your risk of CVD but you will also decrease your risk of developing dementia and Alzheimer's. Heart health is brain health! After a quick walk around the block, come meet me in Chapter 7.

CHAPTER 7

When It Don't Come Easy♪

Brain Health and Alzheimer's

Dear Sis,

The fact that women live longer than men is a good thing. But if your brain health is compromised, you may not even know you've lived longer. Remember that thing we mentioned earlier called "health span"? This is what Alzheimer's robs you of.

Women make up the majority of people living with dementia, and it's not simply because of those three extra years or so that we live. Dementia is the only one of the top fifteen causes of death where the risk for women exceeds that of men. If you're wondering why we don't understand the reason for that, join the club. And if you're wondering why no one ever thought this line of inquiry was worthy of investigation, your guess is as good as mine—although I'm sure we can come up with a few theories.

I know that sounds bleak. But for those of you who think your fate is sealed because your mother and your grandmother had dementia, think again. There is evidence to suggest that as many as 50 percent of dementia cases may be preventable.

Remember the conversation we had in the last chapter about heart health? Well, guess what? The same things you need to do to protect your heart will also protect your brain. You don't need the expensive brain supplements advertised on TV or have to learn quantum physics to keep your brain healthy. The solutions are easier than you think.

So, sit back, keep reading, and by all means, do not despair. As I always say, how well you age requires some effort on your part, but it's doable. And remember, you got this.

xo, Dr. Sharon

Although dementia and Alzheimer's are frequently used interchangeably, they are not synonymous. Dementia encompasses a broad range of irreversible neurodegenerative changes in the brain that can be caused by infections, head trauma, vascular injuries (strokes), alcoholism, and Parkinson's disease, as well as Alzheimer's.

Alzheimer's disease is the most common cause of dementia and accounts for 60 percent of the cases of cognitive decline diagnosed each year. This is a good place to acknowledge that, as common as it is, we still don't actually know what causes Alzheimer's. The diagnosis is typically made clinically (by symptoms) after ruling out other causes. This lack of understanding how and why Alzheimer's affects so many of us as we age has hampered our ability to treat it effectively. And it's way past time that we fix this.

Alzheimer's Disease

According to the Alzheimer's Association, an estimated 6.5 million Americans age 65 and older are living with Alzheimer's disease, and almost two-thirds of those are women. If you are a Black woman, your risk of Alzheimer's is twice that of white women. And if you are Hispanic, your risk is one and a half times higher than white women's. Although we don't know what causes Alzheimer's, the prevailing wisdom is that it has something to do with the deposition of abnormal proteins (amyloid) in the brain. We don't even know if these amyloid deposits are a cause or an effect of Alzheimer's. Is amyloid the chicken or the egg? But we do know what established Alzheimer's disease looks like on brain scans—shrinkage of overall brain volume with thinning of the brain's cerebral cortex (gray matter). Positron emission tomography (PET scan), a more sophisticated imaging test usually done in academic settings, can visualize the neurofibrillary tangles and amyloid plaques characteristic of Alzheimer's. Conventional CTs and MRIs cannot see the amyloid plaques on scans but are useful in ruling out other causes of dementia.

Dr. Lisa Mosconi, a neuroscientist of Weill Cornell Medical Center, who has relied on these sophisticated imaging techniques to study female brains during pre- and perimenopause, has established that both physically and metabolically, women's brains change dramatically during that time. Dr. Mosconi's findings, detailed in her book *The XX Brain,* clearly suggest that these critical changes associated with Alzheimer's occur years, if not decades, before any cognitive changes are clinically apparent. Given the demographics of Alzheimer's cases, Dr. Mosconi asserts that the biggest risk factors for developing the disease are being female and having an affected parent (the risk is higher for those with an affected mother than for those with an affected father), followed by all the exact same risk factors that increase your risk for cardiovascular disease. To date, almost every longitudinal study that has followed patients as they age who subsequently developed Alzheimer's has identified the same factors.

Dr. Mosconi's imaging studies comparing the brains of premenopausal women to perimenopausal women revealed changes in metabolism and brain structure starting in perimenopause. Brain fog, difficulty concentrating, and forgetfulness are all on perimenopause's long list of common symptoms (see Chapter 9). But for most women, these symptoms are a normal side effect of perimenopause and should ease as you transition through to menopause. In other words, the confusion and lack of focus that some women experience during that transition are not necessarily harbingers of future dementia. What we do know is that if you have menopause before the age of 45 (either naturally or due to chemotherapy, radiation, or surgery), your risk for developing Alzheimer's is increased, and some estimates place that risk as much as 70 percent higher than that of women who go through menopause at age 51 or older. It is for this reason that in the North American Menopause Society's 2022 guidelines, hormone replacement therapy (HRT) is recommended for women who experience menopause before age 45. They also recommend that HRT continue *at least* until the average age of menopause. This is especially critical information for Black women, who on average tend to experience menopause almost a year earlier than white women and are twice as likely to undergo hysterectomies, often with removal of the ovaries.

Don't panic if you frequently can't recall names or words that should be on the tip of your tongue, or if it occasionally takes you longer than it should to do simple arithmetic. But don't sleep on it either. Know your family history and your risk factors for developing Alzheimer's. And institute the lifestyle changes early on that will minimize your risk. There is no reason to wait—start now! Pay attention to the evolution of any distressing memory symptoms, and if they become more frequent or acute, talk to your doctor.

It wouldn't be a bad idea to get baseline cognitive testing done if your mother or sister has been diagnosed with dementia. That said, the idea that most dementia is hereditary is false. Remember, a family history reveals a propensity, not a certainty. According to Dr. Mosconi, only about 2 percent of dementia cases are due to genetics, and if your family members who have Alzheimer's were diagnosed after 60, relax, it is unlikely that you have the gene. (The discussion of the Alzheimer's gene, the APOE gene, is beyond the scope of our conversation here. But take some comfort in the fact that the data on the significance of this gene is complicated.)

Race Matters (But Not for the Reasons You May Think)

Why do Black women have twice the risk of Alzheimer's? Really good question. At the threat of sounding like a broken record, Black women have a higher risk for developing Alzheimer's for some of the same reasons that they have a higher risk of cardiovascular disease, strokes, diabetes, and, well, just about everything. But the answer is not simply because they are Black.

We cannot look at health disparities and simply continue to ask the question, what is wrong with Black women? We must ask more in-depth and harder-to-answer questions, like what are we doing *to* Black women? What is it about their lived experiences that increases their risk for these debilitating diseases? Blaming *any* race of people for the disparities they face is far too simplistic. We already know that Black women's socioeconomic class, education level, and insurance status are highly significant factors in determining their health and healthcare outcomes. Yet even when these factors are taken into account, Black women are still at higher risk for Alzheimer's. Why?

One possible explanation circles back to the concept of "weathering," or accelerated aging due to stress, racism, and the social determinants of health (as discussed in Chapter 5). The social determinants of health include all the things that can negatively impact health outside of the individual (poverty, access to healthy food and clean water, safe environment, education access, and healthcare). Weathering, as noted by the University of Michigan's Dr. Arline Geronimus, may be one of the previously unnamed drivers of health disparities and adverse outcomes that underpins everything from increased maternal and infant mortality to cardiovascular disease and increased risk of Alzheimer's.

Simply put, the additional burden of stress experienced by Black people in this country is not only aging our bodies, but it is also aging our brains. Scans done on Black people reveal that their brains appear much older than their chronological age. That means that the damage starts to accumulate earlier and faster. Not only do we need to know why, we need to get answers as to what we are going to do about it. Despite the alarming statistics and their potential repercussions for Black women, studies on the issue are almost nonexistent. We need two things: more funding and research into this topic, and more people willing to participate in long-term studies. Currently less than 2 percent of all subjects in studies of Alzheimer's are Black.

Despite their elevated risks, Black and Latino people are less likely to receive an accurate Alzheimer's diagnosis or to be offered certain treatment options. While this can be one of those areas where patients may tend to avoid or deny symptoms out of fear, another possibility is that healthcare professionals may not be as aggressive in evaluating and treating Black and Latino patients. This is particularly critical, because we do know that the earlier dementia and Alzheimer's are diagnosed, the better. Delayed or inaccurate diagnosis can result in a cascade of deficits, from fewer treatment and care options to a patient's inability to participate in their own planning, and worse health outcomes overall.

Estrogen and Brain Health

Is it the lack of estrogen that affects women's brains adversely at menopause? Let's start with what we know. Dr. Lisa Mosconi's research shows estrogen or lack thereof does appear to play a role in brain health. Whether that relationship is causal or correlated is a matter of debate, but the evidence is highly suggestive of the former. Women's brains are affected by estrogen. We know that during perimenopause, women can experience depression, anxiety, brain fog, hot flashes, and sleep disturbances. Where do all these symptoms originate? You guessed it—the brain. What makes them go away? Estrogen.

Since we know that estrogen affects the brain at each stage of women's reproductive lives, why, you might ask, don't we definitively know the role of estrogen after menopause vis-à-vis Alzheimer's? We don't know because the one large-scale study that might have answered that question, the Women's Health Initiative, was halted prematurely over twenty years ago, and no other women's study of similar scale has been launched to replace it. Don't even get me started on this one. Thanks to Dr. Mosconi's recent imaging studies of the structural and metabolic changes in the brains of women at different phases of their reproductive lives, we may be inching closer to an answer. Every Alzheimer's presentation is different and the older you are when you exhibit signs, the more quality years you have accrued. But as Dr. Mosconi's research has suggested, by the time the cognitive changes associated with Alzheimer's become apparent, the disease is most likely decades in the making.

Why, then, do we spend the bulk of the time, energy, and Alzheimer's research money targeting treatments for the disease rather than focusing on its prevention? This is a fundamental flaw in most medical research (largely resulting from the fact that much of that research is funded by drug companies). We know the risks associated with vascular dementia. We know who is at risk for developing Alzheimer's, and what we can do to minimize that risk. So, why is more not being done to educate members of high-risk communities? The number of campaigns aimed at the prevention of Alzheimer's and vascular dementias should rival those of the antismoking campaigns in the 1970s.

Wouldn't it be better if we could figure out how to prevent cognitive decline rather than try to fix it after the fact? As my mother would say, it's like closing the barn door after the horse is already out. I'm not suggesting we shouldn't be pursuing treatments, just that we should be able to do two things at the same time. Getting the word out on preventative measures will do more than save women's lives, it will also vastly improve the quality of their lives.

Grace

An elegant and extremely well-educated 84-year-old woman, Grace, is at the end stage of Alzheimer's disease. She is minimally verbal but has severe short-term memory loss and is disoriented to time, place, and location. She lives in a memory care facility and has frequent contact with her children and grandchildren, although she does not know who they are.

Despite experiencing memory and cognitive changes for at least a decade, she deftly managed to conceal the depth of her cognitive decline from most people, except those close to her. At first, her symptoms presented as mild memory lapses—forgetting keys and where she parked the car—so subtle as to be chalked up to just normal aging. When being reminded that she had just told that story five minutes ago, she simply laughed it off or made excuses.

Over time, her confusion became impossible to hide. She increasingly misidentified family members, mistaking her brother for her father. Her appearance, which was always a source of pride, became disheveled and she needed help with basic activities of daily living.

Her family realized in retrospect that the signs of Alzheimer's had been there for at least twenty years. Although she has been on medication for over ten years, it is impossible to know whether the treatments have slowed her decline.

The Takeaway: It is never too early to begin your Alzheimer's prevention plan. Do your heart and your brain a favor and get going!

Vascular Dementia

Vascular dementia is the second-most common type, affecting almost 25 percent of those diagnosed with cognitive decline. Caused by diminished or absent blood flow to areas of the brain, vascular dementia has a direct link to high blood pressure (HBP) and stroke. The risk factors for vascular dementia are the same as the risk factors for cardiovascular disease. (Are you beginning to sense a pattern here?) About 55 percent of Black adults afflicted with dementia have HBP.

Ischemic strokes can produce dementia just as profound as Alzheimer's and may not be evident on initial CT scans. The difference between some vascular dementias and Alzheimer's is the period over which symptoms develop. Also, some vascular dementias are not the result of one single stroke, but of multiple small and often silent strokes. Over time, the damage to the brain accumulates and produces dementia gradually.

The good news here is that if you control your blood pressure, you can decrease your risk of stroke *and* your risk of vascular dementia significantly.

Notably, 1 in 14 people over the age of 65 suffers with some form of dementia. Over age 80, it's 1 in 6. No matter what your current age is, you may be anxious about your likelihood of ultimately developing dementia. Even the slightest concern (and we *all* fall under this umbrella) is reason enough to reset your behaviors, starting today (see Dr. Sharon's Rx).

Trust me: You *can* be the change your body, and your brain, need.

Doris

Doris is a vibrant 66-year-old firebrand. She is overweight, but active. On her last visit to her doctor, her cholesterol level was over 300. She has had high blood pressure for as long as she can remember.

Her doctors recently put her on a new high blood pressure medication and a new statin for her cholesterol. Her prescription directs her to take both daily. But since she retired, money has been tight. The new medications are expensive and are not fully covered by Medicare. To make ends meet, she has been alternating the days that she takes her meds. She takes her blood pressure medication one day and her cholesterol medication the next day. She figures it's better than not taking them at all. She hasn't slept well in years and has simply made peace with her constant state of fatigue.

While getting ready to meet her daughter for dinner one evening, Doris started to feel a bit off. By the time her daughter arrived, she was still sitting on the side of the bed, confused and half-dressed. Doris's daughter immediately took her to the nearest hospital. On evaluation, her blood pressure was 260/142. An initial CT scan was unremarkable, but her mental status did not improve.

Once her vitals were stabilized, Doris was admitted to

the hospital. After two days in the hospital and no improvement in her condition, a second CT scan was performed, which confirmed an ischemic stroke. After discharge, Doris's confusion worsened, and it became clear she could no longer live independently. She now lives with her daughter.

The Takeaway: The next time your doctor prescribes a new medication, ask them what was wrong with your old one. New is not always better, but it is almost always going to be more expensive. Expensive, shiny new drugs may sound great, but if you cannot afford them, you are better off taking an older, less expensive medication that you can afford to take as prescribed. If a new medicine is absolutely necessary (there's almost always a less expensive alternative), shop around for the best price. Ask your pharmacist or look online for coupons. And remember, don't let the perfect get in the way of the good.

Beyond Sudoku: Preventing Brain Decline and Alzheimer's

Now that you know that women are the majority of people living with dementia and Black women are at the highest risk of all, think about what that means for the quality of your life as you age. If you think you're too young to be concerned about this, think again. Think about your mother. It's never too late to do better. Being of sound mind is the cornerstone upon which everything you need to do to remain independent as you age is built. Cognitive decline negatively affects your capacity to earn income, to manage your finances, and to perform self-care.

But hang on—you know this is where I slip in some good news.

No one can predict whether you will get Alzheimer's, but we do know that, as with heart disease, you can push that propensity off further into the future. There is significant evidence that at least 30–50 percent of all dementia cases could be delayed or prevented through the same behaviors that heart health demands. Your brain needs exercise the same way your body needs it. And no, I'm not talking about doing Sudoku all day.

The concept known as "cognitive reserve" means that the more knowledge and varied experiences you have stored in your brain, the more you are able to compensate when, and if, cognitive decline begins. For example, if you only know one way to complete a task, be it a route home or a strategy for completing a puzzle, when that avenue is blocked, you're stuck. This is why physical movement is so important for your brain.

You're never too old to learn something new, and it doesn't have to be quantum physics. Brush your teeth or learn to write with your less dominant hand [♪ **"I Can't Write Left-Handed"**]. Instead of relying on directions apps, find your way around, identifying different routes to arrive at the same place. Learn a new language or musical instrument. Change careers. Adopt a new hobby. Memorize poems, song lyrics, and the birthdays and numbers of loved ones by heart (remember when we knew all of those, back in the before–cell phones times?). These aren't just life-enhancing skills. They're Alzheimer's-blockers.

What's on the Horizon for Alzheimer's?

The only treatments for Alzheimer's thus far are pharmaceutical. There are no cures. Once the damage is done, there is no turning back. All medication can hope to do is slow the rate of decline. Clearly a better plan is early intervention.

The medications Aduhelm and Leqembi, recently approved by the FDA, target removal of the amyloid plaques thought to be responsible for Alzheimer's. But as I noted earlier, we don't yet know whether these plaques are the cause or the result of Alzheimer's. It is also not clear that removing the plaques will significantly improve cognitive function.

These drugs were approved on an accelerated basis by the FDA, and Leqembi has now been granted full FDA approval. Aduhelm, although approved first, has not been widely accepted, not only because of its hefty price tag of $56,000 per year, but also because of its unacceptably high rate of complications, such as brain swelling and bleeding. Leqembi, which has a lower rate of complications, still is quite expensive at an estimated $26,000 a year. Medicare has agreed to cover 80 percent of the cost, but an additional $5,200 a year for medication is still beyond the reach of many seniors. As I said earlier, none of these medications reverses or cures Alzheimer's. You only get worse more slowly. Although a 27 percent improvement in cognitive function with Leqembi may sound impressive, the patients who received Leqembi only scored a half point higher on an eighteen-point scale than patients who received a placebo. And the long-term consequences of taking these medications is unknown because they were approved with only eighteen months' worth of data. What happens after that? Your guess is as good as mine.

When you consider that more than 6 million people are living with Alzheimer's today and over 20 million more will be diagnosed by 2050, you can see that the costs of these drugs will cripple an already over-burdened healthcare system—not to mention the financial health of those who need them. So, I wouldn't exactly call these new drugs breakthroughs at this point.

Prevention is still the most effective weapon we have in the arsenal against Alzheimer's. Yet it is the least utilized. I will not cast aspersions on the genuine desire within the pharmaceutical industry to improve the outcomes of Alzheimer's patients and to relieve their suffering, but we cannot ignore the enormous profit motive for breakthrough drugs and technologies. I am not suggesting that we stifle innovation. Quite the contrary. We need innovative research *and* widescale education and prevention efforts. We *can* do two things at once, and we *don't* have to sacrifice one for the other.

We grow up and, God willing, we grow old. But we don't have to grow tired and bored, or sedentary and unwilling to explore new things. You're never too old to make new connections in your brain. Sure, I want to help you avoid a heart attack, a stroke, and Alzheimer's, but I also want you to be able to get out of your chair when you're 80 to do more than use the bathroom. I want you to spend your retirement savings on vacations, not medications. I want you to not just survive, but to thrive. Sorry, I was channeling my inner Jesse Jackson there for a minute.

DR. SHARON'S RX FOR
Brain Health

1. Don't smoke. (Duh. Just in case you need a reminder.)

2. Alcohol is toxic to your brain. Act accordingly.

3. Control and self-monitor high blood pressure and blood sugar.

4. If you have an early menopause or have your ovaries removed before the age of 50, discuss menopausal hormone therapy with your doctor. And remember: Estrogen matters.

5. High fiber, protein (think fish, nuts, legumes, and lean meats), with vegetables and fruits and healthy fats are the way to go to support a healthy brain.

6. In addition to your usual exercise, develop new muscle skills focusing on large muscle groups and your core. Balance exercises are important. Remember that head trauma from falls is not an insignificant contributor to

dementia, and women's brains are more susceptible to trauma.

7. Stay mentally engaged. Keep learning and challenging your brain.

8. Maintain your village. Friends and community matter. Depression is a risk factor for dementia, and people who remain socially engaged experience less depression.

9. Seek out and participate in Alzheimer's studies, particularly if you have a family history or if you are in a high-risk group.

If you're sensing a pattern, or it feels like I'm just blatantly repeating myself, your brain isn't playing tricks on you. I am intentionally, even relentlessly, trying to imprint these same healthy habits onto you—mind, body, and soul—so you can't ignore them. They may seem basic, even boring, but when consistently applied, these behaviors will have a profound effect on your long-term health, the way you age, and your ability to heal when needed.

CHAPTER 8

I Will Survive♪

"Female Troubles" and
Their Treatments

Dear Sis,

Just what exactly are "female troubles"? I bet you've heard of them—maybe you've used the term yourself or have heard your mother use it. But do you know exactly what they are?

If you're like me, you first overheard whispering about this when you were a child and had no idea what folks were talking about. It just sounded decidedly not good. Maybe a little bit dirty, painful. Shameful even.

Did women cause these "troubles" or create them in their own minds? Were there cures or products or secret passwords that could cleanse you or keep you safe? It was all very mysterious and lived squarely in the lane of "grown people's business." So as a child, or even as a young woman, you dared not query. The hushed tones, side-eyes, and gaping silences made it clear: There was something lurking in the female body that was problematic and too mortifying to be openly discussed.

Hopefully, we have not raised the next generation to feel this way. But it's hard to say because we continue keeping to ourselves about too many of the health issues that come along with this thing called "womanhood." We barely discuss our own experiences with one another, never mind with our daughters and nieces. That silence doesn't serve us. It isolates, harms, and even kills us. We need to stop it. Now.

It's time to talk openly and unapologetically about the common things that we all should know could happen in our bodies, and what to do about them if they do. What's more important than knowing what to expect when you're expecting to live a long time?

xo, Dr. Sharon

Have you ever heard anyone whispering about "male troubles" or making offensive jokes about a men's "curse"? Neither have I, which is interesting because men over 40 are as much at risk for a short list of gender-specific health challenges as we are. But nobody couches their stuff in shade and misery.

In fact, have you seen these ads touting solutions to men's particular issues? They somehow manage to put the "fun" in erectile dysfunction, or at least, its treatment. So, why does everybody from your neighbor to your cousin to your doctor (yes, I said it) get all hushed and awkward about the perfectly normal issues we women face as we age?

At least in part, it's because we let them. As with everything else, if we want a different world, we have to make like the actress Lisa Bonet (who is just a few stops from 60, by the way) and create it. Only then can we get what we need to thrive and stop feeling so alone [♪ "I'm Every Woman"].

It's time to name and claim the things we must navigate, without embarrassment or apology or fear, as we get older. Let's start by dropping the F-bomb: fibroids.

Fibroids: The Backstory

All premenopausal and perimenopausal women with a uterus can develop fibroids. These very common noncancerous tumors of the uterus are naturally occurring and predominantly made up of muscle fibers and connective tissue.

The good news: Most "female troubles," including fibroids, do improve once we cross the reproductive finish line into menopause. They are also entirely treatable. If you've been told otherwise, or have simply been avoiding treating yours, let's start your course correction right here, right now, with some facts.

Despite their ubiquity, only about 25 percent of fibroids require medical or surgical attention. In fact, 50 percent of patients who are diagnosed with fibroids were unaware that they had them until their doctor detected them during a routine pelvic examination or an ultrasound for something unrelated, like back pain.

The bad news is that when fibroids are symptomatic, they can seriously disrupt the quality of your life—and here again, the women most affected are Black. According to the 2021 American College of Obstetricians and Gynecologists Practice Bulletin, fibroids occur in up to 70 percent of women generally—and almost 80 percent in women of African descent, who are also twice as likely to be symptomatic.

Black women's fibroids are typically larger at diagnosis, more numerous (fibroids rarely travel alone), and present at younger ages than white women's. It won't surprise you to learn that Black women are also less likely to be offered a trial of medical management rather than surgery. Even when you control for the size of their fibroids, Black women are not only more likely to have surgery, but they are also less likely to have minimally invasive surgery. This puts Black women at a deficit in terms of recovery times and places them at greater risk for postsurgical complications.

While research has not yet pinpointed why Black women are more susceptible to fibroids, our understanding of these uterine growths, as well as their symptoms and how to treat them, has improved. Other than being Black and having a uterus, the risk factors for developing fibroids are: being pre- or perimenopausal; having a family history of fibroids; being overweight; having hypertension; and having had more time since your last pregnancy.

The average woman's uterus is about three inches long and shaped like an upside-down Bartlett pear (we love a good fruit analogy in gynecology, and this one is really accurate). Fibroids can grow in clusters, like grapes, or as a single tumor—clusters are more common. They can range from 1mm to 20cm in diameter. If you're metrically challenged, like me, the translation is from tiny (think pea-sized) to as large as a melon—and by that, I mean watermelon (you can't say I didn't warn you about the fruit). Very large fibroids can enlarge the uterus as much as a full-term pregnancy.

Despite their potential for drama, fibroids can remain small and quiet, and usually do. Their growth is maintained by estrogen, so they tend to grow during your peak reproductive years and pregnancy, when estrogen levels are high, and tend to shrink during menopause, when estrogen levels drop.

Past use of hormonal birth control pills or injectable medroxyprogesterone (Depo-Provera) is associated with a *decreased* risk of developing fibroids. The added progestogens in oral contraceptives and progestin-only contraceptives mitigate the effects of the estrogen. But it is generally believed that unlike with many of the health challenges we've covered so far—e.g., hypertension, diabetes, and obesity—you can neither cause fibroids nor entirely prevent them. In other words, for those who are prone to them, fibroids are unavoidable but can be quite manageable.

I want you to fully understand what fibroids are, the risks they pose, and the many treatment options now available, because too many of you endure a great deal of suffering and go far too long without treatment. If you can easily tolerate your fibroids, fine. But if they are disrupting your routine, your joy, or your peace, you do not have to endure them—nor should you.

The danger of putting off treatment for symptomatic fibroids is that, over time, they can get bigger. As they do, your likelihood of being able to address them with minimally invasive surgeries decreases. The bigger the surgery, the higher the risk of complications and the longer your recovery time. And I'm sure you have things you'd rather do.

When Fibroids Spell Trouble

Let me repeat: Fibroids are almost always noncancerous. Leiomyosarcomas are very rare cancerous tumors occurring in less than 1 in 1,000 masses removed from the uterus. And know this: There is no correlation between having fibroids and developing leiomyosarcoma or any other form of cancer.

That said, I hesitate to call fibroids benign, because while they can be small and completely asymptomatic, there is nothing benign about their impact on your life when they are not. No one should have to take to their bed writhing in pain during their period or bleed so much that they are afraid to leave the house. After thirty years of practicing medicine, little surprises me. But I have seen the full scope of the pain, heartache, shame, and fear these noncancerous tumors of the uterus can cause. And I never cease to be amazed—and heartbroken—by the conditions some women (and their doctors) will normalize rather than address.

Symptoms that should signal you to seek treatment are:

- Heavy bleeding

- Prolonged periods (7+ days)

- Light-headedness/dizziness

- Pelvic pain, back pain, or pain during sex

- Anemia

- Frequent urination or difficulty emptying your bladder or bowels

- Enlarged abdomen and unexplained weight gain

Bleeding (How Much Is Too Much?)

The number one problem that brings women over 40 to the gynecologist is heavy, prolonged, or irregular bleeding. The medical definition of *heavy bleeding* is "loss of more than 80cc (cubic centimeters), or about a half cup of blood, in one entire menstrual period." If you've ever had a period, you know that is not a lot. But many of you with fibroids are saying, "I can lose that much blood in an hour!" If that is your truth, know (no!) that is not okay.

I have patients who tell me that they wear two super-plus tampons together with a maxi pad to prevent leaks. Others wear adult diapers or Pampers to avoid bleeding onto their sheets at night. Y'all, that's not normal! And it warrants not just an evaluation, but a solution.

Understand that when it comes to bleeding, it is not just the size of your fibroids that matters. With fibroids, as with real estate, it's all about location, location, location. The closer the fibroids are to the lining of the uterus (the endometrium), the more bleeding they can cause. I have seen fibroids smaller than a grape cause enough bleeding to necessitate a blood transfusion, and fibroids the size of cantaloupes that didn't make the patient skip a beat.

Many women adapt to living with unpredictable, excessive bleeding (often accompanied by pain that can veer from minor to excruciating), not just for months but years. While it may be understandable to gradually recalibrate one's sense of what is normal, the impact is about more than doubling down on menstrual products or routinely traveling with extra underwear or a change of clothes. When you lose excessive amounts of blood, cycle after cycle, it can lead to anemia, a condition that when chronic can make you feel weak, dizzy, exhausted, and generally speaking, lousy. It's just no way to live.

Yvonne

Eight months into a demanding surgical residency, Yvonne felt tired on her best days. And so, she thought, did all of her peers. The sleepless nights on call, the physical demands, constant pressure, and stress—residency was one long, draining test in every way. So, it made sense to her that she felt bad.

But almost a year later, Yvonne would sometimes get so tired walking to her car, she would have to stop, sit on the curb, and gather her strength before driving home after work.

When she finally saw her doctor and had a complete blood count done, she was already severely anemic. Her hematocrit was 14; normal is over 36. She was walking around with less than half the amount of blood capacity that she should have—and she didn't get there overnight. Because her menstrual bleeding worsened gradually over many months, she didn't realize what was happening— even as a doctor! This gave her an appreciation for how deceptive and sneaky the onset of chronic anemia can be and how you can lose a considerable amount of blood over time and not realize how much it's diminishing your life.

The Takeaway: Any menstrual cycle consistently lasting more than seven days with heavy bleeding is not normal. Imagine having your period ten days a month and living with the constant fear of bleeding through to your clothes. I know some of you don't have to imagine it, you live it. Now I want you to go fix it.

An evaluation for heavy bleeding should always include a complete blood count, iron levels, a pelvic ultrasound, and if risk factors for endometrial cancer are present, an endometrial biopsy. Heavy, prolonged bleeding can also be a warning sign of endometrial cancer, particularly when there are risk factors present—obesity, long-standing history of polycystic ovarian syndrome (long periods of irregular bleeding), or a family history of uterine cancer. So, don't sleep on that. But you know that I believe common things happen commonly, and if you have fibroids and heavy or prolonged bleeding, the source is usually the fibroids.

Sick and Tired: Sizing Up Your Suffering

Large fibroids, even when bleeding is not an issue, can cause symptoms purely related to their bulkiness. What are bulk symptoms? A large fibroid sitting on your bladder (mini anatomy lesson: The uterus sits right between your bladder and your rectum) can cause urinary urgency, increased frequency (due to decreased bladder capacity), and occasional stress incontinence. If you have ever been pregnant, you know how fraught with danger an unanticipated cough or sneeze can be.

When a fibroid sits on your rectum, it can make bowel movements difficult to pass, or it can change the size and shape of your stool (TMI? There's no such thing when it comes to your health). And since your uterus sits right at the apex of your vagina, large fibroids can make penetrative sex uncomfortable or painful with certain positions. But here's the deal: These are symptoms that *can* happen, not that necessarily *will* happen. And let me repeat, fibroid size doesn't always correlate with the severity of symptoms. That is why a perfectly reasonable option for those who are asymptomatic is a wait-and-see approach.

Larger fibroids and their bulk can distend your abdomen in a way that looks like you're pregnant. But remember—and this is an important point—if you have no other symptoms and looking like you're five months pregnant doesn't bother you, then you can decide to do nothing other than buy elastic-waist pants.

However, even asymptomatic fibroids require monitoring. Sometimes a pelvic ultrasound is warranted, not only to monitor growth and check the ovaries, but also to ensure that very large fibroids are not compressing the ureters (thin tubes that connect your kidneys to your bladder). Chronic compression of the ureters can lead to kidney damage. Fortunately, this is rare. But it is yet another reason to keep up with those annual gynecologic examinations.

Darlene

True story: Way back in the days before ultrasounds, legal abortion, and a woman's right to choose (I will *not* veer off course here about the horrors of history repeating itself!), my brother's girlfriend's belly kept getting bigger and bigger. We all assumed Darlene was pregnant, and so did she.

It was a time when the only decent response to getting pregnant out of wedlock was to get married. Told you this was a long time ago.

Not long after the wedding, my brother and new sister-in-law learned they were the proud parents of a bouncing five-pound fibroid. Needless to say, the marriage didn't last . . . and neither did that fibroid.

The Takeaway: Do not make life-changing decisions based on any self-diagnosis. Ever.

It may seem silly (it clearly wasn't to the unhappy couple), but that's what can happen when you minimize and normalize your symptoms or when, as in this case, you assume you know what's happening inside your body rather than go find out for sure. And I will say it over and over: Suffering should not be an expected or accepted part of woman-hood. To paraphrase Fannie Lou Hamer, we need to get sick and tired of being sick and tired. Deciding when or if to seek fibroid treatment is completely up to you, but feeling "kinda okay" as a daily baseline is not okay. I want you to feel great.

Fibroids and Fertility

It's unusual that fibroids are a direct cause of infertility or failed preg-nancy, but depending on their size and location, they can sometimes interfere. That's why in the old days, the prevailing thought was that fibroids should be addressed before a planned pregnancy—not only because they could impede a woman's ability to get pregnant, but they might cause premature delivery or miscarriage. This is no longer what we recommend except in very specific cases.

Brenda

Brenda was a newlywed in her mid-30s who came in for a preconception visit. On physical exam, she had very large fibroids. Since she was planning to have children within the year, I thought her fibroids might be worth removing be-fore she got pregnant, not only to optimize her chances of conceiving but to minimize any potential for complications during pregnancy.

We discussed her options; she listened carefully and chose not to have her fibroids removed before trying to conceive. (TBH, I thought she should have. They were huge!) Well, not only did she get pregnant, she got pregnant with twins!

I was way more nervous than she was—about miscarriage, growth of her fibroids during the pregnancy, preterm labor, pain, and just about every prenatal and postpartum complication in the book. I also worried about just how much room she had in her abdomen to carry all those fibroids and two babies, because she was not a large woman. Let's just say, I was concerned.

But Brenda sailed through and delivered two healthy babies at term. Other than a few more gray hairs for me, the pregnancy, delivery, and recovery were textbook normal. So, you just never know. It was a risk, but it was Brenda's call to make. And this is why we don't treat fibroids just because they're there.

The Takeaway: Sometimes it's better to be lucky than good. However, given the high costs and variable success rates of IVF, for those undergoing assisted reproduction, your doctor may advise fibroid removal first to optimize your potential of conceiving and maintaining a pregnancy. Given the reduced odds of conceiving as you age, the recommendation may be similar if you are over 40 and trying to get pregnant naturally. In either case, your doctor can only advise you; the final decisions are yours to make.

The Untallied Costs of Fibroids and Being Female

Aside from the pain, bleeding, bulkiness, and other symptoms associated with fibroids, they can take a huge psychological toll as well, in the form of stress and the need to plan your life (including sex, major events, vacations, or business trips) around your period. How reasonable is that? Not very.

Let's also take a minute here to discuss menstrual equity as an economic issue [♪**"Only Women Bleed"**]. Did you ever stop to think about how poor women pay for sanitary products? Tampons are not cheap. Did you ever wonder why they cost so much? Jennifer Weiss-Wolf, executive director of the Birnbaum Women's Leadership Center and author of the book *Periods Gone Public: Taking a Stand for Menstrual Equity,* has pushed for pads and tampons to be available free of charge in women's prisons and public schools. Why don't we regard sanitary products for women as essentials? We should make them available the same way we make toilet paper and soap available in public spaces.

Women with heavy bleeding can go through two or three times as many sanitary products. The cost of that is ridiculous. Thanks to Jennifer Weiss-Wolf's advocacy, many states have voted to at least eliminate the tax on menstrual products. It's a start, but we have barely begun to address the many inequities of possessing a uterus.

Whether because of the stigma associated with periods or a lack of understanding about what constitutes "normal," most women don't give great thought to these issues or even the details of their menstrual cycles. They tend not to discuss them with their doctors either, unless asked very strategic questions. When women are simply asked if their periods are "regular" or "normal"—the typical annual exam question—they usually reply, "yes," and leave it at that.

It's always good to ask your doctor questions, like: "Do you sense anything out of the ordinary?" "Is my pelvic exam the same as last year's?" "Do you think I have fibroids?" Fibroids run in families, so if your sister or mother has had them, that's worth mentioning. This is also why having some consistency of care (rather than seeing a different doctor in urgent care every year) is preferable. For the record, I typically mention what I see or feel during an exam, even if it's ordinary. Not all doctors do, and that's not wrong—it's just a style thing. But as gynecologists, we should do better at helping our patients make practical self-assessments by asking questions like:

- How often are you changing pads or tampons in a day?

- Are they soaked when you do?

- Do you ever bleed through to your clothes or bedsheets even though you are wearing adequate sanitary protection?

- Do you feel exhausted during your period?

- Does your period inhibit your activities?

Keep these questions in mind when you see your doctor, whether you get asked them or not. And yes, I do get all up in your business. That's my job.

Hysterectomy and Its Checkered History

Hysterectomies, in which the uterus is removed, have historically been performed too often. But Black women are still steered toward this invasive, fertility-ending surgery at twice the rate of white women.

Vivian, Joyce, Gwen, and (almost) Margie

All four of my sisters had fibroids. Although the timing of their symptoms varied, they all eventually had extremely heavy bleeding, resulting in three hysterectomies and one near-hysterectomy. Funny thing about perimenopause and fibroids, having the two together is not just additive, the effect of one multiplies the effect of the other.

Joyce started having out-of-control periods in her 30s. Her doctor immediately recommended a hysterectomy. In fairness, minimally invasive surgery didn't exist then. It was the 1970s.

Gwen made it as far as her mid-40s before the out-of-control bleeding set in. She, too, went directly to a hysterectomy. Vivian rounded out the trifecta, with heavy bleeding that started late in her 40s, and by 48, her uterus was history. None of them made it to menopause with an intact uterus.

Just when it seemed inevitable that Margie would be next in line for a hysterectomy, the ground shifted. Although her doctors recommended a hysterectomy as the treatment for her fibroids, Margie simply refused.

It was the early 2000s, and patient empowerment was just becoming a thing. She wanted to exhaust her other options before going that route, so she said, "No, thank you. Let's try something else first." Guess what? With careful monitoring and minor procedures, Margie was able to avoid major surgery. But had she not advocated for herself, she would have fallen in line with the rest of the Malone women.

Margie and I beat the clock and made it to menopause. As of this writing, I not only have my uterus, but my one tiny fibroid is steadily shrinking, even though I take hormones.

Another important data point: Margie and I are the only ones in our family who are not overweight and the only two thus far who have not had cancer. I'm not bragging, I'm just reminding you that genetics is not destiny and the more you know, the more you can avoid some of the pitfalls that you see coming down the road. If you see a sign that says, "Bridge Out Ahead," do you keep driving straight at full speed or do you turn the car around and find another route? You are at the wheel of your own life. You get to decide which roads to take.

The Takeaway: Hysterectomy is not the only option today. Nor is it often the optimal option. Given advances in surgical tools and techniques, there are more treatments available, and many are less invasive with faster recovery times. Unfortunately, too many women, particularly Black women, are not being offered the full array of possible treatments for their symptoms. So, let's make you aware of what they are.

Fibroid Treatments Today (Nonsurgical)

Expectant Management

Once more so you're crystal clear, just because you have fibroids doesn't automatically mean you have to do anything. This is what we in medicine call "expectant management," which is a fancy way of saying, "Let's just wait and see."

No symptoms? No problem. Minor symptoms that cause you way less discomfort than any surgery? That's your prerogative [♪ **"It's My Prerogative"**]. BUT . . . see your gynecologist regularly to monitor your fibroids' growth. Intervene if and when you become symptomatic, or if your fertility is impacted by their location. And keep in mind, if you make it to menopause, those fibroids will typically take care of themselves, so your age should be factored into your decision.

As my own case illustrates, the overwhelming majority of fibroids stop growing after menopause even if you take menopausal hormone therapy. The amount of hormone used to treat symptoms is a fraction of the amount of hormones that you produce in a normal cycle. Fibroids that continue to grow after menopause (which are rare) are a warning sign for uterine cancer and must be addressed with your doctor. This is *again* why I insist that you must continue to have an annual gynecological exam.

Medical Management

- **Nonsteroidal Anti-inflammatory Drugs (ibuprofen, naproxen), or NSAIDS,** work well for most mild cases of episodic heavy bleeding. For example, if you know the first day or two of your period is heavy, you can take 400–600mg of ibuprofen every eight hours or 440mg of naproxen sodium every twelve hours. This works well if in addition to bleeding you have mild cramping. Make sure not to take either on an empty stomach or for more than 2–3 days. Avoid aspirin-containing products (often present in over-the-counter migraine medications) because aspirin prolongs bleeding. And if you cannot tolerate nonsteroidal medication or have an allergy to ibuprofen, this option is clearly not for you.

- **Tranexamic Acid (Lysteda) and Mefenamic Acid (Ponstel)** require prescriptions but work well for moderately heavy bleeding. Like NSAIDs, they work best when taken before heavy bleeding starts and should be continued through the normal/heavy days. Follow the instructions provided by your doctor.

- **Combination Contraceptives** (pills, patches, or rings) contain both estrogen and progestin and are good options for controlling heavy, irregular cycles in women, regardless of the need for birth control. For perimenopausal women who might be experiencing symptoms such as hot flashes and mood swings, this option can be a life changer because it controls bleeding as well as those pesky menopausal symptoms.

- **Progestin-Only Contraceptives** (minipill or Depo-Provera) can be used for those women who either cannot tolerate estrogen-containing contraceptives or who have contraindications to their use. Progestin-only contraceptives can sometimes help with heavy bleeding but do not typically relieve many of the symptoms of menopause.

- **Progestin-Releasing IUDs (Mirena, Liletta)/Hormonal IUDs** are not only great birth control, but they are also FDA-approved for managing heavy bleeding. Full disclosure—don't be surprised if it takes 3–6 months for the bleeding to settle down. You may initially experience more days of lighter bleeding, but that diminishes within a few cycles. By the end of one year, more than 50 percent of women will not bleed at all. The IUD works best for fibroids that are not in the uterine cavity itself. If there are fibroids in the cavity, there is a higher risk of expulsion of the IUD (and not helping with the bleeding). Pro tip: Make sure your doctor shows you how to check for the IUD string. If your heavy bleeding returns, you need to verify that your IUD is still in the proper position.

- **Gonadotrophic-Releasing Hormone Agonists (Lupron)** I know is a mouthful, but remember when I told you that once you reach menopause, those fibroids, deprived of estrogen, will shrink over time? Well, the bleeding problems disappear as well. Think of GnRH agonists as a medically induced (albeit temporary) menopause.

Why on earth would anyone intentionally induce menopause, you're asking? Good question. GnRH is typically used short-term (3–6 months) in anticipation of surgery. Inducing menopause will stop the periods for women who bleed heavily and are anemic, in an attempt to build up their blood counts before surgery and avoid the need for transfusions.

The other reason to use a GnRH agonist is to attempt to shrink fibroids prior to surgery, increasing the likelihood of having a less invasive surgical procedure (laparoscopy or hysteroscopic), rather than an open major operative procedure (see Myomectomy and Hysterectomy).

Understand that even a medically induced, short-term menopause can produce all the symptoms of natural menopause, like hot flashes, night sweats, brain fog, and sleeplessness. If that is a concern, your doctor can prescribe add-back therapy, giving you a small enough dose of estrogen to treat the menopausal symptoms without interfering with the larger goal of shrinking the fibroids.

Surgical Treatment Options for Fibroids

Good news: Today, there are more surgical options for treating fibroid symptoms than ever. Each has pros and cons that you need to understand fully before making any decisions—particularly major surgical ones—about which way to go and which surgeon to go with. Once more: *You* are your own primary caregiver. And this is an area in which you must take great care.

Ironically, the skill and proficiency of a surgeon matters more for minimally invasive procedures than for traditional open procedures, because minimally invasive surgeries require more technical expertise. Even major surgeries such as hysterectomy and myomectomy, which were once very straightforward, can now be fine-tuned in the ways they are performed. Make sure that you understand all the different surgical options and understand why you are, or are not, a candidate for each procedure.

Even after you do your homework and decide on a treatment, have your doctor fully explain it to you. Remember, you are in the driver's seat. Don't let go of that wheel. It's your body and only you know how you feel. Do not minimize your symptoms to accommodate the options you may prefer—that won't get you the relief you deserve. Remember when I mentioned that sense of interoception, way back in Chapter 2? If not, spin the wheel and read that again. Because you're going to need it now—and forever.

Uterine Artery Embolization (UAE)

This is one of the few procedures that is not done by a gynecologist or a surgeon. UAEs are performed by specialists called "interventional radiologists." A small incision is made in the groin and a catheter is inserted through an artery and maneuvered into the arterial blood supply of the uterus and the offending fibroids. (Don't worry, they're watching this on a screen as they are doing the procedure.) Biodegradable pellets are then injected directly into the artery feeding the fibroid, which cuts off the blood supply, causing the fibroid to degenerate and shrink over time.

This is a great procedure for fibroids that may not be accessible via hysteroscopy (see Hysteroscopic Resection). It is also good for someone nearing menopause who wishes to buy some time and avoid major surgery. It is not as efficient for treating bulk-related symptoms because its effect is gradual, taking months to years for a change in the fibroids' size to become noticeable. Unlike with major surgery (see Myomectomy and Hysterectomy), the recovery time is days, not weeks. But full disclosure, you will experience some discomfort (doctor-speak for *It's going to hurt like hell*) that will most likely require prescription pain medication for a few days [♪ **"This Too Shall Pass"**]. So, don't make any plans for a week or so.

Condi

Yes, *that* Condi (is there any other?). Back when the first Black woman to serve as U.S. Secretary of State lived and worked in D.C., she was my patient. Secretary Rice had uterine fibroids that we had been successfully managing with medication. But as she got closer to menopause, the medication wasn't quite doing as well as we would have liked. In other words, her fibroids kept growing.

With the constant demands of her job's international trips and high-level meetings, and with perimenopause on the horizon, we didn't want to take the chance of creating an international incident. And she couldn't reasonably take 6–8 weeks off for major surgery.

So, after considering the risks/benefits and real-life implications, I referred her to an interventional radiologist who performed a successful uterine artery embolization. Her downtime was minimal. We beat the race to menopause (she was about two years out) and avoided major surgery.

The Takeaway: The treatments you choose should take into account not only the realities of your condition, but your age and the logistics of your life. When it comes to treating fibroids, there is no one right answer, there's just the right answer for you. And don't worry—I'm not violating any HIPAA regulations. Condi was happy to share her story in order to educate women about their fibroid treatment options, and she wrote about it in her memoir.

There's also the long-term versus short-term to consider. One benefit of hysterectomy is that it is a definitive treatment, and you'll never have to worry about fibroids or periods again. Without a hysterectomy, it's not uncommon to need more than one surgery, particularly if you are on the younger end of the spectrum. With these less invasive procedures, even if you remove all visible fibroids, chances are there will still be some left behind. And if you're ten years away from menopause, those remaining fibroids might become problematic before you get there.

Radiofrequency Ablation and Focused Ultrasound

These are two new noninvasive procedures that essentially zap fibroids with radiofrequency or high-intensity ultrasound waves. These high-frequency energy sources heat up and coagulate the fibroids. It's almost like microwaving your fibroids (my own very nontechnical description). These are relatively new technologies and not widely available yet. Give it some time. At the rate medical technology is moving, what's new today can soon become passé [♪"What Is Hip?"]. Quiz your doctors and ask if they personally have had experience with these procedures. I have not.

Hysteroscopic Resection

This is a great procedure for people experiencing heavy bleeding due to fibroids that are inside and impinging on the uterine cavity, which may be problematic for fertility. This is typically an outpatient procedure in which the cervix is dilated and a small telescope-like instrument (hysteroscope) is inserted. After distending the cavity with liquid, and under direct visualization, the fibroids are either shaved down or plucked out. Since there are no incisions (the surgery is done via the vagina and inside the uterine cavity), the recovery time is minimal, and the uterus remains intact.

Myomectomy

A myomectomy is a surgical procedure where the fibroids are removed, and the uterus is left intact. You should expect heavy bleeding to improve after a myomectomy, but you will continue to get your period. Whether that is a good or bad thing depends on how you feel about getting your period. Some people are delighted to never have a period again after these procedures, and others see their period as an essential part of their womanhood, even if they have no desire to get pregnant again. How you feel is how you feel, and that is not to be discounted.

Of course, you would choose myomectomy if you want to have

children in the future, or if it is simply your personal preference to keep your uterus.

Myomectomies can be performed either with a hysteroscope (see Hysteroscopic Resection) or through a few small incisions in the abdomen via a laparoscope (laparoscopic resection) or as an open surgical procedure (laparotomy), which requires a large incision in the abdomen. Factors to consider in deciding which option to choose are the fibroids' size, number, and location, as well as the expertise of the surgeon.

A laparoscopic myomectomy, while less invasive, is technically more challenging than an open one done via laparotomy. A surgeon who does not perform laparoscopic procedures frequently is likely to recommend the type of surgery that they are most comfortable doing. That may or may not be the best option for you.

Whichever option you choose, you do need to understand that with myomectomies there is the possibility of the fibroids regrowing. The likelihood of needing a second procedure is anywhere from 23–30 percent for younger women; for women over 45, the risk of recurrence is 17 percent. Major surgery is a big deal, and since fibroids have a tendency to regrow, unless you hope to get pregnant in the future, why take the chance of having to come back for a repeat procedure later? That sounded judgy, didn't it? But there are some benefits, from the standpoint of hormone therapy after menopause, that might make a hysterectomy a better option than not. We will discuss this in Chapter 10. This is my opinion, and you should take it as such. The choice is yours. Let me remind you again, when it comes to medical treatments, there is rarely just one right answer; there is only the answer that is right for you.

Hysterectomy

Hysterectomies are the most common surgical procedures performed in women and fibroids are the most common reason for performing them. For complicated reasons, some warranted and some not, the decision to have a hysterectomy can be emotionally fraught. But there is no question that the most definitive relief from bleeding problems, back pain, cramping, and the bulkiness associated with fibroids is a hysterectomy.

Good news first. The incidence of hysterectomies has gone down in the past thirty years because of the medications, hormonal IUDs, and less invasive options for dealing with fibroids and bleeding. So, yay! There are also now several different ways to perform hysterectomies:

- Vaginally (TVH or total vaginal hysterectomy), with the surgery performed through the vagina or with laparoscopic assistance, through small incisions in the abdomen, with the uterus being removed vaginally (laparoscopic-assisted vaginal hysterectomy or LAVH).

- Completely laparoscopically, with a small stump of cervix left behind (laparoscopic-assisted supracervical hysterectomy or LASH).

- Robotically done with surgically placed instruments that the surgeon controls via a console—not exactly like an Xbox controller, but it's a similar concept. The surgeon is controlling the robotic instruments, which are performing the actual surgery. This is not available everywhere and requires a technically proficient surgeon and specialized equipment to perform.

- The old-school open surgical way—abdominal incision with the surgery performed under direct visualization.

Interestingly, Black women are more likely to have hysterectomies done the old-fashioned way, even when controlling for the size of the uterus. Once more, we lack ample research to explain exactly why. Okay, we don't have the research, but we do know why now, don't we?

Hysterectomies have been the most performed gynecologic surgery in the United States, but they have a long and complicated history. This is especially true for Black women, as stories have surfaced about the procedure's use as a tool of targeted and explicit control of Black women's reproduction and bodies. As a result, many Black women are suspicious whenever hysterectomy is recommended. So, here is some practical advice: If your fibroids are especially large or plentiful, if you have been bleeding excessively or experiencing pain (cramping and back pain) and you are finished with childbearing, getting a hysterectomy is your best bet for complete relief. You may choose it as your preferred treatment or not. But the more symptomatic you are, the better option a hysterectomy may be—especially if you want to avoid additional surgery in the future.

Regardless of how a hysterectomy is performed, there is almost no risk of the fibroids regrowing or new ones forming. I said *almost* because if a small stump of cervix is left behind (LASH), a fibroid could theoretically grow in the stump, but this is extremely unlikely. If pain, pressure, and heavy bleeding have been an issue, your quality of life will immediately improve. Contrary to popular belief, for most women, sexual function is not impaired. You will not be plunged into menopause if you keep your ovaries, and if they are normal, there is no reason to remove them. For those who keep their ovaries, menopause will be defined by an onset of symptoms (hot flashes, night sweats, etc.) rather than by a lack of periods and can be confirmed by a simple blood test.

As with myomectomy, logistics and surgeon proficiency are key. The larger the fibroids, the higher the difficulty factor in performing surgeries laparoscopically. So, make sure you get all your questions and concerns satisfied ahead of time.

Hysterectomy vs. Myomectomy

Choosing between myomectomy and hysterectomy depends on your age, your outcome and fertility goals, and your personal preferences. Obviously if you are younger and hope to get pregnant, then myomectomy is your answer. But if you've tried other medical interventions to no avail and your fibroids are still wreaking havoc and you are officially over it, hysterectomy is the most definitive fibroid treatment you can get [♪ "i tried everything"].

Studies have shown that there is no higher risk of complications in myomectomy versus hysterectomy, but the general quality of life indicators are higher for women who have hysterectomies.

Endometriosis

Endometriosis affects anywhere from 5 percent to 10 percent of the female population, which means that at any one time, about 5–10 million women in the United States have it—and it can be very painful. Its causes, as with fibroids, are multifactorial, and it runs in families. Women who have a sister or mother with endometriosis have a 7–10-fold higher likelihood of developing it themselves. This is yet another reason why you need to be well versed in your family's medical history. Ask your sisters, mothers, and aunties if painful periods and infertility have been problems in the past. Even if they have not been officially diagnosed, this is a significant data point for you.

As part of a woman's normal menstrual cycle, endometrial tissue grows within the lining of the uterus, thickening it. That tissue sheds each month when you do not conceive.

Endometriosis occurs when instead of being inside your uterus, where it is supposed to be, this endometrial tissue is implanted outside the uterus, on your bladder, ovaries, bowel, or just about anywhere within the abdominal cavity. There are a lot of theories about how it gets there, but no one really knows for sure. What is clear is that without a way to exit the body, this tissue can trigger a range of problems for which pain is the sine qua non (if you are asking what the hell that is, it's doctor-speak for a defining feature).

The predominant symptoms of endometriosis are painful periods, infertility, and ovarian masses (called "endometriomas"). But endometriosis is the great masquerader and can present with symptoms as varied as painful urination or bowel movements, painful sex, and in very rare instances, periodic lung collapses. Unlike with fibroids, where almost 50 percent of women are unaware that they even have them, people with endometriosis are all too aware that something is amiss, because they are hurting. They just don't know what is causing it. A recent survey in the *American Journal of Obstetrics and Gynecology* revealed that in the five years prior to a confirmed diagnosis of endometriosis, 93.7 percent of women had seen their gynecologist; 60 percent had symptoms severe enough for the women to be seen in an emergency room.

The average amount of time from the onset of symptoms to a definitive diagnosis has been reported as anywhere from 3 to 10 years. The delays in diagnosis are as complicated as the variety of symptoms, and as with fibroids, the severity of the symptoms doesn't always correlate with the amount of actual endometriosis present. More often than not, the diagnosis is made based on clinical symptoms or a physical examination, not lab tests or ultrasounds (an ovarian mass is the exception). The only definitive ways to diagnose endometriosis are by visual inspection or by biopsy of suspected lesions via laparoscopy.

Carolyn

Carolyn, 42, came to see me for a routine gynecologic examination. She had no children but hoped to have some in the future. She had a history of heavy, painful periods, starting in her 20s. After prescribing increasingly higher doses of pain medication, which offered Carolyn no relief, her previous gynecologist obtained an ultrasound, which showed bilateral ovarian masses that were consistent with endometriomas (endometriosis implanted on the ovaries with internal bleeding).

She underwent surgery to remove the ovarian cysts and was told, post-op, that there was extensive endometriosis within her abdomen. Carolyn could not remember what organs were involved, but her surgeon had removed as much of the endometrial tissue as she could.

After the surgery, Carolyn was placed on Lupron (the same medication used to temporarily shrink fibroids) for six months to starve the endometriosis left behind. The Lupron put her in a temporary menopause, which was incredibly stressful. She had traded severe pain with her periods for hot flashes and night sweats—all of which made her life miserable.

After stopping the Lupron, her periods returned, and the hot flashes resolved. But gradually, over the next couple of years, all her original symptoms returned. This was no diagnostic dilemma. Her endometriosis had returned, causing pain nearly as bad as it was before her surgery.

She told me, tearfully, that her life revolved around her period. The pain was often accompanied by nausea, diarrhea, and bleeding so heavy that she couldn't leave her house or be more than five feet from a bathroom.

The first thing I asked her for was a copy of her operative report from her previous doctor. I also sent her for another ultrasound to confirm that the endometriomas had returned. Unfortunately, they had. Upon review, the findings from her previous surgery were worse than I expected. She not only had endometriosis on her ovaries, but on her rectum and large intestine; she had small lesions throughout her abdomen, often described as "powder burns," as well as severe adhesions and scarring behind her uterus. On a scale of 1–4, she had stage 4 endometriosis.

So, what to do? The answer is: It's complicated. With endometriosis, as with fibroids, we always try medical options first.

- Prescription-strength nonsteroidal pain medications (Motrin, naproxen), with the understanding that sometimes that is not enough

- Codeine or other narcotic pain relievers, with the clear understanding of the potential risk for dependence

- Oral contraceptives taken continuously—no break for periods

Carolyn could try Lupron again, but going back into menopause, even temporarily, was not high on her list. In the end, we settled on pain relief when needed and continuous oral contraceptives (skipping the placebos) with the hope that, without a period, we could eliminate much of her period pain. This plan wasn't perfect, but it worked for a while.

Here's the problem with endometriosis: Unless you do something definitive, like have a hysterectomy with removal of the ovaries or go through menopause, it is very likely to recur.

Carolyn and I discussed the possibility of a hysterectomy, which would involve removal of her ovaries as well. A hysterectomy would give her the best chance for definitively relieving her pain, but it would also close the door permanently on her chances of getting pregnant—and she wasn't there yet. I understood how difficult the choice was for her, and my job was to support her and do the best I could to relieve her pain.

Don't worry—Carolyn's story has a happy ending, but it took a while to get there, and she suffered. A lot.

She got married and stopped taking the pills in the hope that she would get pregnant. She didn't. Her endometriosis worsened, and even though she was clearly in the perimenopausal age range, menopause didn't look like it was on the immediate horizon either. So, she made her peace. She adopted a beautiful baby girl and finally had that much-needed hysterectomy, and she's doing great! She made it across the menopausal finish line and is now taking menopausal hormone therapy without problems, for relief of her menopausal symptoms. She has no more pain.

The Takeaway: Sometimes decisions are easy, more often they are not. When there is not necessarily a right answer or a wrong one, the best you can do is understand what your goals are and find a doctor who will support you in that journey.

Endometriosis is hard to diagnose in some cases and obvious in others. Because the face of endometriosis is often portrayed as a college-educated, thin white woman with no children, the diagnosis is not top of mind when dealing with women of color. But even when the diagnosis is clear, knowing when and how to intervene is a collaborative and iterative discussion between doctor and patient.

The message I want to leave you with is one that you've heard in other chapters and that I will repeat every chance I get. Suffering should not be your default mode. It is quite okay to choose you. Just remember that. You are way more than the sum of your parts. Hold on to your uterus if that is your choice, but make no mistake about it, you are no less of a woman without it.

Adenomyosis

If fibroids and endometriosis had a baby, that would be adenomyosis.

Adenomyosis occurs when endometrial tissue (yep, the same type that causes endometriosis) grows into the wall of the uterus itself. Whereas heavy bleeding and bulkiness are often present with fibroids, and pain is more of a defining feature of endometriosis, adenomyosis combines all the above.

Symptoms include heavy, painful periods. The uterus can be minimally or markedly enlarged. On physical examination, an enlarged uterus due to adenomyosis feels very similar to a uterus with fibroids, so the diagnosis is typically made with a pelvic ultrasound or pelvic MRI. The image will reveal a uterus that is thickened and enlarged but without discrete masses like with fibroids. This distinction is important because, unlike fibroids or endometriosis, which can be removed, adenomyosis is frequently global, affecting all or significant portions of the uterus. Thus, the minimally invasive procedure (hysteroscopy) that works well for fibroids tends not to be as effective with adenomyosis, but the drill is the same. Heavy bleeding, which can be severe, is most effectively treated with a hysterectomy.

Before You Decide How to Treat, *Talk* to Your Doctor!

Before you choose any particular surgery or surgeon, there are some important questions to ask. If you're too uncomfortable to speak up yourself, bring a trusted advocate or your health proxy to a pre-op doctor visit to do it for you:

- *When was the last time you did this procedure?* "Yesterday" is always a better answer than six months ago. Practice makes perfect, and it requires constant practice to keep a surgeon's skills sharp.

- *How many procedures of this type do you do in a typical month? In a year?* The more procedures a surgeon performs not only keeps their surgical and technical skills up, it also means that they probably have encountered and dealt with many of the complications that may arise. In minimally invasive surgery, it is not uncommon for new techniques and equipment to show up in the OR. I've always considered it bad form to ask a scrub nurse or the surgical assistant how to use a new device. But it happens—and you don't want to be on the operating table when it does. It takes a lack of ego to know what you don't know and to cede that space to those who do. High-volume surgeons are more likely to keep current.

- *On average, what percentage of your cases that start as laparoscopies end up converting to open procedures? Barring an unforeseen complication, what is the likelihood that a case like mine can be successfully done laparoscopically?* Your surgeon should be able to give you a sense of whether your surgery is successful 90 percent of the time or 50 percent of the time. This helps you plan the timing of the surgery as well as the length of a possible hospital stay (open procedures have longer recovery times). A lower likelihood of completing the surgery as planned is not necessarily the sign of a poor surgeon. More experienced laparoscopic surgeons will attempt more difficult cases and a 50 percent chance of having a less invasive procedure is generally better than a 100 percent chance of not having one.

- *What is your complication rate? What complications am I most at risk for?*

Good surgeons won't be put off by these questions. If they are, find another doctor.

DR. SHARON'S RX FOR
"Female Troubles"

1. Keep a menstrual diary. A plain old calendar or daily planner will do. There are online menstrual trackers, but make sure you know what they are doing with your data. Make a note of how frequent your period is, how long it lasts, and how many pads or tampons you use per cycle. Note any non-period bleeding that occurs throughout the cycle. Be able to explain what a typical period is like. But

be assured, your doctor is probably not going to want to hear about each and every one of them.

2. If your cycles last more than seven days or you are changing pads or tampons hourly for more than twenty-four hours, know that this is not normal. Even if you are not symptomatic, you should get a complete blood count and iron level at least once a year. Take a woman's formula multivitamin with iron. Eat dark green leafy vegetables. My mother would say, "Eat some liver," but that's a hard pass for most folks. An occasional steak wouldn't hurt.

3. If you are consistently bleeding heavily on the first few days of your cycle, try to anticipate your bleeding. It is easier to ward off heavy bleeding than to try to stop it when it is in full swing. Take 400–600mg of ibuprofen every eight hours on those days. Remember not to take this on an empty stomach. Do not take aspirin or aspirin-containing medications, as aspirin prolongs bleeding.

4. If you are experiencing pain, persistent urgency, or frequency not related to a UTI or associated with your menstrual cycle, ask your doctor if a sonogram would be appropriate.

5. Heavy periods with associated extreme fatigue, light-headedness, or dizziness are no-wait situations. These are signs of anemia. Call your doctor for instructions on how to proceed.

6. Don't normalize discomfort. Demand to be heard, to be seen, and to have your complaints addressed.

7. Remember, surgery should be the last option, not the first.

8. Enroll in a study. We need answers and solutions for *all* women, particularly Black women and other women of color.

CHAPTER 9

Hot in Herre ♪

Welcome to Perimenopause, Fertility's Final Frontier

Dear Sis,

If you're not familiar with the term perimenopause or you don't have any idea what it means for you, you're not alone. It's one of the million things that we don't talk enough about—not on the on-ramp leading to it and not even when we're in the midst of it and afraid we're losing our minds.

Maybe you've heard your mother or aunties whispering about The Change and found yourself wondering what is changing or when—and what in the world are we changing into? Their whispers (much like their hushed chatter about "female troubles") may cause you to be curious or fret, but not openly or without judgment. Why are we conditioned from girlhood to feel ashamed of the natural things our bodies do, and to experience them in isolation? The costs of all that secrecy are greater than we dare calculate, beginning with our lack of knowledge about our bodies—even when we're Grown with a capital G.

I'm a believer in the power of answers, no matter what they are. Give me the facts any day over being left to wonder, "What's going on?" (Can you hear Marvin Gaye crooning?) So, let me say this as plainly as I can:

What's going on once you're over 40 (and in some cases earlier)? Perimenopause.

What happens next? Menopause. Guaranteed.

There is no preventing this or putting it off. There is no sidestepping or short-circuiting it. Vitamins, supplements, herbs, sage burning, exercise, penance, or prayer is not going to keep you from going through it. So, sit with that for a minute.

You may have your period right now or get pregnant, like my mom did, at 44. But if you're over 40, whether you have symptoms or don't, you have entered the perimenopausal phase of your life. Even if you're 54, still menstruating like clockwork, and praying for an end to cramps and tampons, hold on, because the big M is coming . . . eventually. For now, though, you are still perimenopausal.

The list of potential symptoms is long and sobering and few of us will escape them. If you're Black or Latina, buckle up and grab an extra-sturdy fan, because you will likely begin this transition earlier and experience more severe symptoms. But there can be great joy in this part of the journey too. Let's not forget that.

Our goal here is to make sure you are not blindsided by these changes. I want you to know what's coming and what to do about it. So, grab a tall, cool glass of water (and that fan if you need it) and let's learn.

xo, Dr. Sharon

First things first. *Perimenopause* literally means "around menopause." If your response to that is a glassy-eyed stare, I'm with you; it's one of the most unhelpful definitions ever. The store may be "around the corner," but is that a block or half a mile? Same thing with perimenopause. *Around* is a relative term, which makes knowing when and where it will show up confusing.

We're already in a tailspin when it starts, living at the intersection of our most demanding career, parenting, and eldercare years. Those "sandwich years," when we're stuck between managing children and aging parents? No one warns you that it's a triple-decker club sandwich!

If you don't believe perimenopause and menopause correspond to one of the highest stress phases in a woman's life, consider this: Women are more likely than men to file for divorce. The so-called "gray divorce" rate (divorce after 50) has doubled in the past two decades, and Black women have the highest divorce rates between the ages of 50 and 59. Here's another little tidbit: Most people file for divorce during the spring and summer. August—typically the hottest month—has one of the highest rates of divorce filings. Coincidence? I don't think so. I can't prove it, but I have a strong suspicion that perimenopause and the turmoil it creates certainly don't help the situation.

Since most of you have been caught flat-footed by the changes associated with perimenopause, having a common rubric under which to place them as well as the proper language to describe it are keys to understanding the process. There are essentially four stages of a woman's reproductive life: premenopause, perimenopause, menopause, and postmenopause. Unless you're under 35 (giant kudos for seeking this info early if you are), you may be just entering perimenopause, smack-dab in the throes of it, or on the glide path to menopause [♪ "Everything Must Change"].

Premenopause begins with puberty, when your ovaries begin to secrete hormones, most notably estrogen, progesterone, and testosterone. Together, these hormones facilitate your physical transformation from girl to woman. The estrogen and progesterone produced with each menstrual cycle prepare your body for possible pregnancy and lactation. The testosterone produced is responsible for sexual desire, pubic hair growth, and those newfound body odors that show up at puberty. The ovaries are the repository of all the eggs you will ever have. Unlike men, women are born with about a million eggs, and you don't make any new ones. That number decreases each year, but not for the reasons you think. Only about five hundred will be ovulated in your lifetime. The rest are lost to *atresia,* which is just a fancy medical word for "the slow degeneration over time of the eggs remaining in your ovaries." This atresia, or natural loss of eggs, accelerates with age. Premenopause represents the period of a woman's peak fertility, which typically lasts for twenty or more years.

Perimenopause, also known as "the menopause transition," is the time between a woman's peak reproductive years and menopause, when fertility permanently ends. As your available reserve of eggs declines in number and quality, there are accompanying changes in the secretion of estrogen and progesterone that can disrupt your menstrual cycle and your fertility. Since your eggs are as old as you are, in addition to a general decrease in fertility, there is also a concomitant increase in the rate of miscarriage and chromosomal abnormalities. Just as significantly, your changing hormone levels are thought to be responsible for many, if not all, of the symptoms that show up in perimenopause—the intensity and duration of which are unpredictable. These symptoms can last anywhere from a few years to more than a decade.

Menopause begins with your last menstrual period but is confirmed after you've gone twelve consecutive months with no bleeding. If you're born with ovaries, you will be menopausal. Period. (Pun intended.) If your ovaries are removed for any reason prior to natural menopause or you undergo chemotherapy or radiation for cancer treatment, menopause can be precipitous. Likewise, taking medications to shrink fibroids or treat endometriosis (GnRH agonists such as Lupron) can also plunge you into menopause. The menopause induced by medications may be temporary or permanent, depending on your age. Once you are officially menopausal, you will be menopausal for the rest of your life, with all the rights and privileges therein.

Postmenopause encompasses the phase of your life after those twelve months of no periods have elapsed and lasts until the day you leave this earth. I often use the terms *menopause* and *postmenopause* interchangeably. To my way of thinking, *postmenopause* implies that at some point you are over menopause. I assure you, you are not. Menopause, like a diamond, is forever. Even if your most bothersome symptoms have subsided and your period is a distant memory, you are still not done with menopause, because menopause is never, ever done with you. The ramifications of these persistent low estrogen, progesterone, and testosterone levels will continue to affect you and every major system in your body for the rest of your life. With the proper care and attention, that could be a very long time. Women will spend a third of their lives in menopause/postmenopause. Now, that's something worthy of your attention.

Perimenopause: The Middle Years

Imagine if we entered puberty with as little information as most women have when entering perimenopause (frequently described as "puberty in reverse"). The sudden onset of vaginal bleeding, pain, strange body odors, and tender breasts that accompany puberty would scare you half to death if you didn't know what to expect. Normalizing this experience and celebrating our changing bodies is the goal that we have set for educating our daughters. (Thank you, Judy Blume, for educating those of us of a certain age.)

So, why do we as perimenopausal women not get the same treatment? Where's our perimenopause party? The hormonal changes that accompany the profound changes in our bodies are every bit as consequential as puberty and pregnancy, and yet many of us are left to fend for ourselves. We don't talk much among ourselves, and we in the medical community (okay, not me) have failed to prepare you for what to expect. This, I think we can all agree, has got to stop.

You already know I come from a long line of women who did not live long enough to impart the wisdom of menopause to their daughters. But I am the youngest of five girls. Surely I should be familiar with the menopause journeys of my older sisters, but we are no different from most families. We simply didn't discuss it. When you add to this the fact that three of my sisters had hysterectomies before menopause, I'm not sure that even they connected the dots. This places many of us in the ridiculous position of navigating a sometimes difficult experience that each and every one of us will go through in relative isolation. Not knowing what to expect, not knowing what is normal and where to go to get relief, has hampered our ability to be our best selves in what should be our most productive years. So, let's fix that.

What Can I Expect?

If you don't have any of the following thirty-four concerns, good for you. Skip this chapter and we'll talk about something else. But pause for a second first and take an honest personal assessment of what you're dealing (or have already dealt) with. I'm guessing you'll quickly recognize that some of what you've probably attributed to stress, thyroid problems, teenage children, or simply growing older can be explained by perimenopause.

- Allergies

- Anxiety

- Bloating

- Body odor

- Brain fog

- Breast tenderness and changes in size and shape

- Burning/Dry mouth syndrome

- Depression

- Digestive issues

- Dizziness

- Electric shock sensations

- Fatigue

- Feelings of dread

- Formication (feelings of bugs crawling on your extremities)

- Hair changes (thinning, changes in texture)

- Headaches/Migraines

- Hot flashes

- Incontinence

- Irregular heartbeat

- Irregular menstrual cycle

- Irritability

- Itchy skin

- Joint pain

- Libido changes (higher or lower)

- Mood swings

- Muscle aches

- Night sweats

- Panic attacks

- Paresthesia (tingling or numb extremities)

- Sleep challenges

- Vaginal dryness

- Weakened fingernails

- Weight gain

- Wrinkles

Dare I mention that *mood swings* can include bouts of irrepressible rage? And by *hair changes,* I mean hair loss where you want to keep it and hair growth where you don't. So, now would be a good time to invest in a magnifying mirror and some tweezers. Since your period has become difficult—if not impossible—to predict, you might want to keep tampons and pads handy at all times. This is one more reason why menstrual products should be widely accessible. And those periods that used to last for 3–4 days can drag on for 10.

The amount of bleeding you can do during perimenopause can be so heavy that it is worthy of crime scene photos. And have you noticed how many ads there are on TV for incontinence medications and undergarments? Who exactly do you think they are talking to? Ah, that would be you—and your soon-to-be menopausal friends. I could go on, but I won't, because it really doesn't have to be all bad.

Right about now, you're probably thinking, *If this is so huge, why didn't anyone warn a sister?* Better late than never. Now that I've thoroughly depressed you, take heart and hang in there. There's a light at the end of this tunnel.

What on Earth Is Going On?

Perimenopause has an end, but like all good stories, it also has a beginning and a middle. What symptoms you are experiencing at any one time will depend on where you fall in this timeline. It ends when you've had your last period plus twelve months of no further bleeding. Then menopause officially begins. And for those of you who might be asking, "Why do we care?" The significance of that somewhat arbitrary twelve-month marker is so you will know what is typical and when you might reasonably expect to be able to wear white pants again with reckless abandon. If you go six months with no period and then in the middle of your much-needed beach vacation, you get your period—chalk it up to perimenopause. You're simply not done yet. However, any bleeding that happens after twelve contiguous months of no bleeding should be reported to your doctor. It may not mean that anything is wrong. You just need to let your doctor tell you that. As I frequently used to tell my patients, not everyone's body has read the book.

Although there is a somewhat distinct line to signal the end of perimenopause, there is no bright line that signals its beginning. It can start as early as your mid-to-late 30s and as late as your late 40s. The fact that it corresponds to a stretch of life that's already a bottleneck of emotional, physical, and work–life stress is like adding insult to injury. Could we have picked a worse time for our hormones to go haywire? Not likely. That's why so many of the symptoms, particularly the mood-related ones, are confusing. Do you not want to have sex because you hate your partner, or do you hate your partner because you've been experiencing irritability or rage, and you haven't had a good night's sleep in a year? Good questions, and perimenopause probably plays a role. How big? I'll leave that one to you to decide, but you get my drift.

So many of us end up walking around untreated—sometimes for years—enduring symptoms that are misdiagnosed, uncomfortable, and upsetting, wearing out our very last nerve or, worse, making us think we're just falling apart. The range of symptoms is so broad, it's easy for you—and even your doctors—to think they're unrelated. Which only adds to your stress as you think, *What the hell is happening to me?*

In rare—and I do mean very rare—instances, you will experience nary a hot flash or sleepless night. But whether you have all, none, or some combination of symptoms, if you are 40-plus, *you are perimenopausal.* So, while you're experiencing everything that goes with being a natural woman, dial down the thermostat if you need to and relish this newfound phase of womanhood [♪ "(You Make Me Feel Like) A

Natural Woman"]. This is a big shift and your ability to make the best of it begins with being prepared.

Although the actual moment of perimenopause's onset is impossible to predict, armed with the proper information, it's easy to detect, based on:

- Your age (over 40)

- Changes in menstrual-cycle length (typically shorter—every 23–25 days rather than 28–30)

- Changes in menstrual flow (heavier and/or more unpredictable)

- Any of those other thirty-four symptoms

Symptoms from that long list can occur as one-offs or in combination, coming and going with a mind all their own. These are indicators that your reproductive life has taken a definite turn. But that's only if you recognize them for what they are; if not, these symptoms can be confused with myriad other health conditions and not treated or dealt with appropriately. Attitude and preparation aren't everything, but they help.

As with everything else our bodies go through over our lifespans, there are patterns, but no singular "here's what to expect" profile. Even within families, each woman is different. Symptoms may ebb and flow and can range from the benign to the wild and crazy—as in, you think you are losing your mind. But you're not. You're just perimenopausal.

Shawna

Shawna is a 45-year-old marketing executive. She is, in short, a boss. She has two teenage children, one of whom will be applying to college soon. She has a stable drama-free marriage. Sex, which used to be a big part of her relationship, has become infrequent, not because she doesn't love her husband, she just doesn't feel like it. Still, she has no major complaints. She is up for a big promotion and has a presentation to the board of directors. She's worked really hard on it and is super-prepared. Here is what perimenopause can do:

- Minutes before her presentation, she breaks into a full sweat. I mean a makeup-melting, hair-drenching sweat. Heat quickly rises from her core into her face until she literally feels like she's about to turn into the Wicked Witch of the West and dissolve into a puddle on the floor.

- Seated at the long boardroom table, she senses that little bit of warmth that signals a vague wetness in her underwear. She thinks, *That's just discharge or sweat, right? It couldn't be my period. I just had it last week.* Within minutes, she gets that sickening feeling where the warmth has now spread onto the seat of her chair. "Please, God," she silently prays, "make it not so."

- Shawna's in the middle of her presentation, and she is killing it. All of a sudden it feels as if someone just came in and shook her brain like it was an Etch A Sketch. She has forgotten what she was saying. It's not like a minor digression. She literally has no idea what she was talking about.

- John, who she finds only mildly annoying on most days, asks her a question, and her usual level of annoyance boils over into a rage as she thinks, *How dare he try to show me up in front of the board!* Now Shawna is envisioning walking across the room to confront him directly and slapping the crap out of him for good measure. Instead, she excuses herself for a couple of minutes and regains her composure in the ladies' room. She returns and, cool as a cucumber, replies, "Yes, John. Lunch will be served after the meeting." Okay, so maybe it wasn't personal.

The Takeaway: If you have experienced something similar, you, too, may be perimenopausal. If you have not but you are over 40, don't gloat. You're perimenopausal too.

There is not a straight line in the decline of your hormones during perimenopause. Unlike men, whose testosterone levels decline with age in a gentler fashion, our hormone levels fluctuate wildly during this period. Your estrogen levels can be too high one day, only to plummet the next. Your brain and body are in a constant state of recalibration in response to these hormonal shifts. The fluctuations often result in symptoms such as weight gain; mood swings; persistently swollen, tender breasts; and headaches or migraines, as well as hot flashes, depression, and insomnia. Here's the thing about libido during perimenopause: Remember when I told you that changes in libido are a common symptom? Well, because your hormones are fluctuating wildly—sometimes lower and sometimes overshooting the mark—it is not uncommon for women to report bursts of renewed sexual interest. So, it's not all bad news.

Hot flashes are the symptom most associated with menopause, but most women are unaware that hot flashes can begin years before their last menstrual period. And for the record, although hot flashes can be easy fodder for comedians, there is nothing funny about them.

Although we don't know the exact mechanism for hot flashes, think of it as having a faulty internal thermostat. Your HVAC system is not the problem. The cooling mechanism that normally kicks in when you are overheating can just start up at any time, irrespective of the ambient temperature. So, it can be 55 degrees outside, and you can break out in a full sweat like you were sitting in D.C. traffic in August with the windows rolled up and no air-conditioning. If you don't recognize what I'm talking about, give it time, you may soon be joining the over 80 percent of women who do.

Scientifically termed *vasomotor symptoms,* hot flashes are more than just annoying and embarrassing, they are often the canaries in the coal mine—harbingers of more serious health issues. Women who experience the most severe hot flashes (and Black women are overly represented in this group) are also at a higher risk for developing cardiovascular disease later in life. Hot flashes at night, better known as "night sweats," are potent disrupters of sleep—which not only increase your risk for weight gain and elevate your blood pressure, but also increase your risk for cardiovascular disease.

While there's some anecdotal evidence that ambient heat, spicy foods, and alcohol may increase the likelihood of hot flashes, the triggers for initiating them vary from person to person. So, be on the lookout for what precipitates yours and try to minimize those triggers. And if your hot flashes are significantly disrupting your sleep and your life, don't make light of it. Get them treated.

The Study of Women's Health Across the Nation (SWAN), the longest longitudinal study of women as they progress through perimenopause and menopause, released results in 2019 that showed women of color (both Black and Latina) tend to enter perimenopause and menopause at earlier ages than white women. Having tracked a cohort of Hispanic, Japanese, Chinese, Black, and white women in seven U.S. cities for more than two decades, the study found the average duration of hot flashes and night sweats in non-Hispanic white women was 6.5 years compared to 8.9 years in Latina women and 10.1 years for Black women. The duration was just 5.4 years among Chinese American women and 4.8 for Japanese American women. Separate data published in *Menopause*, the journal of the North American Menopause Society (NAMS), suggested that Native American women may have the worst menopausal experience of all. Regrettably, they haven't yet been studied enough to know for sure.

The SWAN results made clear something that I and some of my OB/GYN colleagues who were paying attention saw but couldn't broadly prove—that Black women have a higher prevalence, longer duration, and more intense hot flashes than others. This evidence is in direct conflict with what we were taught in our training. We were taught that Black women, because they tend to be heavier than the general population, experience fewer hot flashes. In actuality, the observed data from the SWAN study shows just the opposite.

Nicole

Nicole is 58 and, after twenty-one years of marriage and nine years divorced, she had a date!

She had met Julian at an entrepreneurs' conference on a Thursday. Within minutes, he asked if she had plans for that Saturday—and she did. But she said she was free because he was fine and kind, and she needed this.

Juggling her clients, an ailing mother, three kids, two dogs, and weekly duties at church had filled every second of her time since her divorce. Now, with her kids away in college, life was calming down just as her libido—which she thought died with her marriage—was heating up. Tall, dark, and charming Julian had appeared right on time, so she would make herself available.

When Nicole walked into the restaurant and saw his face light up, she knew the extra hour she took getting ready was worth it. Nails, hair, makeup, cute new top—check! They ordered wine, talked easily, and flirted a lot. He told her she looked beautiful. She said, "Thanks," then took refuge behind her menu so he wouldn't see her blush. It had been a long time since she'd seen a man look at her that way.

Suddenly, as she scanned the appetizers, she felt a rush of heat sweep through her chest, overtaking her shoulders, back, neck, and face. She shut her eyes and prayed for it to pass, resisting the urge to fan herself with the menu. She'd been dealing with intense hot flashes for a decade and knew what they could do.

Just as she felt her inner inferno start to ease, the waiter appeared, ready to take their order. "Ladies first," she heard Julian politely say.

Slowly, Nicole lowered her menu and watched Julian's sweet smile disappear. Her blouse was stuck to her back and chest, her forehead was drenched, her mascara had smeared, and the bouncy curls she'd so carefully arranged an hour earlier were frizzing and falling, defeated, which is exactly how she felt.

"Are you okay?" Julian asked, looking genuinely concerned.

Nicole tried to pull herself back together in the ladies' room and made it through dinner without another flash. But she was mortified, her confidence was shot, and she couldn't wait for the date to end.

The Takeaway: Don't be embarrassed by a natural process. Perhaps this could have been a teachable moment for Julian. Or as my friend Michelle Obama would say, "There's no shame in my menopause game." The only tragedy here is that Nicole suffered for ten years unnecessarily with hot flashes that could have been addressed.

TV journalist Gayle King has talked openly about having similar meltdowns on the red carpet. She's great at making light of these experiences in hindsight, but such moments can have you saying no to even the most coveted ticket in town. Hot flashes won't kill you, but they won't make you stronger either. In fact, they have zero upside, so you shouldn't hesitate to seek medical help to alleviate them (see Yes, Virginia, There Are Treatments).

As I mentioned previously, although we don't know the exact causes of hot flashes, we do have a sense of who is at an increased risk of developing them. Women who smoke tend to have more hot flashes and at earlier ages. Women who have their ovaries removed or who undergo treatment for cancer, either via chemotherapy or radiation, also have more severe symptoms, because they do not have the luxury of years of transition. They are literally falling off a hormonal cliff. Black and Hispanic women also experience hot flashes at earlier ages, more intensely, and for longer periods of time. Some of that increase may be due to an overall higher weight than white women when entering perimenopause. We do know that women who weigh more have more hot flashes. But there are other yet-to-be-determined factors, such as stress, accelerated aging, or overall poor health when entering the perimenopausal space that may put Black and Hispanic women at increased risk.

Another important but little-discussed finding is the fact that Black women are half as likely to report the symptoms of menopause to their doctors, even though SWAN has shown that they are more severely affected. Worse still, even when they complain, they are half as likely to be offered a prescription for hormone treatment for their symptoms and half as likely to take the medication when it is prescribed. The net effect is that those who suffer the most get the least relief. That is patently unacceptable. Lack of treatment can have profound implications for your long-term health, no matter your race. You can help change that by being more informed and making your doctors aware of the SWAN results. Encourage them to become better informed about menopause and to be more effective in counseling and treating *all* of their patients.

Here again, the dismal lack of clinical research on midlife women, and the fact that much of what does exist centers on middle-class white women, handicaps the treatment of women of color. This is yet another reason why more women of color *must* volunteer to participate in clinical trials. They should seek out reputable studies aimed at answering many of the questions still unanswered about health disparities in communities of color. While there are some cultural and racial distinctions, the experience of perimenopause is universal. We just need better strategies for addressing the symptoms that are a significant part of the lived experiences of all women.

Untangling Our Body's Ball of Confusion

If you're taking all of this in but are still confused, that's *not* brain fog creeping in and you're *not* alone. Erratic by nature, perimenopause routinely frustrates and confounds patients and doctors alike.

You might wrestle with a few symptoms, have them fade, and think it's over. If they return or swap themselves out for new ones, you could think perimenopause is finally over and you've officially entered menopause. But unless your period has stopped for a full year, you have not. Anything short of a year is fair game.

In the absence of clear symptoms, how do you know when perimenopause has snuck up on you [♪ "How Will I Know"]? There is a very simple answer, so don't let your doctor or girlfriends overcomplicate it. Do you have ovaries? Are you between the ages of 40 and 50? Are you having any one of those thirty-four symptoms? Congratulations. You're in perimenopause.

If you have had a hysterectomy, have a hormonal IUD, or have had an endometrial ablation (a procedure used to treat heavy periods), hormone tests can be helpful in diagnosing menopause—but not perimenopause, because on any given day during perimenopause, your hormone levels can be normal, slightly abnormal, or off-the-charts abnormal, only to return to normal the next week. While you don't need blood tests, sonograms, soothsayers, or an endocrinologist to know that you're in perimenopause, you might need a healthy dose of humility and good ol' self-acceptance. And no matter where your symptoms are on the spectrum, keep a written record of any changes you experience so you can keep your doctors apprised at your regularly maintained appointments. (Yes, that's me, reminding you again—are you due for a checkup? If so, I'll wait here while you handle that.)

Given the wide age range during which symptoms may show up and the sheer number and variety of them, it is easy to mistake the symptoms of perimenopause for something else. The fact that you may experience them in any combination, in no particular order, and—here's the kicker—all while you are still having relatively *regular* periods? This isn't just an inconvenient truth, it can feel like an irrational one, leading to a common scenario that plays out in doctors' offices every day.

Belinda

Belinda is a 44-year-old woman in relatively good health. She takes no medications. She notices that she has started to gain weight without any change in her diet or activity, and she is starting to experience bouts of anxiety and nervousness unrelated to what's going on in her life.

She has also been having difficulty going to sleep and staying asleep at night, which leaves her incredibly fatigued during the day. In short, she doesn't feel like herself.

Her periods are like clockwork. Every month. Right on schedule. She sees her gynecologist because she doesn't have a primary care doctor (most young women don't, by the way), and her gynecologist orders blood tests, all of which come back normal. She even does tests to check Belinda's hormone levels, which are also normal.

Her doctor tells her, "It can't be menopause-related."

Hold up! Wait a minute! *What?*

The Takeaway: Don't be surprised if doctors don't always recognize the signs of perimenopause. Although irregular bleeding is a feature of perimenopause, it need not be present for the diagnosis. Many women with regular periods are indeed perimenopausal.

Basic awareness of perimenopause *before it begins* won't help you prevent symptoms, but it will at least help you feel more competent and less stressed as you move through it. That said, if you weren't already knowledgeable about perimenopause, the good news is that there have never been more conversations about perimenopause and menopause than there are today. If you don't believe me, check out TikTok and Instagram. The menopause warriors are out there, and that's a beautiful thing. Even if you're past it, you can pay it forward by sharing what you know with your younger friends.

Your mother probably didn't talk to you about this stage, because no one had schooled her either. She, like the generations of women before her, has normalized suffering. You may have seen her going through it and thought her inexplicable crying jags and flashes of temper were what a midlife crisis looks like—or that she was just upset because you were making her life miserable (and let's face it, you probably were). You might have also thought, as most daughters do when they witness Mom struggling, *That will never be me.* So much for that. I've always said, like it or not, if you live long enough, you'll turn into your mother.

Given what you now know about the importance of family medical history, if you're lucky enough to still be able to ask your mother about her journey with perimenopause and menopause, do! It's never too late. This goes for your sisters and aunts too. Knowing what your elders experienced may give you a road map of what you might expect.

Being grown and sexy [♪"Grown & Sexy"] (thanks, Babyface) is achievable, but not effortless. What you should most want to be is empowered. That begins with owning the stage of life you're in and trusting that whatever it brings, you can handle it. Too many of us only see the negatives of getting older. Our value is not tied to our fertility, and neither is our sexual appeal or vitality. Perimenopause should be a time for celebration. We've successfully negotiated phase one of our reproductive lives and can show off some of that wisdom that only comes with age.

While perimenopause can be disruptive, it will feel less unsettling if you keep reminding yourself that it is temporary and part of your body's natural life cycle. In the meantime, as with any other health issue, if you need help, get it!

So, You're Perimenopausal. Now What?

When you go to see your doctor, you're ready for some solutions. You might even be at the end of your rope. I understand. But be ready for some unevenness in the quality of advice you might receive. The best doctors mean well, but truth be told, they don't know everything. Until very recently, most medical schools did not include post-reproductive care in the training of medical residents, so much of what doctors know about how to treat perimenopause and menopause comes from on-the-job-training fueled by their patients. OB/GYNs and family practice physicians are the logical doctors to address peri-menopausal and menopausal symptoms, but according to a 2017 Mayo Clinic survey of young doctors, more than 20 percent reported never having experienced a single formal lecture about menopause while in medical school. To make matters worse, only a third of them would prescribe hormone therapy to symptomatic women—even without any contraindications. Worst of all, a mere 7 percent of those surveyed felt adequately prepared to manage menopause in their patients. I know what you're thinking (insert personalized exploding head emoji here), but stay with me.

As for my OB/GYN colleagues, the sheer volume and breadth of what they handle on a regular basis is overwhelming. These same doctors treat adolescents and midlifers, menstrual problems, sexually transmitted infections, birth control, infertility, teen pregnancy, and high-risk pregnancy, while also delivering babies and tending to postnatal care. At times OB/GYNs are called upon to provide primary care, give mental health counseling, and do minor and major surgeries. I'm not making excuses for our shortcomings, but that mix consumes a lot of time. What routinely goes missing in this robust lineup is the stretch between when you're done having babies and when you're ready to sign up for Medicare. It's an important gap—and a long one—that patients and doctors must address together and make a priority.

Because the typical OB/GYN practice is geared toward fertility, pregnancy, childbirth, hysterectomies, and other surgeries, most doctors are focused on *doing*. Treating perimenopausal and menopausal women requires *listening*. I've always believed that if you ask the right questions, patients will eventually tell you what's wrong. But this requires time and patience, both of which are in short supply in medicine these days.

The older I've gotten, the more interesting this phase of life has become, both personally and professionally. It is frustrating to see how sorely lacking in research midlife women's health still is today. We don't have answers to questions we've been asking for decades. But we are finally starting to gain some traction. By advocating for yourself and demanding that more attention be paid and more research be done, you will help make a positive difference in the quality of our last and, hopefully, most fulfilling chapter [♪ "The Best Is Yet to Come"].

How we age and, most importantly, how we age healthily requires forethought and daily attention. It simply cannot be left to chance if we truly want to look good and feel good. And make no mistake, all roads lead to menopause. Accept that. Embrace it. That doesn't mean you should stop pushing for answers—quite the opposite. Who gets answers and who doesn't is a very self-directed exercise. And when it comes to your health, no question is too dumb or too small, so ask them all. Without apology.

Making the Most of Your Doctors' Appointments

For doctors to "see you" in the proverbial sense, they have to first see you in the literal sense, and too many women stop going to their OB/GYN once they stop having children. After the many years women spend largely focused on others, perimenopause and menopause represent a time to shift the focus inward. It's time for you to take care of you. A great first step is continuing to see your OB/GYN, even if you've had your tubes tied or you no longer need birth control. As you can see, we've still got lots to talk about.

So, if your OB/GYN retires or no longer meets your needs (even after a long relationship, it's fair to ask your doctor about their expertise in post-reproductive health), get a new one *tout suite* (that's French for "at once," because we're fancy). A gynecologist (just an OB/GYN who no longer delivers babies) will have more time and more experience with women of a certain age and is more likely to be of a certain age herself. So, she gets it. And yes, it's almost always "she" these days. Over 85 percent of practicing OB/GYNs are female. And for the record, if your OB/GYN has taken the place of your internist during your childbearing years, it's time to establish a relationship with a good internist and begin those more comprehensive annual physicals *in addition* to your regular gynecological exams. But don't ditch your OB/GYN. They know you. They've watched you age, and they will be more likely to notice changes in your weight, movements, and demeanor that could signal a health issue worth exploring. And let's be clear:

Even with their lack of dependable knowledge about how to deal with perimenopause, your best bet for getting those answers is still your gynecologist.

That said, more than 10 million women in this country don't have access to an OB/GYN in the towns where they live. In fact, over 50 percent of the counties in the United States do not have an OB/GYN. If you're lucky enough to live in a part of the country where there is a certified national menopause practitioner (you may check at menopause.org), you are in a distinct minority, as there are fewer than 1,200 certified menopause practitioners for an estimated 55 million menopausal women. So, here is where we have got to start thinking out of the box. If you are one of the millions of women who has no convenient access to an OB/GYN, or if you have a doctor who has not kept current with new guidelines, telehealth may be your best option. As long as you have access to a primary care doctor to handle your other healthcare needs, menopausal care and prescription services work very well in the telehealth environment. There is little point in trying to deliver twenty-first-century medicine with a nineteenth-century delivery model. We can and should do better.

If your doctors are not interpreting your panoply of symptoms within the context of your reproductive stage in life, you may find your care parceled out to a dermatologist for skin and hair issues, a rheumatologist or an orthopedist for joint pains, a psychologist for mood swings, a cardiologist for palpitations, etc. Each doctor will treat the symptoms most common in their particular specialty, perhaps never thinking that they are part of a bigger picture. *So, bring it up! After reading this book, you're going to have the receipts!*

Don't hesitate to initiate the conversations you need to have with your doctors. And lead with affirmations ("This might be important . . ."), not apologies or disclaimers ("I'm sorry, this probably doesn't mean anything, but . . ."). Let your doctors figure out what's useful and what's not. Don't minimize your concerns. I always used to say to my patients, no matter how small the concern, if it bothers you, it bothers me. Let's figure out a way to fix it. And to be clear, your doctors may not have all the answers, but she sure should know how to find someone who does.

Talk liberally and in detail about your symptoms and concerns. I'll say it again: Keeping a detailed written record of the problems you may be having is essential. When the doctor offers you the routine opener, "How have you been feeling?" don't say, "Not bad," and move on. That's your cue to respond with the list you've been keeping of anything out of the ordinary.

Really smart doctors learn as much from you as you learn from them. The higher the quality of your input, the better the outcomes your doctors will be able to effect. You are critical to that vast body of cumulative knowledge that we doctors call "experience." And this is sometimes more important than anything we can read in textbooks. So, don't deny your doctor the opportunity to learn from you directly. And remember, communication is a two-way street. So, don't pretend to understand things you don't. We're doctors, and sometimes we use words or explain things that are clear only to us. Make us make it plain.

Facing Fertility's Final Frontier

Perimenopause is more than challenging symptoms and irregular periods; it's a time to take your fertility very seriously, because *it will end with menopause*. And there's no going back. That is why in my patients' early 30s, I start discussing their plans for when they would like to start their families. No judgment or pressure, but I'd rather *you* decide when to have children rather than let your biological clock decide.

The median age of women giving birth has steadily increased throughout the industrialized world over the last three decades. In the United States, it's risen from age 27 in 1990 to 30 in 2019, according to the U.S. Census Bureau. That's the highest in recorded history.

During that time, birthrates declined by almost 43 percent for women between 20 and 24 years old, and by 22 percent in those between 25 and 29. While the number of births among premenopausal women have steadily decreased, births increased by about 67 percent for women between ages 35 and 39, according to the 2019 Census Bureau analysis of National Center for Health Statistics, and (hold on to your hat!) by more than 132 percent for women between 40 and 44. In other words, more perimenopausal women gave birth in 2019 than ever.

The growing choice to delay motherhood has mostly been attributed to the prioritized pursuit of higher education and professional careers. But the availability of a suitable partner and the economic anxieties associated with raising a family cannot be ignored. The largest increases in the age of giving birth have been among immigrant women, where the median age has risen from 27 to 32. For Black women, the median age rose from 24 to 28. For both of these groups, the median age for becoming a first-time mother still falls within premenopause, or the height of their fertile years.

The relative explosion in the birthrate among women aged 35 to 44 corresponds to a steadily increasing demand for options in the fertility services market, which is estimated at $8 billion annually. Its offerings—which include in vitro fertilization (IVF), genetic testing, egg freezing, reproductive tissue storage, and donor services—are not only on the rise but also may be covered by employers who are competing for female talent.

The fact that there is more assistance available for a perimenopausal woman to bear a child does not change the simple fact that your fertility in your 40s is not what it was in your 30s. Seeing Hollywood stars getting pregnant in their mid-to-late 40s may be a beautiful thing, but trust me, it was most likely no easy road to get there. The reality is, the chances of getting pregnant with your own 50-year-old eggs, even if your periods are as regular as clockwork, lies somewhere between slim and nonexistent (unless your eggs were frozen when you were much younger). And that's not being harsh. It's being real.

Now, maybe your grandmother had a baby when she was 49. My mother had her last child (yours truly, here) when she was a month shy of her 45th birthday. But I was baby number eight, and my mother's last prior pregnancy was eight years before. Now, I can spin it any way I like, but I'll bet you a dollar to a donut that neither your grandmother nor my mother was *trying* to get pregnant, they *happened* to get pregnant. In fact, most women *can* get pregnant at 40; but with every passing year, the likelihood that they *will* declines. While the health risks for mother and child increase with maternal age, most of those risks are not insurmountable. The biggest obstacle to overcome post-40 is fertility.

So, the choice to delay pregnancy until you could require medical assistance to achieve it should never be made haphazardly. Try to consider your options while they are as plentiful as possible. As you carefully evaluate each one, realize that no matter how innovative the technology, how high the price tag, or how successful the specialist, there are zero guarantees. Recognize also that FemTech is the wild, wild west of fertility—the science is way out ahead of the regulations around it, so take extra care.

Jacqueline

Jacqueline was 39 years old. She had always wanted to have children because she absolutely adores them. But life doesn't always come at you the way you expect it to.

Although she yearned to become a mother, she was not interested in being a single parent. So, she was vigilant about preventing pregnancy until finally, at 40, she met the man of her dreams, and after a brief and very romantic courtship, they married.

Even before the wedding, Jacqueline and her husband agreed that they wanted to have a child together but hadn't set a timeline. As newlyweds, they wanted to get settled in the marriage first.

At 42, she felt ready. She wasn't worried about getting pregnant because she'd had two unplanned pregnancies before. But here's the reality: 42 is not 22, and prior pregnancy is not a guarantee of future pregnancy.

Jacqueline and her husband tried for six months with no success. They then sought help from a fertility specialist. Two years, thousands of dollars, and many fertility shots, pokes, and prods later, she was still not pregnant. Ultimately, Jacqueline and her husband had to accept that they would not be able to conceive.

The Takeaway: If you are over 35 and you have a partner identified, sooner is always a better choice than later if you wish to conceive naturally. Otherwise consider IVF with embryo freezing (if you know with whom you would like to conceive) to maximize your chances of having a baby.

Jacqueline just happened to be heterosexual, but her journey wouldn't be much different if she had a same-sex partner or if she chose to become a single mother. Every woman who wants to get pregnant has to confront the same biological truths and make informed timing decisions when seeking to answer that fundamental question: When do I start trying to conceive [♪ "Nick of Time"]?

Although we do not have the technology today, there are a growing number of biotech companies seeking to slow down the aging process of the ovaries. To be sure, there may be certain circumstances under which this would be helpful, but we should at least consider the implications when it comes to fertility. We can argue later about whether or not that's a good idea, but just consider this scenario—a 60-year-old with a toddler? I'll let you decide.

For now, any planned pregnancy must begin with an unvarnished view of your age and where you are in your reproductive life. It has to take into account your personal health risks, your financial ability to pay for expensive procedures and medications if not covered by insurance, and your likelihood for success before pursuing pregnancy. Most risk factors are not insurmountable, just know what resources you need to have available. If you are not sure about the timing, make a simple list of the pros and cons. (I'm a big fan of lists.) Each person will have their own personal issues to weigh, but I always ask my patients this: If you wait and can't get pregnant later, will you regret it? And will your reason for waiting have been worth it? You decide. Not your doctor. And not your mother, who's pining for a grandchild.

There is no ideal time to have a child, so get that notion out of your head. If it comes down to trying to get pregnant now or two years from now, from a fertility point of view, now is always better. Now would also be a good time to talk to your mother. How old was she when she went through menopause? How old was she when she had each of her children? Did she ever have difficulty trying to conceive? Did she ever miscarry or have a high-risk pregnancy or birth? These are really important data points that may affect your decision.

That said, there are options, and I want you to be clear-eyed about what they are—and what they cost. As a patient once said to me, "I always thought that raising a child would be crazy expensive, but I didn't think that trying to conceive one would be."

Make Like Nike and Just Do It

Your first option is the simplest and cheapest. Go ahead and try to get pregnant the old-fashioned way. Because you know your fertility is not what it once was, give yourself a few months. You might also use one of the many over-the-counter ovulation predictor kits to be more precise about the conception timing.

Depending on your age, you may want to see a fertility specialist, who can suggest ways to further improve your odds, usually by incorporating fertility drugs, timed ovulation, and/or timed inseminations. And while you are planning to see the fertility specialist, feel free to continue trying on your own. It is quite all right to get pregnant on your own while you are waiting for your appointment.

What if you've made the decision to have a baby but you don't have a male partner or you've decided you want to be a single mom? Aside from the obvious (recruit a healthy volunteer), you can ask a friend to donate some sperm (people do it all the time) or see a fertility specialist and try artificial insemination with donor sperm. A vial of donor sperm generally costs $900 to $1,000, and the insemination procedure runs $200 to $400. Of course, there are some cautionary tales to consider if you choose this path. Perhaps you saw the *Dateline* episode featuring the guy who "donated" sperm to more than 130 women. That's a bit extreme, of course.

On the other hand, a *New York Times* article reported that there is actually a shortage of Black sperm donors. The wide availability of DNA testing pretty much voided the idea of truly "anonymous" donors, which might have put a chill on the donating market. Oh, and that guy who "altruistically" has been impregnating women all over the country? He's been successfully sued for child support for at least five of his children so far. I guess it's true what they say—no good seed goes unpunished. (I simply could not resist.)

In our modern world, these are just points to consider. It can be easy to make light of them, but they're important. And keep in mind that you may have to try more than once to be successful, repeating those costs each time. Check your insurance coverage to see what is and is not covered under your current policy.

Freeze (Mother) Time!

If you are still holding out hope for a partner, or are not ready to commit just yet, there's the option of egg freezing. Coined the catchy "mature oocyte cryopreservation" by fertility centers, the cost—typically $13,000 to $17,000 per retrieval—allows you to literally buy time. Perhaps.

The procedure involves harvesting eggs from your ovaries in the same way as in a typical IVF cycle. But instead of fertilizing them before freezing, the eggs are frozen and stored, waiting not only for the suitable time, but also for some yet-to-be-discovered sperm. Before you do your happy dance and delight in the notion that modern medicine has solved everything, there are a few things I want you to consider. To have a reasonable shot at conceiving when the time comes, you need to have as many eggs stored as possible. This is because some of the eggs will not survive the freezing and thawing process. To get the requisite number of eggs necessary to have a reasonable shot at success may require more than one round of harvesting. For women over 35, the average number of retrievals needed is 2.1. In addition to the costs of possibly multiple rounds of harvesting, there is the annual storage fee for keeping your eggs on ice.

Be careful when interpreting the statistics around the success rates of frozen eggs versus frozen embryos, because it can be quite confusing. Make sure they are comparing apples to apples. A recent study out of the NYU Langone Fertility Center reported a 70 percent success rate when using frozen eggs from women younger than 38; however, here's the kicker—that statistic is only true if you froze your eggs before age 38 *and* you collected twenty or more eggs. The true rate is somewhere south of this.

Here is the conundrum—the younger you are when you freeze your eggs, then the more eggs you are able to collect, but the less likely you will be to need them. And when you add to this the fact that most women with frozen eggs do not use them, it turns out to be a very expensive proposition. For young women who have these costs covered by their employers, it's a benefit worth exploring. If you don't have coverage for those costs, financial constraints can easily be prohibitive.

While healthy babies have reportedly been born from eggs stored for more than fourteen years, the current consensus is that it's best to use your eggs within ten years. Keep in mind, this is still a relatively new procedure, so long-term data is scarce and ever-changing. Do your homework. Only consider centers that share their statistics on *actual* pregnancies and *actual* live births, rather than stoke your hopes with theoretical odds and best-case scenarios. Make sure they have a track record of success and that they have been around long enough to ensure that they will still be in business years from now when you are ready to conceive.

Think of egg freezing like fire insurance: Most people never need it, but it sure is a godsend if your house burns down. While limited, the data available puts the overall chance of a live birth from frozen eggs after age 35 at 39 percent. (I think this is rather optimistic—especially since only about 6 percent of people with frozen eggs have come back for them.) So, in broaching the subject with patients, I often echo Dr. Marcelle Cedars, former president of the American Society for Reproductive Medicine, who famously said: "There's not a baby in the freezer. There's a chance to get pregnant."

High-Tech Babies

In vitro fertilization is the most commonly used form of assisted reproductive technology. It involves retrieving mature eggs from your ovaries and fertilizing them using previously retrieved sperm in a lab (*in vitro* means "in glass").

The embryo(s) are then implanted in your uterus. One full cycle of IVF takes three weeks, or more. Expect to be quoted a price of $12,000 to $18,000, not including medication. And expect to wrangle with your health insurance provider—many don't cover it.

If necessary, IVF can involve eggs, sperm, or embryos from known or anonymous donors. Your chances of success depend on several factors, including your age, general health, and cause of infertility.

What if you've seen a fertility specialist, tried multiple rounds of IVF, and endured countless episodes of frustration and disappointment, and still nothing? Now might be a good time to discuss donor eggs with your doctor. If you really want the experience of being pregnant and giving birth, then egg donation is a good option.

Instead of your egg, the donated egg is harvested from a younger woman who has proven fertility. The likelihood of success with a donor egg is much higher because fertility follows the age of the donor—i.e., a 25-year-old's egg will have the fertility of a 25-year-old, not yours.

Surrogacy

For some women, being a parent is an experience that they'll pursue at almost any cost—physical, emotional, or financial. If carrying a pregnancy to term is medically not an option for you, you can hire a surrogate. Although the price tag for this option can vary significantly, once you factor in agency fees (for vetting and helping you manage the surrogate relationship), legal fees (for preparing the key documents you will need both pre- and post-birth), surrogate compensation and contingent fees, and insurance costs, you're easily talking six figures. In the United States, experts put the total at anywhere from $100,000 to $200,000 or more.

The surrogate option is typically used in one of two ways: with your partner's sperm and either your egg (if viable) or with your surrogate's or a donor egg.

If you use a surrogate with both donated egg *and* sperm, that's basically a premium-priced in utero adoption. But it's your money, and your call. While surrogacy is highly successful, it carries with it the same risks for potential miscarriage and stillbirth as any other healthy pregnancy. That is to say, this route to motherhood is still not 100 percent guaranteed.

Motherhood: Guaranteed

The one pathway to motherhood that all but guarantees you will end up with a child is adoption.

There are three main ways to adopt children in the United States: through the foster care system; a local adoption agency or private attorney; or internationally. All three require a home-care study where you, your home, and your life are vetted by a social worker for safety and suitability. Outside of that, the three avenues are quite distinctive.

International adoption is becoming less common and more difficult, but there are U.S.-based agencies that specialize in it and can assist you.

Private adoption can cost around $50,000, and the wait for a healthy infant can take months to years. But it depends on what kind of baby you want. The single most significant factor in the wait for a newborn is the race of the child. If you want a white baby from two white parents, be prepared to wait as long as three years. Mixed-race and Black babies are easier to adopt. The more stipulations or preferences you have, such as the sex of the baby, the lack of drug use of the mother, or the health of the baby, the longer the wait. Now, we could write a dissertation on how messed up that is, but this is the reality of adoption in America.

Adoption through the foster care system is virtually free, and on any given day, there are more than 100,000 children in U.S. foster care who are in need of permanent new families and homes. Black children age 9 and older, and children with special needs, are disproportionately represented in this group, so those adoptions can proceed more quickly.

The only point I'm trying to make is that there are many paths to motherhood; choose the one that feels right for you.

Finally, if you love children but are unsure about committing to parenthood, perhaps becoming a foster mother is for you. Many children need temporary homes because of situations in their current homes. Just remember that mothering involves a much more complicated skill set than giving birth. And be assured that if you have a burning desire to be a mom, there is always a way to make that happen.

Yes, Virginia, There Are Treatments!

Now that we've tackled the hard stuff, let's get back to the issue at hand—perimenopause and what can be done about it. To treat or not to treat, that is the question. There's no perfect time to seek treatment, but a difficult perimenopause can seem to go on forever—and forever is way too long to be having a heat wave [♪ "Heat Wave"]. Although we use the one-year-of-no-periods marker for menopause, you do *not* need to wait until then to treat your symptoms. Nor should you if you are miserable. Your doctor can help you assess your risk factors for conditions that may benefit from early intervention, like diabetes and osteoporosis. But only you can decide when or if to seek treatment.

Low-Dose Birth Control Pills

Yes, plain old birth control pills work beautifully to control perimenopausal symptoms. Especially for women still having relatively regular periods who, in addition to symptom relief, also need birth control. There are enough surprises in this transition, and a baby shouldn't be one of them. Birth control pills contain estrogen and progestin, the same components that are menopausal hormone therapy. However, the doses of estrogen and progestin in birth control pills are higher doses than what you would take after menopause. Also, the estrogen and progestin in oral contraceptives are not bioidentical. The pill can be taken continuously (which just means skipping the placebos, allowing you to bypass your period altogether) or in a fashion that gives you a monthly period. Continuous use of birth control pills is preferable for women who are symptomatic on the placebo week or just simply prefer not to have a monthly period.

Low-dose birth control pills are also a good option for women with heavy and/or unpredictable periods due to perimenopause. During perimenopause, the bleeding can sometimes be difficult to manage, and if you have fibroids, the effect of the two together is a multiplier, not just simply additive. With pills, your periods can be lighter, more predictable, or if you prefer, skipped altogether. Yay!

Now, you might ask, if I'm getting my period with the birth control pills, how will I know when perimenopause is over and menopause has begun? You won't. You will continue to get a period monthly (if you choose this option), because the bleeding you get is caused by the pills you take, not the hormones you make. If you are healthy and don't smoke, you can stay on your pills until you are menopausal. You can stop them briefly each year, have bloodwork done to see where you are in the menopausal spectrum, and transition seamlessly to hormone replacement if you choose to do so.

Laura

Laura was 47 years old, and like a lot of women in Washington was overworked, managing a high-stress job and a brood of teens and tweens. I had been seeing her for over fifteen years. I took care of her through three uneventful pregnancies. After the birth of her last child, she used birth control pills as her preferred method of avoiding pregnancy. It also helped with PMS and cycle control. She had no problems on the pill, and other than mild, well-controlled hypertension, she had no other health issues.

Laura saw her internist, who suggested that maybe she should come off her birth control pills. Why, you might ask, was her internist giving her advice about her birth control? Good question. I wasn't making suggestions about her blood pressure medication. But I digress. She came to me to see if she should stop. I asked if anything in her health history had changed since her last visit. The answer was no. I checked her blood pressure and it was well within the normal range. Given that she was 47 years old and was very likely to be right in the middle of perimenopause, I suggested that now would not be a good time to stop her pills. You see, Laura was a very high-ranking government official. She frequently advised Cabinet members on issues of national and international importance. She and I decided that as long as everything was going well, she should stay on the pill. Neither she nor I was interested in finding out whether she was going to have hot flashes or bouts of rage while she was in her current job. She needed her wits about her at all times. Brain fog for her was not an option. She stayed on the pill until she was 52, when she had the time and the bandwidth to assess her menopausal status

and symptoms. After confirming she was indeed menopausal, she started hormone replacement. America, you're
welcome.

The Takeaway: You don't have to be a high-ranking government official to know that there are effective treatments during perimenopause that allow you to function at
your peak. Birth control pills are a good way to transition
seamlessly from perimenopause to menopause without
skipping a beat. If you are already on birth control pills and
doing well, you can continue them until the age of menopause and reassess. And no, you don't have to wait a year
to confirm your menopausal status to start hormone replacement therapy. A simple blood test will do.

Progestin-Only Pills/Progesterone

There are a few people who cannot take estrogen, such as those at high
risk for developing blood clots. Progestin-only pills provide birth control and some degree of cycle control, although they are not as effective
as estrogen-progestin pills in controlling the other symptoms.

Alternatively, micronized progesterone, which is the same type of
progestin used in menopausal hormone therapy, can help with some
bleeding issues and some menopausal symptoms, particularly hot
flashes and sleep. However, micronized progesterone does not provide
any birth control.

Hormone-Releasing IUDs (Mirena, Liletta)

This is a great option if you need birth control and have heavy, unpredictable periods, but relatively few other menopausal symptoms. In
my experience, most women with an IUD will not get a period at all,

and those who do report much lighter bleeding. Bear in mind, since there is no estrogen in the IUD, the other symptoms of perimenopause will not be treated. However, if you have or develop other menopausal symptoms, a simple solution is to add back a low dose of estrogen either orally or topically. The progestin in the IUD is more than sufficient to protect the uterus.

The good news is that the IUD can be kept in place for up to eight years, which conveniently is about the length of perimenopause.

Low-Dose Antidepressants

When your predominant symptoms are hot flashes, and either you cannot or choose not to take estrogen and progestin, there is only one FDA-approved option: paroxetine. Paroxetine is an SSRI (selective serotonin reuptake inhibitor—now you know why we call them "SSRIs") that has been used for years as an antidepressant. The dose used to treat hot flashes is lower than what is typically prescribed to treat depression. Paroxetine has been proven to be only about 50 percent effective at relieving hot flashes, and it does not specifically address any of the other thirty-plus symptoms of menopause.

Fezolinetant (VEOZAH)

As of this writing, the FDA has approved a new medication for the treatment of hot flashes. This medication targets the area of the brain (the hypothalamus) involved in temperature regulation. Its cost is estimated to be $550 a month. The target audience for fezolinetant is women who either (due to contraindications) cannot or choose not to take hormones. Aside from the high price tag, the downside is that we have no long-term data on its use. The studies cited in its approval process included only one year of safety data. Since I have zero clinical experience with this medication, I'll let you decide if it's worth it.

Non-Pharmaceutical Options

Now, I'm not going to call any product out by name, but here's the bottom line: Vitamins, supplements, herbs, and nutraceuticals are not regulated in the same way as medications. These over-the-counter or internet-marketed products have no duty to prove effectiveness, consistency of dose, or purity. Let that sink in for a minute.

In fairness, they do have to prove safety; that is, they have to at least demonstrate that they won't kill or harm you. That's it. Most of what is going on here is marketing. So, since we are now all crackpot internet sleuths, before committing, ask to see the data behind the miraculous claims that many of these products make. I'm not talking testimonials here, but real data. You know what you'll likely hear? Crickets. If there are studies available, they usually involve small numbers of patients for relatively short periods of time. If that's enough for you, I've said my piece—just proceed with caution and immediately stop taking anything that affects you adversely.

Charlene

Charlene is 52 years old. She teaches yoga and has always considered herself to be in control of her body and her health. She takes no medications and exercises regularly. She has been having severe hot flashes since she was in her mid-40s and hasn't had a full night's sleep in over a decade (before the hot flashes started, she had a toddler who wouldn't sleep through the night).

She has eliminated red wine (her favorite) and every other thing in her life that she thinks might be triggering these gnarly flashes. A few years back, I raised the option of her using hormones, but she politely declined, saying she prefers to do things naturally. Since then, she has seen an herbalist and an acupuncturist, changed her diet, and tried every over-the-counter remedy known to womankind—to no avail.

Her recent purchase (recommended by her most trusted healthcare advisor, her hairdresser) is this "amazing" herbal concoction that includes vitamins and nutrients in a special proprietary blend. The packaging is beautiful, and for a mere $100 a month she has a guarantee of success from the company who sells it.

When I see her for her physical a year later, she proudly proclaims that since she has been on this new supplement, she is down to only three or four hot flashes per day instead of her usual ten.

Hold up, wait a minute!

Girlfriend has been having symptoms for about seven years. They are starting to improve, and although she is happily crediting the expensive treatment she just tried, the reality is that what she is experiencing is the amazing power of the tincture of time.

The Takeaway: Most hot flashes will eventually recede, even if you do nothing. The real question is—and everybody will have a different answer—How long are you willing to wait? Whatever you decide, on this and all health matters, be decisive!

Why Do We Choose to Suffer?

I went to medical school to figure out how to alleviate suffering, not simply to observe it. So, in my many years of practicing women's medicine, it's been frustrating to note that for women, and for Black women in particular, suffering is a default mode. This is magnified during perimenopause and menopause. And by avoiding potential treatments, not only are you suffering, you're increasing your risks for menopause's most damaging effects on your long-term health. We'll address those in the next chapter.

Let me repeat: Menopause is mandatory, suffering is not. For generations of women, especially for women of color, that latter part wasn't true. Now that we have a choice, we need to work up the nerve to *choose not to suffer*! Speak up, ask questions, share your experiences and coping tools. We need to demand more and better treatments, more studies into minimizing risk, and we need to keep demanding until we get them.

The one thing none of us can justify anymore is helplessness. Passive acceptance of the status quo in women's health is no longer an option. Not when it comes to unnecessary suffering, not when it comes to perimenopause and menopause, and not when it comes to figuring out how to get the healthcare you need so you can live your best life—no matter what age the calendar says you are.

DR. SHARON'S RX FOR
Perimenopause

1. Keep a detailed diary of your menstrual history and document symptoms and when they are occurring relative to your period. Also, make note of what triggers your menopausal symptoms, and try to eliminate those triggers. Always know the date of your last period. *Any* vaginal bleeding that occurs after one year of no bleeding needs to be investigated.

2. Your diet matters. Weigh yourself at least once a week. Know that most women will gain *at least* a pound a year during the menopausal transition. It is far easier to not gain a pound every year than it will be to lose ten pounds a decade from now.

3. Eliminate processed foods from your diet . . . okay, reduce them. There still must be some joy in the world, and I'm a doctor, not the food police. That said, starting in peri-menopause, your gut microbiome changes, so ultra-processed foods, which increase inflammation, disrupt your hormones, worsen your mood, and make you fat, should find their way out of your diet.

4. Exercise. Exercise. Exercise. I know I sound like a broken record, but the purpose of exercise is not to lose weight. Its purpose is to preserve your muscle mass, improve your mood, and improve your cardiovascular health. I could go on, but the bottom line is, *do it!* Call your friends, do it together. Make it fun.

5. Stop smoking. Smokers have earlier menopause, more symptoms, and a higher risk of developing osteoporosis.

6. See your doctor regularly and make sure your blood pressure and blood sugar are under control. Get cancer screenings.

7. If you have done all of these things and you are still both-ered by the symptoms of perimenopause, then for good-ness' sake, talk to your doctor about hormone therapy. You do not have to wait for a full year of no periods to get relief. Remember, for most women the benefits far out-weigh the risks.

CHAPTER 10

Finally!♪

Menopause and Beyond

Dear Sis,

I can't tell you the number of patients who have walked into my office after not having had a period in ten years, and proudly reported that they didn't go through menopause.

Wait, what?

News flash—you did.

Just because you either a) can't remember what it was like, or b) didn't have the typical hot flashes and mood swings, doesn't mean it didn't happen. I assure you, it did.

Menopause is like parenting. Once you're in it, you're in it for life. There is no turning back the clock on that one. Whether your journey is easy or hard depends not only on your attitude, but also on your physical and emotional health, your habits and family history. Don't be ashamed if you are having a hard time, and don't pat yourself on the back if you're not. Once you cross that perimenopausal finish line, we are all in the same boat.

You can now officially say goodbye to pregnancy worries and periods—forever! And this newfound freedom may create a resurgence of creativity and energy that you haven't felt in years . . . or not. Either way, I want to get you on the right track to making the best of what we hope to be the next thirty-plus years of your life. Even though your hot flashes and brain fog may have abated, menopause is still doing its thing. So, we're going to go to a few places that you may not have expected, but that are equally important to your menopausal journey.

I want you to know what to look for and how to deal with it when the time comes. Why? Because you deserve to be your best, healthy self all day, every day.

xo, Dr. Sharon

So, it's been twelve months since your last period. You are now one of the estimated 2 million women in the United States who enter menopause each year. Congratulations! You've officially crossed over.

The average age for becoming menopausal in the United States is about 51. But who's average? About 5 percent of women experience what is considered an early menopause, defined as having had your last period between the ages of 40 and 45. Whether early menopause occurs naturally or because of surgery, medication, or certain medical conditions, it puts you at higher risk for the long-term consequences of menopause, which we will discuss in a bit. Fortunately, only about 1 percent of women go through menopause before the age of 40. But as we discussed in the last chapter, the symptoms that we associate with perimenopause/menopause can show up as early as ten years *before* the final menstrual period. This means that about 6 percent of women can become symptomatic and experience suboptimal fertility in their 30s! Thus, knowing the signs and symptoms as well as your family history is extremely important in not only making an accurate diagnosis, but in effective family planning.

There are currently over 55 million menopausal women in the United States alone. The latest CDC provisional life expectancy statistics (2021) report that the life expectancy for white women is 79.2 years; for Black women, that figure is 74.8; for Hispanic women, it is 81; and the ethnic groups with the highest and the lowest life expectancies are Asians at 85.6 and Native American/Alaskans at 69.2. Of note, all of these numbers have decreased by almost two years since COVID. Let's hope and pray that these numbers will soon return to pre-pandemic levels. Whether they do or not, most women in this country will spend on average 25–30 years in menopause. Think about that: You are likely to spend as much time in menopause as you have spent in any other reproductive phase of your life [♪ **"Always and Forever"**]. So, why do we talk so little about it? We've explored some of the "why" in other chapters. And we've touched on the "when" and the "where" of menopause. At this point, inquiring minds want to know, what now?

This may not be your favorite answer, but as with most things in life, it depends. For starters, what are your menopausal symptoms? And how severe are they? Although your hot flashes, mood swings, and brain fog will likely get better after your hormones settle down, some of those other thirty-four symptoms will not. (Think dry skin, dry vagina, thinning hair, and low libido, to name a few.) And for a few unfortunate souls, intense hot flashes can persist for years, even decades.

Any of these symptoms can and should be treated if they are diminishing your quality of life. But the bigger health issues, the ones that can exact a heavy toll for many years after menopause, these are the ones I want you to pay special attention to. I'm talking about cardiovascular disease, osteoporosis, and Alzheimer's disease, which can snake their way in, uninvited and under the radar.

Now that I've got your attention, you should also know that 80 percent of women will also experience the genitourinary syndrome of menopause (GSM), which is a constellation of symptoms, such as vulvar and vaginal dryness, painful sex, and urinary problems that tend to worsen if they're not addressed. So, don't sit idly by "dealing with it." This is no surrender-Dorothy, woe-is-me situation.

Now more than ever, women are speaking out about menopause openly and honestly, and are demanding answers. We are setting new standards for what aging gracefully and healthily looks like. Michelle Obama, Tracee Ellis Ross, Maria Shriver, and Oprah Winfrey have shared their menopause stories, changing the face of what health and strength look like at 50, 60, and 70. This is not your grandmother's menopause! Nor should it be.

Understanding and taking better care and control of this time in your life matters. So, let's be good stewards of our health as we age. That means knowing what your objectives are, what your particular risks are, and what to do about them once you've identified them. There is no one-size-fits-all solution, but there are options—all of which are going to require you to be your own best advocate. Start by going to your doctor to discuss how to create a plan for healthy aging and disease *prevention*. Doing so can be a challenge when menopausal specialists are few and far between. I firmly believe that you deserve access to quality care, whether you live in Yazoo City or New York City. But you and I have lived long enough to know that people are not always going to give us what we deserve, we're going to have to go after it [♪"You Can't Always Get What You Want"]. No matter where you live, be unrelenting in your pursuit of the information you need to make good choices.

The Resurrection of Menopause Relief

Now that you understand that menopause is a hormonal issue, it won't surprise you to know that, as with perimenopause, its most effective treatments involve some form of hormone therapy. In an excellent review entitled "The History of Estrogen Therapy," Dr. Grace Kohn writes about the colorful history of the use of hormones for relief of menopausal symptoms. We may have just started having discussions about menopause, but believe me when I say women have been complaining about it for as long as we've lived long enough to experience it. Aristotle described the symptoms of menopause in the fourth century B.C.

I know you're probably thinking, if we've known about menopause and women have been suffering for centuries, what took so long to figure it out? But to be fair, we hadn't figured out a lot of things about how the body works, and living to and much beyond menopausal age was a rarity. Dr. Kohn chronicled how the extraction and use of biologic compounds to treat the symptoms of menopause began in the late 1800s. The extracts (estrogen wasn't even identified then) from cow's ovaries were injected into German women in an attempt to relieve menopausal symptoms. By the 1900s, a succession of cows and pigs sacrificed their ovaries (and their lives), which were desiccated and pulverized into powders to treat menopausal women. In fact, Dr. George Papanicolaou (yes, the same guy who invented the pap smear) was the first person to describe how estrogen interacted with the areas of the brain that regulate the menstrual cycle. Now, don't worry, he didn't experiment on humans, he used guinea pigs. But given that he did his research in the 1920s, I can see how you might have had concerns.

Once the substance we today know as estrogen was identified, doctors still had no way to manufacture it. They had to kill an awful lot of cows and pigs to get enough ovaries to grind up. This wasn't the most efficient manufacturing process.

Now, this is where the story gets interesting. The first commercially marketed product, Emmenin (pick your favorite Eminem song 'cause I don't have one) was actually collected from pregnant women's urine. Finding all those pregnant women willing to collect, save, and sell their urine was difficult and expensive—as well as, uh, gross! So, the friendly people at the pharmaceutical company Ayerst thought to themselves, *If only we could find someone who pees like a race horse? How about a race horse?* Thus, in 1941, Ayerst introduced Premarin, which, in case you didn't know, stands for "pregnant mare's urine," and admittedly has a better ring to it than *prewomenin,* right?

Once scientists identified the substance that treated the symptoms of menopause—estrogen—and figured out an unlimited source (pregnant mare's urine) that didn't require sacrificing the animal to produce it, they were off to the races. (Sometimes I crack myself up.) Still, the widespread use of estrogen to treat the symptoms of menopause didn't get a huge boost until the 1960s, when a gynecologist, Dr. Robert Wilson, wrote a rhapsodic ode to estrogen in his book, *Feminine Forever.* He full-throatedly endorsed the use of estrogen for women to preserve their femininity and desirability. After all, who wants a cranky, old, wrinkly woman with no desire for sex?

My favorite chapter in Dr. Wilson's tour de force begins, "At the risk of seeming paradoxical, I should like to launch into the subject of menopause by discussing its effect on men." Need I say more? Nonetheless, the book was a national bestseller, and the use of Premarin skyrocketed. It was only after Wilson's death that his son admitted the book had been paid for by—you guessed it—the pharmaceutical company that made Premarin.

Estrogen use increased steadily throughout the 1960s and '70s until a marked uptick in the rate of endometrial cancer was observed in estrogen users. Women who still had their uteruses and who had been using what we now call "unopposed estrogen" (estrogen without progestin) had an alarming increase in endometrial cancer. And in case you're wondering what took them so long to figure it out, a good percentage of women entered menopause without their uteruses.

Hysterectomy was the most common surgical procedure in women in the United States. The use of estrogen decreased until doctors finally figured out that the increase in endometrial cancer could be counteracted by adding a second hormone, progestin, to the regimen. By the mid-1980s through the 1990s, estrogen was back in the mainstream, with progestin added for those with an intact uterus, and estrogen only for those who'd had a hysterectomy.

By the early 1990s, we had amassed considerable information about the use of HRT. Hormones had been used in some form or fashion for over eighty years. Premarin was still the most frequently prescribed estrogen in America. Fueled in large part by the Nurses' Health Study (NHS), a large observational study launched in 1976 by Dr. Frank Speizer to look at health outcomes of nurses over time, newfound interest in women's long-term health started to emerge. One of the most interesting findings was the fact that nurses who took hormones after menopause had about a 50 percent decrease in the rate of cardiovascular disease. Although compelling, an observational study can only show correlation, not causality. This is where the idea for the Women's Health Initiative (WHI) was born.

In 1991, the WHI, a randomized double-blind placebo-controlled study (which I introduced to you earlier), was designed to definitively answer the question of whether hormone therapy did, indeed, cut the risk of heart disease in half as suggested by the NHS. If proven, this would have been an incredible boost to the already-known benefits of hormone therapy in relieving menopausal symptoms. Not only would the quality of women's lives be improved, but by reducing the risk of heart disease, hormone therapy had the potential to save lives as well.

By 1993, women were enrolled in the study in forty medical centers around the country. Over 27,000 women participated in the estrogen and estrogen-progestin arms of the study, which was slated to run for eight years. At the five-year check-in, things began to go off the rails. After a preliminary analysis of the study results, a study-monitoring group at the NIH did not see the anticipated decrease in risk of heart disease. Without consulting the investigators around the country who had been collecting data from their medical centers, the study was abruptly halted. It was not stopped simply for the lack of benefit in cardiovascular reduction, but primarily because of a slightly increased risk of breast cancer. In a jaw-dropping, paradigm-shifting press conference convened by the NIH monitoring group, two reasons were cited for halting the study—lack of benefit (the investigators did not show HRT reduced the risk of heart diseases) and excess harm (there was a slight increase in the risk of breast cancer, blood clots, stroke, gallstones, and dementia in hormone users versus nonusers). A reported 26 percent increase in the risk of breast cancer in women who used estrogen and progestin stole the show.

When the highly anticipated, and might I add very expensive, Women's Health Initiative released the findings of "No cardiac benefit and increased risk of breast cancer," hormone therapy went from being a godsend for symptomatic women to being a turd in a punch bowl. One infamous and well-attended press conference convened at the National Press Club, at the behest of the study regulators at the NIH, altered the landscape in the use of hormones and research in menopause overnight, and more than twenty years later, we are still trying to correct the record.

The news landed like a nuclear bomb. Headlines ricocheted around the world before we in the medical profession even had a chance to review the full report. In fact, the article in the July 2002 *Journal of the American Medical Association* (*JAMA*) announcing the findings was written and in the can before any of the doctors in the participating medical centers even had a chance to weigh in. After this study was released, hormone use plummeted from nearly 40 percent to less than 6 percent almost overnight. Women promptly abandoned their hormone treatments, no matter how good it made them feel. It was game, set, and match for HRT.

There was no follow-up explaining to the media or medical community that this 26 percent increase in breast cancer in real numbers translated into less than one additional case of breast cancer per 1,000 women per year—and only in the group who took estrogen and synthetic progestin. Want some further perspective? According to a review article in *Climacteric,* Dr. Howard Hodis and Dr. Philip Sarrel estimated that the increased risk of getting breast cancer while on estrogen-progestin therapy (EPT) was less than the risk associated with drinking two glasses of wine a day, being overweight, or being physically inactive. Have you seen the press conference about that? Me neither.

Also, the fact that the estrogen-only arm of the study did not cross the safety protocol (i.e., no increase in the risk of breast cancer) and continued for another two years after the estrogen and progestin arm of the study was halted did not get much pickup in the press. For women who had hysterectomies (a category which, as you now know, includes a higher percentage of Black women) and took estrogen alone, the risk of being diagnosed with breast cancer actually *decreased*. After follow-ups at ten and twenty years on the original data from the WHI, the WHI investigators reported not only a 22 percent decrease in the incidence of breast cancer, but a 40 percent decrease in the risk of dying from it. Where was that headline, you ask? I'm still waiting.

Today, the most effective treatment for the symptoms of menopausal women with uteruses is estrogen-progestin therapy; for women who have had a hysterectomy, it's estrogen-only therapy. Full stop. (Notice I didn't say "period" again. You're welcome.) This isn't just my opinion. The North American Menopause Society (NAMS) and more than thirty other medical societies agree with this statement. And full disclosure: I have personally been taking HRT for more than fifteen years despite a family history of breast cancer, and that's *my* choice based upon *my* personal risk factors and expectations. The North American Menopause Society's 2022 guidelines for hormone use plainly state that a family history of breast cancer is *not* a contraindication for taking hormones. In plain English, your risk of getting breast cancer is unchanged by whether you take hormones or not. The overwhelming majority of women who get breast cancer each year are *not* on hormones and do *not* have a family history. And in this you should take some comfort: Even if you do get breast cancer while on estrogen and progestin, your risk of dying from breast cancer is unchanged. And in the population of estrogen users versus nonusers, the risk of dying from any cause is 30 percent lower.

After two decades of languishing in purgatory, there is renewed support of HRT. The American College of Obstetrics and Gynecology endorses it, the North American Menopause Society endorses it, the Endocrine Society and thirty other national and international medical societies endorse it. They agree that for women who start hormone therapy before age 60 and within ten years of their last menstrual period, the benefits outweigh the risks. That's real progress. But this consensus still hasn't fully restored the confidence around HRT that women and their doctors once had. Whether or not you choose to use systemic menopausal hormone therapy, almost without exception, all women can and should use some form of topical vaginal estrogen to prevent thinning of the vagina, painful sex, vulvar discomfort, and urinary frequency, urgency, and urinary tract infections.

And let's be clear, estrogen is not for everybody. There are some legitimate medical and personal reasons why estrogen may not be right for you. But every woman should get the information they need to decide what's right for them based on facts, not fear. According to the North American Menopause Society's 2022 guidelines, the only contraindications for hormone use are:

1. Personal history of breast or estrogen-dependent cancer

2. Undiagnosed vaginal bleeding

3. Active liver disease

4. Personal history of heart attack or stroke

5. Personal history of unprovoked blood clots in the legs or lungs, or a genetic susceptibility for increased clotting (even this has some exceptions; talk to your doctor)

That's it. Almost. I would be remiss if I did not mention that some of these contraindications like breast cancer are not absolute. For an excellent review of the scientific data on breast cancer and estrogen, I would recommend the book *Estrogen Matters* by Dr. Avrum Bluming and Carol Tavris, PhD. The conversation around estrogen use in cancer survivors is a nuanced one and should be discussed with your doctor—after which, remember, *you* get to decide [♪ **"Sisters Are Doin' It for Themselves"**]. The North American Menopause Society affirms that with informed consent the ultimate decision is yours. Even for women who have a history of deep vein thromboses (DVTs) or blood clots, there are ways to benefit from HRT and still minimize the chance of a recurrence. For these women, transdermal estrogen is preferable to oral estrogen.

For everyone else, the discussion to take hormones after menopause should be on the table. The decision about whether to take or not to take hormones should be based upon a conversation between you and your doctor that assesses your personal risk factors, treatment goals, and risk tolerance. You may also talk to trusted friends who can share real-life testimony about its use, but remember that their experience is *their* experience. It has nothing to do with yours. And let me repeat: There are real-life consequences at stake. If you are flashing and sweating; dressing and undressing; not sleeping—*for years*—understand that there are significant long-term health effects from that.

Hot flashes, night sweats, and sleeplessness increase your risk of cardiovascular disease and decrease your ability to control your weight. Menopause can affect your mood, your attentiveness, your ability to do your job and care for your family. When we're hot and bothered, it impacts not only our lives, but commerce, economics, our communities, and ultimately, society. A recent survey by Dr. Stephanie Faubion and her colleagues at the Mayo Clinic estimates that the cost of symptomatic menopause due to lost productivity and absenteeism in the workplace exceeds $1.8 billion a year. Their estimate for associated medical expenses clocks in at a whopping $26.6 billion. So, now you know why employers are beginning to address menopause in the workplace—because not dealing with it is expensive and figuring out how to keep their most experienced employees in the workforce just makes good business sense.

HRT/MHT: Is There a Difference?

Modern medicalese is full of acronyms. Designed to make things simpler, they unfortunately sometimes create confusion. Case in point: You may see HRT (hormone replacement therapy) referred to elsewhere as MHT (menopausal hormone treatment). HRT is kind of old-school and MHT is au courant. But they're essentially different terms for the same thing, or as you might say, "SSDD (same 'stuff,' different day)." So, with that bit of context, let's look at your HRT options. And remember if you have a uterus, you need estrogen and progestin; no uterus, estrogen alone is all you need.

Estrogen

Estrogen is the key ingredient in the special HRT (because I'm old-school) sauce. The female body has over four hundred different tissues/cell types that have estrogen receptors. We have estrogen receptors not just in our reproductive organs, but also in our skin, brains, blood vessels, eyes, bones, gut . . . just about everywhere. It is the estrogen component of HRT that is responsible for symptom relief, as well as for the maintenance and protection of our many other organ systems.

Systemic Estrogen

Systemic estrogen simply refers to estrogen given at a dose necessary to control the symptoms of menopause throughout the body (the entire system, get it?). It can be taken as an oral pill, a patch, gel, vaginal ring, or spray. In the proper dosages, all are equally effective in relieving the symptoms of menopause. Because of the higher doses of estrogen needed to affect the entire body, unless you have had a hysterectomy, systemic estrogen is prescribed with a progestin to protect the uterine lining.

To choose between the many ways to take estrogen, consider several factors—ease of use, personal preference, cost, and certain personal risk factors. For example, if you smoke or are at risk for developing blood clots due to your family history, the transdermals (patch, gel, spray, or ring) may be preferable to the oral option, because the estrogen goes directly into the bloodstream through the skin or vagina and does not pass through the digestive system or the liver. I won't bore you with the details of liver function. Once more, you're welcome. If you don't smoke or have any additional risk factors, you can use oral or transdermal. Your choice. Oral estrogen is typically the less expensive option.

Local Estrogen

Local (or vaginal) estrogen is used for prevention and treatment of genitourinary syndrome of menopause (GSM), described in detail in its own section), delivering a much smaller dose of estrogen directly to a target area—vagina, labia, urethra, or vulva. It does not travel far beyond its target tissues and hence it does not address symptoms impacting other areas of the body.

It can be delivered vaginally as either a cream, a suppository, or a ring (not to be confused with the systemic vaginal ring). The reasons for choosing one over the other are similar to those for systemic estrogen—ease of use, cost, and personal preference.

Unlike systemic estrogen, which has clear contraindications, local estrogen can be used by almost anyone. The dosage is so low that no progesterone is needed even in people who still have a uterus. If you have had breast cancer, topical estrogen can be used without harm, just inform your oncologist.

Progestin/Progesterone

If you have a uterus and seek broader relief than a local estrogen will offer, a progestin is added to the estrogen regimen to protect the lining of the uterus. The progestin can be delivered together with the estrogen in a single pill, as separate pills, in a progestin-releasing IUD, or in a vaginal gel—not a very popular option but it can work well for some women who are intolerant of oral progesterone.

For those who use transdermal estrogen, the progestin can be provided three ways. There is a combination patch (CombiPatch) which contains both estrogen and progestin. If you choose estrogen-only patches, gels, sprays, or the ring, progestin can be given as an additional daily pill. And here's some news you can use: A progestin-releasing IUD such as a Mirena or a Liletta is quite effective at protecting the uterus and can be used in lieu of a progestin pill—and the IUD can be left in place for eight years.

Quick Menopause Treatment Q&A

- *When should I start hormones?* You should start hormones when you are bothered by the symptoms of perimenopause/menopause or when you reach menopausal age and are at risk for conditions that HRT is known to protect against, such as osteoporosis. Bear in mind that most women are symptomatic for years—if not a decade—before their last menstrual period. Also remember, if you are in your 40s, you are perimenopausal even if you are still getting your period regularly. The strategy for how to take hormones differs somewhat during the menopausal transition and after menopause (see Chapter 9), but the goal is to get you symptom-free. The decision of when and what to do should be a collaborative one between you and your healthcare provider, based on your symptoms and personal risk factors. Do not let answers like "This can't be menopause" deter you from getting the relief you need.

- *I have a family history of breast cancer, so I can't take hormones, right?* Wrong. First of all, only about 5–10 percent of all breast cancers are thought to be due to genetic or hereditary factors. Second, although 1 in 8 women will be diagnosed with breast cancer in her lifetime, that is a population statistic, not an individual risk. (See Chapter 4 for a complete explanation.) So, most of us have had at least one family member with breast cancer. The North American Menopause Society in their 2022 guidelines states that when comparing nonusers with hormone users, "there appears to be no additive effect of hormone therapy with age or elevated personal breast cancer risk factors on breast cancer incidence." In normal-person-speak, your risk of developing breast cancer is the same whether you take hormones or not. Adding hormones does not increase that risk.

- *Wait, but are you sure estrogen doesn't cause breast cancer?* Estrogen alone does not cause breast cancer. In a twenty-year follow-up from the Women's Health Initiative, the women who took estrogen alone had a 22 percent *decrease* in the incidence of breast cancer and a 40 percent decrease in the risk of dying from breast cancer. For the women who took estrogen and progestin, the increase in the risk of breast cancer in estrogen users was less than one additional case per 1,000 women per year, which is less than the risk attributed to drinking two glasses of wine per day or being overweight. In the Danish Osteoporosis Prevention Study, where women were followed for sixteen years, women who took estrogen and bioidentical progesterone at the time of natural menopause and continued for ten years had no increase in the risk of breast cancer.

- *What is the difference between synthetic progestins and bioidentical progesterone?* All pharmaceutical progestins are synthetic. *Synthetic* simply means they are made in a lab and not naturally occurring (as they are inside your body). All progestins perform similar functions. Their only role in hormone therapy is to serve as a counterbalance to the estrogenic effects on the uterus. Without progestin, the uterine lining, under the influence of estrogen alone, can overgrow. Over time, this overgrowth can lead to a risk of endometrial cancer.

  The progestins may be bioidentical, which means that if you drew the molecule on a chalkboard (yes, now I'm taking you back to chemistry class), it would be structurally the same molecule as the one your ovaries make. Non-bioidentical progestins are modified versions of the progesterone molecule, altered for stability. It is one of these non-bioidentical progestins, medroxyprogesterone, that was used in the Women's

Health Initiative and was associated with the *slightly* elevated risk of breast cancer. Other non-bioidentical progestins—like norethindrone, levonorgestrel, and norgestimate, to name a few—are used in birth control pills. Norethindrone acetate is the progestin used in combination estradiol/progestin hormone replacement medications, such as Activella. Levonorgestrel is the progestin component in Mirena and Liletta IUDs. There are many different types of progestins, and each is used in different medication formulations. Bioidentical progesterone, the one we just drew on the chalkboard, is also used in hormone replacement, but not in birth control pills. The good news is that most studies using bioidentical progesterone in hormone replacement have shown no increase in the risk of breast cancer. There are no head-to-head randomized controlled studies comparing the different types of progestins in HRT. In medicine as in life, we know what we know until we learn something new.

- *What are compounded hormones?* Okay, so here is where it gets a little confusing. Typically, all compounded hormones are bioidentical, but not all bioidentical hormones are compounded. So, what is the difference? Compounded hormones are typically made in small, often bespoke, batches by compounding pharmacies. A pharmacist can create nonstandard doses in combinations not available from standard pharmaceutical manufacturers. Here's the problem: Because they are made, in some cases, by pharmacies that are not subjected to the same testing and verification processes as FDA-approved medications, the quality and safety of compounded medications is not assured. However, to be fair, some compounding pharmacies are regulated by states and adhere to United States Pharmacopeia regulations. The compounded medications are only as good as the compounding pharmacy, and these medications are almost without exception more expensive and often not covered by insurance. They also do not carry the black-box warning that commercially manufactured hormones are required to use, warning of possible increased risks. This omission could give the misimpression that compounded hormones are safer.

In reality, there is no way for you to be sure that what a compounded product label says is in it actually is, in the correct amounts and free from contaminants. For this reason, the North American Menopause Society and the American College of Obstetricians and Gynecologists do not recommend the use of compounded hormones unless there is a compelling reason to do so, such as allergies or the need for nonstandard doses.

There are FDA-approved bioidentical hormones that are commercially available at your local CVS, Walgreens, or Costco. That being said, are all compounded hormones bad? Probably not. But think about it. Would you want to eat in a restaurant that *never* gets inspected by the health department?

- *What about testosterone?* For menopausal women with hypo-active sexual desire disorder (just a lot of words for the low libido that plagues so many of us), there is ample evidence that supplementing with low doses of testosterone is effective. Here's the problem: There are no FDA-approved testosterone prepara-tions for women in the United States. Okay, here we go again. There are FDA-approved testosterone medications for men because, well, of course only men need their sexual desire issues addressed. Right? (Use your powers of deduction here and you can probably feel my head about to explode.)

  So, what can you do? You can ask your doctor to prescribe the FDA-approved medications for men and titrate the dose downward. The recommended dose for women is typically one-tenth of the dose prescribed for men. But it is difficult to figure out how to dispense one-tenth of a patch or gel that most testosterone preparations come in. This might be the one instance where a compounded testosterone medication could be preferable. However, again, know your pharmacy.

Unlike with estrogen, you'll be required to have baseline blood tests before and after treatment to make sure that you are not exceeding the blood levels of testosterone that are normal for women. And, if you opt for a compounded testosterone medication, ask for a daily cream or troche that can be easily discontinued or adjusted if need be. Compounded testosterone pellets are not recommended because once a pellet is injected into your butt ('cause that's generally where they're placed), there is no way to remove it or adjust your dose. So, if it causes unwelcome side effects (acne, weight gain, and mood swings are a possible few), you'll just have to wait until it wears off, which could take up to six months. That's right: I said six *months*.

The Fight for Equity, the Need for Agency

In the UK, there's a huge grassroots movement of women, led by Dr. Louise Newson, the founder of the Newson Menopause Clinic, which has successfully advocated for access to doctors and hormone replacement therapy for all who want it. The tireless UK menopause advocates Kate Muir, author of *Everything You Need to Know About the Menopause,* and Davina McCall, maker of the documentary *Sex, Myths and the Menopause,* have brought menopause into the national spotlight. In fact, Parliament even appointed a hormone replacement czar to deal with the unprecedented demand for hormone therapy and the resultant shortages. The successes spearheaded in the UK targeting access to hormones, education, and issues in the workplace have provided the template for our advocacy here in the United States.

As we have now had two decades to unpack the limitations of the WHI, we have come not only to understand the problems with the study's design, but also the damage done by generalizing the complications and outcomes to all women, regardless of age.

The WHI was the genesis of the thinking that hormones are bad. And that mindset persists, not only in patients but in doctors as well.

It has stuck for twenty years. And during those two decades, a generation of women has suffered unnecessarily.

Many governing agencies—the American College of Obstetrics and Gynecologists, the North American Menopause Society, and the Endocrine Society, to name a few—amended their cautions about HRT in the 2022 guidelines. But you may have to swim upstream on this one and buck your doctors, who might still be making recommendations based on 2002 data. This is about having agency and being an advocate for yourself, and each woman must decide, *What is my quality of life worth to me?* Even if there is a treatment that is proven, but not perfect, I'm in favor of giving women all the information we currently have, then trusting them to decide for themselves.

There are huge movements now for menopause equity in the workplace. Women are saying that attention must be paid and accommodations must be made. There is now a veritable cottage industry of menopause consultants and HR specialists who are looking to "solve" this issue. But I add this caution: Women don't need fans and menopause leave. They need what their compatriots in the UK have been advocating for—access to healthcare, affordable treatments, and education on this important life stage. And to that, I say that it's about time [♪ "About Damn Time"].

Women who are on hormones tend to do better throughout menopause, in part because of the consistency of engagement with medical professionals that HRT requires. They keep going to their doctors, getting their mammograms, rectal screenings, and bone density tests as a part of their regular HRT monitoring.

I'm not preaching just for hormones; I'm preaching for agency. I don't want women to discount something (or allow their doctor or girlfriends to turn them away from an option) that might help them, not without learning all about it first, doing a risk-benefit analysis, and then leaning into their own instincts for deciding how to best address their needs.

Deciding among options requires a clear understanding of your medical history as well as your expectations and treatment goals. The

North American Menopause Society has affirmed what those of us who have been practicing OB/GYN for many years already know. For the majority of healthy symptomatic women, the benefits of hormone therapy far exceed the risks. But what I want most for all of you is to make a choice that feels right for you. Suffering cannot be your resting place.

If you feel good and have no issues as you make this transition, I'm truly happy for you. But don't let your menopausal good fortune influence how you speak to those who are not having an easy time with menopause. And for those of you choosing the "natural" route, if that is working for you, great. But you know what else is natural? Discomfort, disease, and death. I'm not judging, I'm just saying that "natural" has its limits.

My job is, and always has been, to educate my sisters about their choices, to clearly explain the risks and benefits, and to ensure that they can make informed choices. That's it.

The North American Menopause Society 2022 guidelines unequivocally state that for women who start using hormones before age 60 and within ten years of starting menopause, the benefits outweigh the risks. The guidelines also state that women should be partners in this decision, based on their own treatment expectations and risk profiles.

I know this may seem glaringly obvious to you, but it's major!

Let's compare this to medicine's approach to the lifestyle drugs for men, Viagra and Cialis, and for goodness' sake, there is now an over-the-counter gel for erectile dysfunction. (I think the directions say, apply to the penis and rub in briskly.) The potential side effects of Viagra and Cialis include facial flushing, headaches, stomach pain, nasal congestion, dizziness, rash, diarrhea, and urinary tract infections. These are just the nonserious ones. The more serious side effects, though rare, include heart attack; stroke; an erection lasting for more than four hours, leading to permanent damage to the penis; low blood pressure; fainting; and blindness. Fainting may seem like a minor side effect, but it's most assuredly not if you hit your head on a porcelain sink as you fall.

Have you seen any campaigns urging men to stop these potentially dangerous drugs? Me neither. Has there been a study that looked at what that wonder gel that men can buy over the counter does to a woman's vagina? My guess is no.

Medicine treats men like adults with agency. They get to weigh risks and benefits for themselves, and the annual sales of erectile dysfunction meds tell us what they are choosing. But when it comes to women, across the entire lifespan our right to govern our own healthcare decisions is continually under attack. For menopausal women, doctors have acted as gatekeepers, restricting the use of medications known to alleviate their suffering, and for what? Doctors and the media have used fear like a bludgeon to steer women away from the most effective and life-altering solution for symptomatic menopausal women. Given what is happening more broadly for women regarding our reproductive rights, can we be surprised? Meanwhile, we have been complicit, choosing to suffer because, culturally, that is what we've been conditioned to do.

Calculating and Managing
Your Menopausal Risks

After 50, as you firmly enter your menopausal years, it's time to reprioritize. Up to this point, you may have put yourself on the back burner. You've been tending to relationships, your children, your career, and you've been more or less successfully juggling it all. But at whose expense? Most likely yours. Now is the time to put yourself front and center [♪ "Love on Top"].

Before 50, we may have gotten away with murder—too little sleep, less-than-healthy diets, and too little exercise, with very little ill effect. But the things you might have gotten away with at 30 will extract a heavy price now, or as my mother would say, "You can pay me now or pay me later, but you gonna have to pay me" [♪ "Bitch Better Have My Money"]. *Everyone* at this stage should get enough sleep, exercise regularly, eat a healthy diet, limit alcohol intake, and see their doctors regularly for cardiovascular as well as cancer screenings. Easier said than done, I know. But if you do these things, you will be surprised at how much control you can exert.

Cardiovascular Health and Menopause

Tina

Tina is a healthy 52-year-old woman who had her last period at 50. Her menopausal transition was mild by most standards. She had some hot flashes and a few months of night sweats that kept her from getting enough sleep. Mercifully, most of her symptoms have subsided. She typically walks to her office each day, but since COVID she has shifted most of her work to her home. Her biggest complaint is her weight. Tina has put on twenty pounds during perimenopause and now, thanks to sitting all day on Zoom meetings, she has added another ten.

She has cut back on her alcohol and tried every fad diet, but the weight won't budge. She joined a gym, worked out religiously for two months, and didn't lose a pound. So, she stopped going. What she finds most distressing is this new weight has settled between her boobs and what used to be her waistline. She is desperate and is considering a tummy tuck and possibly a breast reduction. She is miserable and can't fit into any of her clothes.

The Takeaway: A tummy tuck and breast reduction may make you feel and look better temporarily, but they will do nothing for the fat that is accumulating on the inside. If you don't address the root cause of the problem (menopause), in another ten years or so, you will be right back where you started—and less healthy, to boot.

Remember when I told you that women tend to gain about ten pounds between the ages of 40 and 50, or those years during the menopausal transition? Okay, so sometimes it's more. (And for the record, I totally believe you when you say you haven't changed your diet or your exercise routine, but you are still gaining weight.) Typically, after menopause, the average weight gain of about a pound a year continues, not necessarily because of your hormones, but simply because of aging.

The fact is, menopause (or more specifically, the lack of estrogen) alters your body's composition. The loss of estrogen triggers a loss of lean muscle mass and an increased accumulation of fat. Less muscle not only makes you weaker, it also makes it more difficult to maintain any weight loss that you are able to achieve. Couple that with inevitable changes in your metabolism and a concomitant decrease in activity, and you may find yourself with a weight issue you never had before.

Weight gain is also associated with lack of sleep, which may be why women who take hormone replacement after menopause (effectively treating their night sweats) gain slightly less weight than those who do not.

Focusing on *not* gaining that pound a year is a start—necessary, but not sufficient. The best offense is still a good defense. And to launch that offense, you have to understand that not all weight gain is created equal. Increased weight in your midsection (closer to your heart) is more dangerous than in your hips and thighs because it can boost your risk for type 2 diabetes and heart disease. An increase in fat around your abdomen—regardless of weight increase or decrease—places you at risk for cardiovascular disease.

The more vigilant you are about controlling your weight gain, particularly near the end of perimenopause, the easier it will be to continue those healthy habits into menopause [♪ "The Weight"].

But here's the bottom line: I care more about how well you function than what you look like at this point in your life. By exercising regularly, specifically to maintain your muscle mass and strength, you are doing yourself a world of good even if you don't lose an ounce. And if you do manage to lose some weight, this newfound muscle mass will make that weight loss easier to maintain. Billy Crystal's classic impersonation of Fernando Lamas was not correct—it is *not* better to look good than to feel good. I want you to feel "mah-velous." Young people, if you don't know what I'm talking about, check it out on YouTube.

Genitourinary Syndrome of Menopause

To say that vaginal dryness is a bummer is an understatement. Many of you may already be experiencing a downshift in your libido after menopause. To add vulvar and vaginal dryness and pain to this mix is adding insult to injury. But it is pretty easy to see how a low interest in sex leads to less arousal, and less arousal leads to less lubrication, which leads to painful sex, which makes you even less interested in sex, and so on. This self-perpetuating cycle can quickly spiral into sexlessness. Oh, and did I mention that the low estrogen state of menopause can also cause thinning of the vulva (outer lips) and labia minora (the inner lips), which can make even nonpenetrative sex extra painful as well?

Vaginal dryness; itchy, dry vulvas; and painful sex are all part of the genitourinary syndrome of menopause (GSM). This syndrome encompasses a wide range of conditions involving the vulva, vagina, and urinary system that can affect up to 80 percent of women after menopause. These symptoms can show up early in perimenopause or years after you thought you were all done with menopause. Although some women are able to manage with over-the-counter moisturizers or vaginal lubricants, these products only treat the symptoms. Vaginal estrogen repairs and restores the vaginal mucosa itself. Topical/vaginal estrogen is FDA-approved for the treatment of GSM. But to be effective, it needs to be used consistently.

Urinary Tract Health

Menopausal women experience more urinary urgency, frequency, and incontinence, as well as an increased incidence of urinary tract infections. These urinary changes also fall under the GSM rubric. Urinary symptoms are more than just annoying and inconvenient. Urinary tract infections are the second-most common cause for hospitalization in older people who live at home and the most common cause for hospitalizations for the elderly in nursing homes. The cost to the healthcare system each year is $2–3 billion per year. You know what is a primary cause of all these infections? The urinary tract and vaginal changes that accompany long-term estrogen deprivation and the changes in the vaginal ecosystem—all of which make elderly women more susceptible to infections. Know what will prevent them? Vaginal estrogen.

Osteoporosis: Careful, Don't Fall!

Wouldn't it be the ultimate bummer if you did everything you were supposed to do to stay healthy during menopause—managed your weight and blood pressure, avoided diabetes, kept intellectually active and socially (and sexually!) engaged, only to trip over an extension cord, hit your head, and develop dementia as a result? Or break your hip and end up hospitalized with a permanent loss of mobility? It happens more than you realize.

In the realm of what's important for you to know about aging and menopause, one of the greatest risks to your long-term independence and well-being is one that we least talk about, think about, or do anything about: falls [♪ **"We Fall Down"**]. Consequently, 1 in 4 adults over the age of 65 will experience a fall within the year. And the fallout (forgive me, I'm just trying to keep things light) could be life-altering.

Falls are not just embarrassing, like the TikTok reels you scroll through late at night. They can be the source of permanent disability or even death. Falls that result in head injury are one of the more common causes of dementia in the elderly. Head trauma is one of the top five reasons for cognitive decline. And for reasons that are not entirely clear, women's brains are more susceptible to damage after head trauma. Even if you are mentally vibrant and young at heart, here is the reality: 95 percent of hip fractures are due to falls, and a hip fracture is often the first medical event in a cascade ultimately leading to death.

Women make up three-quarters of all hip fractures, most likely because we make up a disproportionate share of those with osteoporosis. Osteoporosis is a systemic disorder that causes bones to become brittle and weak, leading to an increased risk of fractures, particularly in the spine and hips. Women are four times more likely than men to develop osteoporosis and your risk steadily increases after age 50.

In the year before your final menstrual period, and continuing for about five years after, bone loss accelerates (after that, bone loss continues, albeit at a slower pace). But this isn't something you're likely to notice or even think about until you experience a fracture. A study led by Juan Blumel, published in the September 2022 issue of the journal *Menopause,* followed a group of midlife women for thirty years. The purpose of the study was to see which health-risk factors were more predictive of death. They found that a personal history of a fracture was more predictive of dying within the study period than a history of cardiovascular disease, diabetes, and hypertension. This should underscore how important osteoporosis and fall prevention are. So, if you have a family history of hip fractures or other risk factors, including rheumatoid arthritis, smoking, and alcoholism, or if you have had a fracture (and I don't mean from a ski or car accident), ask your doctor about getting a bone density test. There is also an online tool called

FRAX that will estimate your fracture risk in the next ten years, based on your age, gender, BMI, alcohol and medication intake, and smoking habits.

Hormone therapy is FDA-approved for the *prevention* of osteoporosis, not treatment. If you are a smoker or have had an early menopause, your risk of osteoporosis is increased. The earlier you start hormone therapy after menopause, the more bone density you save. Remember, the goal is to preserve your bone density, not to try to regain it later.

There is a misperception in the medical community that Black women don't get osteoporosis. This is a dangerous myth that can prevent Black women from getting the information, screening, and treatment they need. While Black women do have a lower incidence of osteoporosis, it is not that being Black lowers one's risk, it is the size of one's bones that matters. Smaller bones are at greater risk for osteoporosis than larger bones. Thus, a thin Black woman with small bones carries the same risk of developing osteoporosis as a similarly sized white woman. So, be wary if your doctor says you are not at risk simply because of your race. When in doubt, just get a bone density test.

What is not commonly known is that Black women are more likely to suffer ill effects from hip fractures. In fact, Black women are more likely to die or be permanently disabled within the first year of a hip fracture than white women. Why are hip fractures so dangerous? Because of the high likelihood of complications that ensue from them, such as an increased risk of blood clots, pneumonia, and progressive, debilitating weakness. Hip fractures are one of the most common reasons for older people's loss of independence. They can cause older menopausal women who are otherwise healthy and vibrant to lose their independence and require in-home or inpatient nursing care. Almost any significant fall injury can lead to temporary or long-term loss of function, autonomy, and dignity.

I know that sounds grim, but let this be an incentive for you to avoid the pitfalls that could lead down this road. Hopefully, you are decades away from having to deal with these issues. But whether you are or not, don't turn away; get serious about what you can do to reduce your fall risk. If you are fortunate enough to still have parents, this information will be helpful for them as well. The simplest way to avoid trauma-associated dementia or a loss of independence, which may lead to death? Don't fall! As your own primary caregiver, your goal always is to confront issues before they happen, not after.

Time feels like it speeds up as we age, and the changes can come at a rapid clip too. The more you can anticipate those changes, the better off you'll be. God willing, we will all live to be old one day. And you know by now that I never give you bad news unless I've got some good news to share. The take-home message is that many falls are indeed preventable, and yes, there are things you can do to minimize your risk [♪"Help Me"]. You can start by becoming hyperaware of the three most common contributors to heightened fall risk: impairment due to medication (or overmedication); vision problems (stay on top of your annual eye screenings and any resulting prescriptions and visual aids); and muscle weakness (see Dr. Sharon's Rx).

Also, incorporate these tips on how to reduce your risk of falling into your daily life:

- Check your medications and their interactions with your doctor (antihypertensive medications and diuretics are notorious for causing weakness, dehydration, and fainting).

- Secure loose rugs, keep pathways in your home and office unobstructed (pay special attention to extension cords and chargers).

- Use nightlights if you frequently get up to go to the bathroom at night.

- If you use bifocals, be aware that when descending stairs, your depth perception is compromised because when you look down, you are likely looking through the reading portion.

- Get your eyes checked annually. Your vision naturally changes with age.

- Walk, don't run, down stairs. Counting stairs as you go helps you pace yourself safely.

- Never walk down stairs with your arms full. Always hold the handrail, even if you don't need to (and especially if you're wearing slippers, mules, or high heels).

- Avoid walking while you are on your phone. While you are talking, you are not situationally aware.

- Check your footwear. Only you know for sure when you should give up those Manolos, and for goodness' sake, toss those flip-flops. There are plenty of options to keep you cute and safe. (It's never too late to become a sneakerhead.)

- Stay off ladders or footstools unless you have a spotter. Better still, have a young person reach what you need, just like you used to for your mom. (There's no shame in that game.)

- Apple and Google watches have fall-prevention and fall-detection features (and their competitors won't be far behind). A sudden change in your motion metrics will trigger a loud alarm to alert those around you, followed by a series of displays that require your responses. Without them, the watch will automatically call 911 and your emergency contact if you specified one.

The Takeaway: Pay attention! Being situationally aware is key to avoiding unnecessary mishaps [♪ "Same Thing It Took"].

DR. SHARON'S RX FOR
a Mah-velous Fourth Quarter

1. **Exercise regularly.** Remember our exercise goals after 50 are different. Do not exercise because you are hoping to lose weight. You will be disappointed. Exercise after 50 is to preserve your muscle mass and strength as you age. Include resistance and core exercises to improve balance. Maintaining a strong core will decrease your risk of falling and increase your chances of being able to get yourself off the floor if you do.

2. **Mind your cardiovascular health.** This begins with eliminating the things that increase your risk. Treat hot flashes and sleeplessness. Watch your weight. Take your medications for hypertension . . . every day!

3. **Maintain a calcium– and vitamin D–rich diet.** You start to lose bone mass after menopause if you do not take estrogen. Although calcium and vitamin D do not prevent osteoporosis, they are key nutrients that are necessary for bone health, as well as many other bodily functions. Your calcium intake after 50 should increase to 1,000–1,200mg daily with vitamin D 600–800 IU daily. Dietary sources are *always* better than supplements. Now I know why my mother made me take cod-liver oil in the winter. My mother was a genius! Get your vitamin D levels checked if you are lactose intolerant, are darker-skinned, use total body sunscreen, wear a hijab, or don't like the outdoors. Your body can make its own vitamin D, but only if you have exposure to sunlight at least twenty minutes a day.

4. **Don't smoke!** Smokers have a higher incidence of osteoporosis and more severe menopausal symptoms.

5. **Know your bone density.** I recommend getting a baseline DEXA Scan as soon as you're menopausal, especially if you have a family history of osteoporosis, have had a fracture in the past, smoke, or have poor dietary calcium intake—e.g., are lactose intolerant—or if you are currently taking thyroid medication. The standard recommendation is 65, but don't let that be your guide.

6. **Consider menopausal hormone therapy.** Estrogen is FDA-approved for osteoporosis prevention and is the most effective medication for relief of menopausal symptoms.

7. **Use topical vaginal estrogen.** It not only prevents vaginal dryness and preserves sexual function, but also decreases the risk of UTIs as you age.

CHAPTER 11

Here Comes the Sun♪

Live Your *Best* Menopausal Life

Dear Sis,

You made it!

You've learned tons of valuable lessons and have a stack of strong moves to stand on. Sure, you have a regret (or a few), but regrets keep us humble, don't they? And they make us wise.

You've survived some deep losses and disappointments, and guess what: You're still here! And with no more time or patience for the nonsense, I'm sure. So, I'll keep this short.

Whatever your "it" is, it's time to use it. Not because you'll lose it, necessarily, but because if not now, *when*? And that applies to your good jewelry and your good dishes and whatever else good that you think you've got. If nobody else ever eats off that plate but you, you deserve it!

You're not just getting older, you're increasing in value, so refuse to drift into the background; make your favorite age *now*. Then do it again next year. And the next, and so on. Never, ever, ever give up! More than any life stage before it, this really is *your* time. So, lean all the way in, smile (it's a great workout for your face), and keep reminding yourself that it ain't over till it's over.

Final tip: When all else fails, vibrate! And don't act like you don't know what I'm talking about.

xo, Dr. Sharon

n medicine, we have specific, reliable means for monitoring your four primary vital signs: body temperature, heart rate, respiratory rate, blood pressure. We can also test your blood and urine to gauge the condition of vital organs, like your kidneys and liver. At the height of the COVID pandemic, the CDC encouraged people to add a pulse oximeter to their collection of handy health aids. So, we can now measure our own blood oxygen levels at home. And anybody who works out regularly probably already wears a fitness device that keeps constant track of everything from their daily steps to their heart rate and the length and quality of their sleep.

Yet we still have not figured out how to definitively track one of the most critical components of your vitality—dare I say, your vital signs. And that's your state of mind.

Why is the quality of your mental health as important as your more quantifiable vital signs? Because how you feel about getting older, and life in general, will help determine how you handle everything that aging brings.

That list I keep repeating like you didn't hear me the first fifty times is a big part of keeping not only your body strong, but also keeping your moods stabilized. Keep in mind that physical illness is often a threat to emotional wellness, and vice versa. This is especially true as the years creep up. So, staying as well as you can is more than worth the effort.

Killing it as you age requires you to get good at the DIY practice of guarding your mental state. This could mean limiting your intake of headline news or friends who do nothing but complain or criticize. Or your children's struggles, which they will have (and have to get through) whether you wrap yourself up in them or not. Try to master the ability to empathize without allowing yourself to get consumed, even when those you love are involved.

Better yet, master the art of saying no. Without excuses. Without apology. Without blinking. You've earned that right. The late PBS journalist and my dear friend Gwen Ifill was brilliant at this. Her trusty response to anything outside of her yes zone was, "No, I couldn't possibly," followed by silence. How do you even respond to that? The deal was always sealed.

The good news is, saying no to the people, places, and things that you know are going to literally wear you out gets easier as we get older. But that doesn't make staying mentally fit a layup. It requires you to routinely self-check:

- **Your Moods:** It is normal to have highs and lows that may not always directly correspond to what's happening in your life. But when bad moods stretch into days, pay attention. If your moods interfere with your sleeping, eating, or ability to get things done, don't dismiss the issue. Attempt to course-correct and seek professional help if you feel you need it.

- **Your Emotions:** Humans are emotional beings, and our range of emotions is complex and highly changeable. Thus, our ability to control those emotions is highly sophisticated—and necessary. Your daily behavior should not be governed by your feelings. Neither should your work or relationships. If your feelings are literally out of control and getting in the way of your life, you need to develop better skills for managing them. And yes, sometimes medication helps.

- **Your Thoughts:** The truth is often as simple as what we tell ourselves, so if you tell yourself your best days are behind you, they probably will be. It's also true that whatever we focus on multiplies. So, practice gratitude—and learn to short-circuit negative thoughts before they take hold and spread.

- **Your Stresses:** In American culture, retirement is lauded as "the good life," invoking levels of ease that life never really delivers. The sources of your stress and anxiety may change over time, but you will always need healthy stress-management tools to use, daily. Seek calming, comforting, or uplifting activities. Always have a purpose that motivates you. Keep affirmations—and affirming individuals—at hand. Generally, make like that old song and accentuate the positive [♪ **"Ac-Cent-Tchu-Ate the Positive"**].

- **Your People:** Not much holds more power over you than the people to whom you are closest. There's a quote from *Othello* that says, "Thou hast not half that power to do me harm as I have to be hurt." The point being, you can't control those around you—even those who love you. You can only control you. Feed your positive relationships, starve the bad ones, and the rest will take care of itself.

- **Your Soul:** As influential as others may be, nothing has greater impact than how you treat yourself, how you see yourself, and what you tell yourself about yourself. As trite as it sounds, forgive yourself, learn to silence your inner critic, and love yourself. In a culture that may be quick to diminish or dismiss your value as you age, you've got to become your own best hype-person. (If needed, cue up Sheryl Lee Ralph at the 2022 Emmys for a quick how-to.)

- **Your Future:** If you nurse a belief that the best is yet to come, all gates will stay open to that possibility. Just as I advised you to learn to say no, learn to say yes to the things that bring you joy. And don't look for excuses as to why you can't or won't or shouldn't.

Be Resilient, Like a Ross

"I do feel like so many doors are open to me now. And it started for me in my 40s. I'm really grateful I have a mom [Diana Ross] who's 75 . . . gorgeous, sexy, and full of agency. So that's what I long to walk toward."

—Tracee Ellis Ross, 51, *Variety,* June 2019

Gorgeous and sexy at 75 is a great goal. But mental strength and emotional resilience are going to come in a lot handier in your day-to-day. These traits fuel confidence and self-worth, which in turn fuel agency. Agency has a beauty and power all its own. And at this stage of your life, you'll need it more than ever.

Self-worth can take its sweet time developing, can't it? Luckily, you've now had that time. The time to understand yourself, what you want, and what you need is one of the blessings of age that no surges or dips in estrogen can touch. And it's not the only one.

At the age of 64—classically known as retirement age—the great entertainer and beauty Lena Horne conquered Broadway with her eponymous show, *Lena Horne: The Lady and Her Music.* It became the longest-running solo performance in Broadway history and launched another twenty-year stretch of her career. Not just any old stretch, by the way, a spectacular one! Arguably the most successful and fulfilling of her life.

When Horne died in 2010 at the age of 92, her obituary in *The New York Times* quoted her at 80, reflecting on it all. "My identity is very clear to me now," she said. "I am a black woman. I'm free. I no longer have to be a 'credit.' I don't have to be a symbol to anybody; I don't have to be a first to anybody. I don't have to be an imitation of a white woman that Hollywood sort of hoped I'd become. I'm me, and I'm like nobody else" [♪ **"Beautiful Life"**].

If ever there was a healthy goal to reach for, it's that: being fully at peace with yourself, who you've been, and who you have become. Nobody gets there without taking some tough hits along the way. No woman, especially, gets there without having fallen down and gotten back up—on repeat. That getting up builds muscle and resilience. And thank God, because getting old demands both.

Resiliency is defined by the *Oxford English Dictionary* as "the capacity to withstand or to recover quickly from difficulties." We often refer to it as toughness or the ability to bounce back. It's that old Timex watch tagline about being able to "take a licking and keep on ticking." Not limping, not masking, or suffering in silence, but actually recovering. And while some of us may be more practiced at resilience than others, we all have the capacity to develop this skill.

Mission Critical: Connectedness and Community

I absolutely love the community of women. You might enjoy solitude, but most of us prefer to have someone around to share our joys and our grief. Some recent studies contend that having a solid sense of belonging and community is as essential to your well-being as healthy eating habits and a good night's sleep.

I have been extraordinarily blessed in that I have friends from every phase of my life—elementary school, high school, college, and work. I have parenting friends, couple-friends, and once-new friends who have become old friends. The point is this: Don't be afraid to find friends wherever you are in life. And don't stop just because you've gotten older [♪ "Count on Me"].

I like to think of my network of friendships as a Venn diagram. Many of the circles intersect. Some never do. Just because I like a person doesn't mean everyone has to. Trust me, sometimes separation reduces the drama.

My oldest friend, Karen Michelle, moved in around the corner from me in Mobile when she was 5 and I was 7. After three years, her family moved and what started out as a friendship of convenience flourished,

The 7 C's of Resilience*

1. **Competence**—the ability to face, process, and accept challenges.

2. **Confidence**—the belief in yourself, your strengths, and your ability to thrive, no matter what.

3. **Connection**—having close, dependable ties to others who will encourage and support your efforts to persevere, as well as a connection to yourself and how you operate under pressure.

4. **Character**—having a solid, healthy set of values that underscores your treatment of others and your approach to life.

5. **Contribution**—having a sense of purpose, along with a strong commitment to that and to what you have to offer the world, helps to steady you when other things fall apart.

6. **Creativity**—mindfulness, humor, hobbies—it's important to have a set of healthy go-to coping skills and strategies for helping you navigate difficulties rather than succumb to them.

7. **Control**—staying clear and intentional about what you can always control—your decisions, actions, words, even your thoughts (with some effort) help you overcome anxiety and fear.

*Compiled from the work of several human-development experts who have tweaked them over time even though it wasn't as easy to get together. Over more than five decades, that has never changed.

Dede and I met the first week of freshman year in college. Have you ever met a person who you knew you liked immediately? Well, that's Dede. I loved her at first sight even though I hated just about everything about our school. She was responsible for talking me into transferring after freshman year. I was just prepared to grumble for the next three years. Dede and I would not live in the same city again for over a decade. But distance has never been a hindrance to our closeness, which has only deepened over time.

My first true adult friend, Bonnie, and I met in IBM training classes in Dallas, Texas. She lived in Boston. I lived in Atlanta. We, too, did not live in the same city for over twenty years, yet in every way that mattered, we were never apart.

Darya, my Iranian soul sister, and I met in the trenches of my OB/GYN residency. I was new to D.C., with no family, and Darya helped fill that void. One might wonder what a girl born in Iran and a girl born in Mobile, Alabama, would have in common. Turns out a lot, including being die-hard Earth, Wind & Fire fans. After one really tough night on call, Darya volunteered to go with me to pick out my wedding dress. Short on time and money, we went to one store and picked out The Dress in less than an hour. To this day, she is one of my dearest friends [♪ "September"].

My oldest and dearest friends are a life force for me, and we've stayed close because we put in the effort. No matter what has gone on in our lives—moves across the country, career changes, marriages, child rearing, divorces, deaths—we've always found ways to prioritize our connection. I often think of how bereft I would have been to not have them. After all, they have been at the center of my life for most of it. They know where all the proverbial bodies are buried (I said *proverbial*!). When we see one another, we can still see the 20-year-old girls that we once were. We can never be old in one another's eyes.

Our small circle is tight as a drum and as dependable as the sunrise. Along with the other circles of friends in my world, they have made me smarter, calmer, saner, braver—and they grow more precious and essential to me with every passing year. We see one another for exactly who and what we are, and we love one another anyway. And don't even get me started on the things we have seen one another through! These women have held me (or put me back) together on days when I felt so broken, I made Humpty Dumpty look like Superman.

I'm hoping you can relate and have a great friend group of your own. If not, it's time to get one. If ever there was a life-hack worth the effort, it's this one. Nurturing your connections and sense of community does more than fill your social calendar, it strengthens your health.

Understand that you can have different categories of friendships, each filling a particular need at a specific time in your life. And no, that's not being opportunistic, it's being realistic. No one person can be expected to fulfill all your needs—not even your spouse or partner.

Friendships can be based on a common mission, such as raising children or carpooling for sporting events; or a shared passion, like travel, reading, or music. The keys are mutuality and authenticity. Strong friendships require intention and careful tending until they take root. Even the best friendships can die on the vine if left untended. You might also have to occasionally pull some weeds, but that's the exception rather than the rule. Sometimes you just have to "Marie Kondo" some folks. Pay attention to how your friends treat others, not just you. Let me urge you again to keep in mind what Maya Angelou said, "When someone shows you who they are, believe them the first time." Truer words have never been spoken.

Friendships, like partnerships or marriages, may last a lifetime, peter out with a whimper, or go up in flames. Your best bet, health-wise, is to cultivate an ability to roll with them without growing cynical about the value of connectedness, even when it goes wrong.

In Making New Friends, Does Age Matter?

The short answer to that question is yes. And to those of you who think it's easier to make friends when you're young, you may be right. But so what? Having sex may be easier when you're young, but that's no reason to stop (more on that coming up). Life is less complicated when you're younger and likely to have more time, less stress, and fewer expectations—and scars. As we age, we become less open and less willing to be vulnerable. We start to question the motives of our adult relationships as we get older, and that can be limiting—right at a time when making new friends is possibly more important than ever.

True friendship requires vulnerability. Don't be afraid to take a chance, especially on new people. Trust your gut. You'll be right more often than you're wrong about them. Age and experience give you an advantage here.

While you're assessing others, don't forget to take a hard look at yourself. Ask yourself: Am I trustworthy? Am I kind? Am I generous of spirit? If the answer to any of these questions is no, then you have work to do. Be the friend you want to have. And your mama's advice in first grade still works: smile, introduce yourself, be kind, and share. A few other things to try:

- Join a club or reengage with one that you've let lag (sorority, book club, social club).

- Take a class—especially an interactive one like cooking, quilting, martial arts.

- Join or become more involved in a spiritual home.

- Volunteer around a cause that excites you.

- Learn a new team sport or game (pickleball or bridge, anyone?) or a language.

- Invite acquaintances to do things you're already doing or invite each of your friends to bring a friend the next time you gather.

- Say "yes" to the invitations that come your way—especially those that involve new people.

Beyond that, as Michelle Obama says in her book *The Light We Carry*, to form new friendships later in life, we sometimes need to do something we unconsciously did as children: step out on faith. I learned a lot from Michelle as I watched her make new friends—myself included—when she first moved into the White House.

Michelle

When Michelle and I met for the first time, Barack was a new senator in D.C., and she was still living in Chicago. We were seated across the table from each other at one of those interminable dinners where people were constantly approaching our husbands for glad-handing and photos.

One of our dinner companions said something ridiculous, and Michelle and I exchanged a glance that if put into words would have been an essay. Our mutual understanding of the situation was immediate. She smiled. I smiled. Our shared look said it all. I wouldn't see her again for a couple of years, but we both remembered that moment.

When she moved to D.C., before she had even moved into her new home, someone from her staff reached out to arrange lunch. We scheduled an hour. We talked for three. Michelle trusted her gut and chose to take a chance to bring me into her circle. And I wasn't the only one.

She defied the mantra "no new friends" that can easily come with age, visibility, or status—especially in a place like D.C., and most especially in a vulnerable position like First Lady.

Michelle assembled what she calls her "kitchen table," a core circle of old and new friends, several of whom would become my good friends as well. We were late-in-life friends who laughed together, cried together, rejoiced in one another's successes, and lifted one another up in our failures. We gave one another advice and shared stories of our careers, our children, and our health crises in what became a circle of total trust.

When she started this journey sixteen years ago, Michelle wasn't just building new friendships, she was building a new chapter in her life. A lot was beyond her control, and she became very focused on controlling what she could. That didn't just mean identifying who she trusted and spent personal time with, but how we spent that time.

When she introduced the idea of our going on these girlfriends' retreats at Camp David, I was thinking lounging, cocktails, and massages. So, that was an easy *yes*! In actuality, they turned out to be more like Marine boot camps. Our schedule went something like this: morning cardio before breakfast, followed by group exercises and another workout after lunch. If you're keeping count, that's exercise three times a day. I ain't gonna lie. I was more of a three-times-a-week girl. But once I was in, I was all in.

I have never worked out as hard as we did in those boot camps. And now I know why they call them "suicide drills." (Trust me, if I can do them, you can too.) But the physical strength we developed during those weekends was not the most durable effect. It was the psychological boost and emotional support those gatherings provided. These "retreats" offered an opportunity to improve our health and stamina, and to decompress from the stresses of our daily lives. But what made it all doable and, I have to admit, fun, was that we did it together, as friends.

The Takeaway: There is an African proverb that says, "If you want to go fast, go alone. If you want to go far, go together." Michelle really showed me that getting and staying healthy is something we are far better off doing together.

Longer, Better Life: That's What Friends Are For

Recent studies have flipped the script on the science of relationships in ways that are both enlightening and encouraging, especially for women of a certain age, since most of us are without a partner or will end up there due to divorce or widowhood (harsh, perhaps, but true). Those of us with a community of friends will likely endure those life changes—and others—more easily.

Maybe you've seen the meme: Sisterhood Is Medicine. It's true.

While romantic love was long celebrated for all sorts of health benefits, including lower stress; better diet; lower blood pressure; and longer, happier lifespans, there is evidence today that people with strong platonic friendships enjoy better physical and mental health as they age than those who don't. Furthermore, those with large social networks do better than those with just a partner or small network [♪ "That's What Friends Are For"].

There are several theories about the correlation between friendship and better health. Some are practical. For example, it's easier to make friends if you're healthy than if you're disabled or sick. Large social networks also offer a broad support system for both medical care (e.g., rides to the doctor, help with medical advocacy, and short-term home care) and emotional well-being.

Other benefits are less obvious, even less explicable, but that doesn't make them any less meaningful. Take the study that found those with strong networks to have stronger immune responses to the cold virus. Say what? True.

For years, the belief was that married men outlived single men by a fair margin. But a six-year study of middle-aged Swedish men found that having a life partner had no measurable effect on their risk of heart attack or fatal coronary disease, but having friends did. (Why were only men studied, you ask. Why was there no parallel study done on women? Clearly, gender disparities in medical research is a problem not limited to the United States.)

One study of more than 1,000 Australians over the age of 70 found that those with lots of friends were 22 percent less likely to die during the ten-year study period than those with few friends (even if those same people had children and other relatives).

The CDC has connected the dots between isolation and higher rates of depression, anxiety, and suicide. NIH-funded research has linked social isolation and loneliness to high blood pressure, heart disease, obesity, a weakened immune system, cognitive decline, Alzheimer's disease, and even death.

Women who find themselves alone due to the death of a spouse or partner (or even a longtime pet), or who experience a loss of mobility or lack of transportation, are particularly at risk. According to the CDC, loneliness can increase the risk of heart disease in older women by as much as 27 percent. It's important to note that although about one-third of older adults live alone, according to the Administration for Community Living's Administration on Aging, that does not in and of itself correlate to chronic loneliness. It is also possible to live with others, including a spouse, partner, roommates, or within an entire community designed to offset such concerns, as in assisted-living settings, and still feel intense loneliness.

The pandemic gave way to what some have described as a loneliness epidemic in this country. In fact, one of the pandemic's lesser-known costs was not just in actual friendships lost due to COVID deaths, but in the lost ability to simply spend time with friends, sharing experiences, making memories, and nurturing those relationships. In a 2021 American Enterprise Institute poll, 12 percent of Americans said they had no close friends, and roughly half admitted to having lost touch with one or more friends during the pandemic. The heightened risk of getting COVID among older adults put them in a prolonged state of higher alert than most, which only intensified their isolation.

Some of us not only became used to our pandemic-imposed solitude, we became comfortable in it. But comfortable doesn't mean optimal. Research done at UCLA's Social Genomics Core Laboratory has found that the loss of a sense of connection and community changes a person's perception of the world, which then changes their interactions with it, making them distrustful, even paranoid. That can lead to a defensive posture that only creates further isolation and loneliness, triggering a vicious cycle that's easier to avoid than to break. So, guard against it. Never stop expanding your circles of friends. It's doable, once you're aware.

Amy

Other than being parents of children at the same school, I couldn't imagine that Amy and I had anything in common. She was a stay-at-home mom who grew up in a Chicago suburb and had lived all over the world. I was an often-overwhelmed working mom from Mobile.

She was the classroom parent always bringing the creative decorations and tasty, homemade treats. I was always forgetting it was my turn to bring snacks after the soccer games.

That's all I knew when she approached me one day at the school drop-off to invite me over for coffee. *Coffee?* I sniffed inwardly. *Who's got time for coffee?* Okay, I did have a day off during the week to make up for a 24-hour on-call day. But still. I politely declined.

Then Amy asked me again . . . and again . . . and again.

Just as I was about to write her off as a well-meaning stalker, I relented and showed up at her house. I cannot tell you how surprised I was when assembled around her kitchen island was the most diverse, interesting group of women I had seen in a long time.

There were a few people I knew and many I didn't. When I asked, "How do you know Amy?" the answers covered everything from "I met her in the grocery store" to "She read my book and wrote to me and invited me over." Amy routinely went out of her way to approach people she thought were interesting, and it wasn't about who was famous or powerful, it was simply about who piqued her curiosity. It turned out that they piqued mine too.

After that first coffee, I was hooked. If I didn't have time, I made time. And we had some of the most fun and interesting conversations around her kitchen island that I've ever had.

The Takeaway: Sometimes, you just have to say yes. And if you're lucky, you might find yourself an Amy.

Cultivate and Celebrate Intimacy
(and yes, that includes solo sex!)

Lower libido, dryness, pain. So much of the later-in-life sex narrative for women is just sad. Deflated by terms like *vaginal atrophy* and statistics that show our odds of finding and keeping a mate shifting, almost literally, from under-40 slim to over-40 none, many of us quit. We give up wanting, expecting, even hoping for a satisfying love life, no less sex life. I urge you: don't.

For starters, there are all kinds of love. And the love of friends can, in the long run, prove more dependable, satisfying, and even healthy than romantic love. It's worth adding that the more open you remain to new friendships, the more you improve your chances for new relationships of all kinds to enter your orbit.

As for sex and intimate pleasure, they're more in your control than you think, assuming you are—here's that word again—*open* to seeking it, with a partner or without [♪"Sexual Healing"]. There are a couple of medications on the market for female libido, but we're not where we should be. Why, you might ask? It's because no one is really looking that hard. This is yet another area where we need more research and more solutions. It's taken this many years for Dr. Rachel Rubin, a sexual medicine specialist and self-proclaimed clitorologist, to point out that no one has bothered to study the clitoris. Ever. Not only have medical educators and researchers ignored it, most of them didn't even know what it actually looked like. Hint—it's way more than meets the eye.

In a 2018 article published in the *Archives of Sexual Behavior,* Dr. Talia Shirazi found that, when asked specifically about orgasm frequency, less than 30 percent of women reported being able to have an orgasm with intercourse alone. Did anyone tell women's magazines and the movie industry? Did anyone tell women? Do you have any idea how many women have felt inadequate and have faked orgasms for years to appease their partners while thinking that something must be wrong with them?

Why did no one tell women that this is not only normal, it's common? Given the state of our current knowledge, it shouldn't surprise us that we don't have surefire solutions to our sexual issues at any age, much less at any advanced age. But as you know by now, there's always some good news and advice I'd like to share—if you don't own a vibrator, go get one. Seriously, it will change your life. Whether you have a partner or not, if you would like some reliability to your sex life, there's your answer. The most important thing to remember here is that intimate pleasure does not require anyone's willingness but yours.

Get Your Vagina Together

Mindfulness is a valuable tool for good health, but when it comes to sex, mind over matter will only take you so far. Menopause may affect every woman differently, but it absolutely impacts every woman sexually (see Chapter 10).

Sex after 50 can be a lot of things, but one thing it's not is sex at 20 or 30. Sex after 50 is something you plan for and create, not something you sit idly by waiting for, because you could be waiting forever. It's like that popular definition of insanity. If you're unsatisfied sexually and you want different outcomes, you have to do things differently. Start by realizing that you have plenty of options. Understand what they are and discuss them with your doctor—and your friends!

When you're 30 or 40, you can have sex now, and then a year from now, and you won't notice much of a difference because your vagina is still good to go. It's healthy, supple, and elastic, and is just waiting for the proper motivation. That changes once your estrogen starts to retreat during perimenopause and then disappears completely after menopause. The vagina thins. It becomes less pliable and has a diminished ability to lubricate on its own. The hormonal downshift in estrogen also alters the pH of your vagina. For those of you who slept through that part of chemistry class, pH determines whether something is acidic (like vinegar) or basic (think baking soda). For the record, your vaginal pH should be on the acidic side. Different bacteria grow in an acidic environment than in an alkaline one. Just like your gut, your vagina has an entire ecosystem living in there. And no, that's not gross. It's good. Because the bacteria that thrive in an acidic environment protect you from the bad types of bacteria that can cause odor, itching, discomfort, and discharge. Antibiotics may help temporarily, but a better solution is to change the milieu, or environment, in which the bacteria live.

But let me be clear, a healthy vagina is a self-cleaning organ. If your mama never said this, take it from me: No woman needs to douche. And you surely do not need to steam clean or put anything into your vagina (other than estrogen) to keep it healthy. Ever. Mild soap and water (only on the outside) works. If it doesn't, see your doctor.

For many older women, pain or discomfort isn't an issue, they simply complain of a lack of responsiveness or arousal, which leaves their level of natural lubrication and/or general interest in sex lagging. If that sounds familiar, don't give up. This is not a close-your-eyes-and-think-of-England situation. It's a get-that-fixed situation, because you can. The tired advice to "use it or lose it" is catchy but not always helpful, especially if sexual partners are not readily available (or are contending with their own sexual challenges). The truth is, you never really lose it. Remember, for many of you, an entire human being came out of there, so let's just say you have the capacity. But if you haven't had sex in a few years, you may have to rehabilitate it. Think of it as physical therapy for your vagina. We have solutions, and many of them are noninvasive and fairly simple. In addition to vaginal dilators (graduated in size) that can help improve the elasticity of your vagina, you can enlist the help of a pelvic floor physical therapist. See, there's more help available than you probably realized. Just ask your OB/GYN for a referral.

The simplest and most cost-effective way to decrease vulvovaginal (say *that* four times fast) symptoms and improve vaginal dryness is with topical, or vaginal, estrogen. Unlike with basic lubricants or moisturizers, topical estrogen repairs and restores the tissue rather than just treating the symptoms. Vaginal estrogen can be used in the form of creams, suppositories, tablets, or vaginal rings, all of which require a prescription. Unlike systemic hormones (HRT), they can be used almost universally and without a progestin, because the dose is extremely low. Which form to use should be based on personal preference and cost. And no, I didn't forget about intravaginal DHEA (dehydroepiandrosterone), which is marketed under the trade name of Intrarosa. DHEA is simply the hormonal precursor from which estrogen and testosterone are made. Its effectiveness is based on being converted inside the cell to the active hormones. I've never prescribed it, and it's not because I think it is ineffective. I don't use it because it's expensive, and by now you know how I feel about expensive medications. If the old one works, why change?

Compliance is key with vaginal estrogen. Because it works to restore the vulvar and vaginal tissue itself by stimulating collagen growth and thickening of the mucosa, it needs to be used consistently. Once you stop using it, within a few weeks to months, your symptoms can return. So, choose what you will, at a price point that works for you, but remember to use it consistently. Also check which products are covered by your insurance.

I cannot tell you how many times I've prescribed a topical vaginal estrogen, only to discover when the patient comes back a year later, and I ask, "How's that working out," the answer is, "Oh, I didn't use it." When I ask why, it is almost always the same: There's a warning on every estrogen product that sounds so scary, many women just say, "Never mind." Which is why many of us are advocating for removal of the warning. In fact, there is even a nascent lobbying effort to make vaginal estrogen available over-the-counter. Okay, I started that rumor, but let's go ahead and speak it into existence.

The most important thing is to not just accept that life goes on without sex. It will, but why let it when you don't have to?

The (Future) Joy of Sex

By the year 2030, according to the U.S. Census Bureau, one out of every five Americans will be 65 or older. Our longer life expectancy and increasing numbers are forcing some really old and offensive tropes about senior sexuality to finally give way to real life.

Where once the older you got, the more *asexual* you were presumed to become, current research is making it increasingly clear that the majority of women and men between the ages of 50 and 80 are still enthusiastic about sex and intimacy. In fact, according to a Duke University study, about 20 percent of people over 65 claim to have sex lives that are better than ever. And that is fantastic, but for the other 80 percent of us, it requires some forethought and planning.

Of course, male sexual enhancement drugs have made a significant impact here. But there's a burgeoning industry supporting female sexuality too; and Black women, eager to change the stigmatizing narratives around our sexuality and pleasure, are at the forefront of a movement to encourage women of all ages to explore and engage in sexual pleasure without shame, guilt, or apology. This movement includes a growing industry of sexuality doulas, sexologists, sex therapists, sex educators, sex coaches, and sexual healers. Dr. Kelly J. Casperson, a urologist with a subspecialty in sexual medicine and the author of *You Are Not Broken,* is bringing these discussions about female sexuality into the public square. Most importantly, she is offering concrete solutions and sound medical advice. Honestly, I am so proud of the young women out there who are posting and podcasting about these issues. The good news is that they are not going to stand for the crumbs that our generation has settled for [♪ **"I Ain't Gonna Stand for It"**].

What is the average older woman actually doing sexually? As usual, we are sorely in need of research in this area that is diverse, well-funded, and reliable. I recently read about a study that is recruiting women for research, to examine what happens in the female brain with orgasm.

I'm not sure, but I think you have to have an orgasm while undergoing an MRI. Good luck with that one. However, a few things are certain. Not only is the need for intimacy ageless, but its potential health benefits increase with time. Note here: Intimacy includes affection, pleasurable exploration, and physically expressed tenderness, desire, and attraction, not just intercourse or oral sex.

Your entire pelvic floor is comprised of muscles. It's like a little basket that holds your internal organs (especially your bladder, bowel, and vagina) in place. As you get older, if you don't exercise those muscles, they weaken. Kegel exercises don't generally work because it's hard to do enough of them to make a difference. To really see a result, you'd have to do ten to twenty at a time, several times throughout the day, every day. Sex does a lot to strengthen your pelvic floor, and a strong pelvic floor helps to ward against urinary incontinence and prolapse. Sex can not only literally add years to your life (and, *yes,* life to your years), it can also:

- Burn fat and calories

- Help you sleep, and stay limber and lighthearted

- Cause the brain to release stress- and anxiety-reducing endorphins

- Strengthen and deepen your connection with your partner(s)

- Offer an escape from life's stress and worry (including the headlines!)

Older women often fall into one of two categories when it comes to sexual pleasure. With the risk of pregnancy gone (although you must still protect yourself against sexually transmitted infections if you have a new partner) and your children likely out of the house, we are sometimes more carefree, confident, and curious about sex than ever. On the other hand, the changes in our aging bodies—internally and externally—can make us more physically uncomfortable, anxious about pain, or self-conscious. This is yet another reason why

staying healthy and fit as you age matters. If you feel bad or are dealing with multiple chronic illnesses, sex may fall to the bottom of
your priority list.

Open communication, patience, and an open mind are really important in postmenopausal sex. Here are a few more tips:

- Be playful. Having a good sense of humor never hurts.

- Be honest. Great sexual pleasure requires mutual trust. Trust
  helps you relax.

- Be supportive. Your partner may be just as, if not more, anxious
  than you are. Support each other.

- Be creative. Explore new ideas, alone or with your partner.
  Novelty is sexy.

- Be independent. Solo intimacy can not only be deeply satisfying, it offers the same health benefits as sexual intimacy with a
  partner. So, don't hold back.

- Be persistent. Women 40 and up were often raised with a sense
  of sexual shame, shyness, and embarrassment. Many of us were
  never taught about sex. Some never enjoyed it (or grew not to
  during perimenopause). And others have lived to be seniors
  having had very little sexual experience. To that I say, there's no
  time like the present. And when it comes to orgasm, if at first
  you don't succeed, don't give up. Ever.

Have Great Role Models and Mentors—
Older and Younger

Gayle King launched *CBS This Morning* as its co-host at 57. Nancy
Pelosi became a congresswoman at 47 and was elected Speaker of the
House at 67. Madeleine Albright finished her PhD after raising her
children, and became secretary of state at the age of 60. At 91, EGOT

(Emmy, Grammy, Oscar, Tony) winner Rita Moreno co-starred in a film alongside a lineup of other female stars, all over age 75. Angela Bassett won her first Golden Globe at 64. Hell, I'm writing my first book at the same age.

I could go on, but you get my point. Life's big, bright swings and grandest possibilities don't end until you stop reaching for them. And I want you to never stop [♪"Never Stop"]!

When you were small, you probably had a ready answer to that question adults love to ask children, "What do you want to be when you grow up?" Well, now's a good time to ask yourself, what do you want to be like as you grow old?

Some of us secretly admire the older lady who's in everybody's business and tends to speak her complete mind, fallout be damned. I always had a girl crush on the late, great Miss Nancy Wilson. Why? Not only was she an incredibly classy and talented jazz chanteuse, she was also a woman who aged beautifully and authentically [♪"Simply Beautiful"]. She was as sexy at 70 as she was at 40, and she wasn't afraid to let you know it. Maybe your yoga- and salsa-loving neighbor is more your speed. Or perhaps you've discovered one of the many fabulous over-50 fashionistas flaunting their silver hair and age-positive posts on Instagram.

Wherever you find them, having role models and mentors who are your seniors will keep you motivated and excited about the future. Seeing women who are (sometimes much) older than you thrive is not just reassuring, it's empowering [♪"Sweetest Somebody I Know"].

Augusta ("Dear")

Dear was my mother's cousin and was one of the sweetest people I have ever known. I'm not sure which came first, her nickname, "Dear," or the temperament that may have inspired it.

Dear had clearly endured her share of hardships and tragedies. Like my mother, she had come of age in the Jim Crow South. She was divorced for as long as I'd known her, and lived in a multigenerational house with other women whose names befit their roles—Mama, Grandmama, and Sister.

Her beloved son, Tyrone, was the only person I have ever known who was killed in Vietnam. Despite it all, Dear was truly the most optimistic person I have ever known. She attracted people with her big heart and generous spirit. She volunteered at her church and mentored the young teachers at her school. She looked after their children, and after my mother died, she looked after me as well.

Her house was always filled with laughter, people—young and old—and love. Whenever you asked her how she was doing, her answer was the same, and it always made me smile. "I'm beautiful," she would say—and she truly was.

Dear left this earth at the ripe old age of 94. Her body failed her, but her mind and spirit never did. She was unerringly kind and considerate until the very end. She became my gold standard for how to grow old gracefully—loving and beloved, and absolutely beautiful.

The Takeaway: Multigenerational mentors and role models can be among the most meaningful you'll ever have. And you don't even have to actually meet these women to learn from, and be inspired by, them.

With all due respect to all the "30 Under 30" and "40 Under 40" lists out there causing a stir, Toni Morrison published her first novel at 40; won a Pulitzer Prize at 58; became a Nobel Laureate at 62; and published her last book shortly before her death, at 89. And it isn't just her—the list of women doing amazing things later in life is growing.

As everybody's go-to sage, Oprah, once said, "We live in a youth-obsessed culture that is constantly trying to tell us that if we're not young, and we're not glowing, and we're not hot, that we don't matter. I refuse to let a system or a culture or a distorted view of reality tell me that I don't matter."

To thrive, surround yourself with others who are equally stubborn in their refusal to be defined or limited by Father Time—and that includes young'uns. After all, as the years go by, we have fewer and fewer natural peers. And no one wants to be the last one standing [♪ "Keep Your Head to the Sky"].

So, connect with younger women over common interests and shared goals—and needs. There is so much that we can learn from one another. Most people want role models and mentors. Embrace that role, which allows you to play to your strengths. But as you do, allow yourself to be vulnerable and engaged in how they can mentor you as well. We have a lot to learn from the youngsters, and not just about social media, blockchain, or how to use our latest devices. Don't be so quick to dismiss young people or the great value they can add to your life.

Have Patience with the Pain of Grief and Loss

Despite the fact that grief is universal and inevitable, it is one of life's challenges that we discuss the least. It also remains largely under-researched and widely misunderstood. What we know is that grief is a complex process of navigating loss broadly. Divorce, a career change, or a geographical move can cause feelings of grief as profound as a death.

Grief has aspects that are emotional, physical, psychological, behavioral, social, and spiritual. There are five well-documented stages of grief: denial, anger, bargaining, depression, and acceptance. But the grieving process is rarely that predictable or uniform.

Some of us suffer in silence, stoic and seeking solitude. Others express their grief openly and often or become excessively needy and unable to bear being alone. And research has shown that seniors tend to grieve differently, experiencing two additional stages: disorganization, or temporary confusion, and anxiety. The bottom line: Grief can be uncontrollable and difficult to diagnose—especially as we get older and experience compounding losses, sometimes at an alarming rate. And unlike other types of recovery, which breed resiliency, we don't necessarily get better at grieving the more we experience it. Every loss is unique.

So, how best to cope when a loss occurs?

- Acknowledge your pain rather than try to distance yourself from it.

- Grief takes time. Take all the time you need.

- Choose what's best for you, not others. You have that right.

- Connect with others who share your loss but understand that your grieving process will be unique to you. They may experience grief differently.

- Communicate your feelings and memories, rather than bottling them up.

- Support yourself emotionally by taking care of yourself physically. Pay careful attention to your eating and drinking habits.

- Seek professional counseling or grief support groups if you feel chronically confused, overwhelmed, or anxious.

- And keep reminding yourself that while grief can go on for an extended time, it does eventually get lighter.

DR. SHARON'S RX FOR

Living Your Life Like It's Golden

1. Maintain a close, broad community of diverse friends and loved ones.

2. Identify inspiring role models and mentors, both older and younger, and aim to be one!

3. Stay open to sexual pleasure and intimate exploration, with a partner or without.

4. Navigate loss and grief with great care and seek support.

5. Actively avoid isolation and loneliness.

6. Eat optimism for breakfast, lunch, and dinner.

7. Stretch in every way, every day. Staying open to new ideas, people, and places will help keep you mentally and physically nimble.

CHAPTER 12

Heaven Bound♪

Be a Benefactor, Not a Burden

Dear Sis,

You know what they say about life: No one gets out alive. And yet, preparing for our inevitable demise is an anathema to most of us. So, it's only fitting that before we come to the end of this book, we talk about the end of your life. I know, not the most lighthearted topic of conversation. But the important ones never are.

Everybody acts surprised that they're going to die one day. Not me. A silver lining of losing my mom early is that I have never had any illusions about where my life is headed. Both in how she lived and how she died, my mom taught me that the greatest inheritance we can leave for our children is not material (although that surely helps). It's what we believed, what we survived, and what we learned. And the more we can model for them how to be, the less guesswork they'll have to apply as they move through the world.

Along with that, I know that the more we do in advance to ease the potential stressors of our own decline and death, the better off we and everyone we love will be.

So, my last cliché before we part is this: Hope for the best but prepare for the worst. I know, it can feel overwhelming. But do it anyway. And as you do, keep reminding yourself of the great value there is in that exercise—and in sacrificing the perfect for the good.

You'll find a handy to-do list near the end of this chapter, where you can literally check the boxes, one by one. The more you check, the better. But I guarantee that anything you do to ready yourself and your family for the end of your life will help make the rest of your life better than it would otherwise be.

xo, Dr. Sharon

ave you ever been preparing to leave on a trip and thought, *What if I never come home?* It's not like a serious, black hole of an idea. It's just the perfectionist or drama queen or mom in you who looks around your place before you head out the door and thinks, *I can't leave things like this.*

So, rather than let the clothes you edited out of your suitcase stay piled on a chair, you hang them back up. Then you make your bed, wash the dishes, put out the garbage, and give the bathroom a quick refresh—all driven by the thought of your children or your neighbor or your parents or friends walking into your home after some tragic event, bereft, without you—then looking around and thinking, *WTH!*

When you finally head out the door, you feel satisfied that should you meet some grisly, unforeseen end, at least you won't have left a mess behind. If the worst happens, you tell yourself, that neatness, *that order,* will be a comfort to your loved ones—a final gift, of sorts.

Returning home again, safe and sound and drama-free, you realize it was a gift you also gave yourself. Because it's enough just to have to unpack your suitcase and do the laundry after a trip; who wants to have to clean the house too?

This chapter is about putting your proverbial house in order. Because illness or grief is hard enough; who wants to have to clean the house too? This chapter is *not* about dying. It is about taking charge of your *entire life,* including who speaks for you if you can't and who speaks at your funeral, if you care.

As a physician, I have seen families torn up over illness. But we have all seen families tear themselves apart over things like who's going to get late Cousin Peggy's prized mink—even though nobody wears her size or lives in a cold place, and putting any political views on the old coat aside, it's outdated and ugly. When you're gone and it's time to divvy up the goods, reason often takes a holiday, leaving those evil twins Greedy and Crazy to run the show. Unless you make a plan.

Once the initial shock wears off, nobody cares if you left your bed made; more likely, some relatives you barely tolerated will be looking under it to see if that's where you kept the box with rainy-day cash and the family silver. Unless you make a plan.

For those of you who say, "Who cares? I'm going to be dead anyway," that is true. But ask yourself: Who do you think will be the first person in your house after you're dead? Do you have personal items (think sex toys, journals, porn collections) that you don't want certain people (think children, parents, your neighbor) to find? Gives new meaning to the idea of dying with dignity, doesn't it? So, let me repeat: Make a plan. And plan to update it regularly.

Diane

All of her adult life, Diane was a vibrant, independent woman, as was her only sibling, Genevieve. The more fashionable, funny, and outgoing of the two, Diane was a pioneering public-school principal, overseeing several schools set aside exclusively for pregnant girls. Genevieve was a highly regarded pediatrician.

Both women loved to travel. Neither married nor had children. And both retired just before age 70.

As soon as she retired, Diane hired a lawyer and got all of her affairs in order. She executed a will, a living will, and a health proxy. She also bought long-term disability insurance and prepaid funerals for both herself and her sister. Genevieve, a type 1 diabetic, became riddled with health problems before doing any of that.

By the age of 80, Genevieve was blind and confined to a wheelchair. Diane, 86, oversaw her sister's care, determined to honor her promise to let Genevieve stay in her own home, despite the financial stresses it created. Only after Diane suffered a major stroke and died two weeks later did her loved ones gain a sense of the burdens she'd been shouldering.

Because Diane hadn't updated her advance directives in more than a decade, her health proxy, a dear friend around her age who was also in decline, wasn't well enough to even visit her in the hospital, no less make medical decisions on her behalf. While Diane's will left some funds to her godchildren and a few charities, her primary beneficiary was her sister, who was moved to a nursing home after Diane died, and then died herself within weeks.

Because Genevieve didn't have a will, after her nursing home bills were paid, all of her estate and much of Diane's reverted to the state in which they'd lived.

The Takeaway: Handling your affairs is not a one-and-done exercise. The consequences of not updating your advance directives can be as serious as never preparing them in the first place. Here's another piece of good advice: If you're lucky enough to live a long life, make sure the person you put in charge could reasonably be expected to outlive you.

Defining Your Options

Death is the one thing we all know is coming that too few of us prepare for—especially when we're in the best position to do so, which is when we're healthy and sitting around the kitchen table, not sick in the ICU.

Only 1 in 3 adults has completed any sort of advance directive, according to CDC reports. Many more admit to starting the process but never completing it. Partial measures (maybe you think about it, discuss it with your relatives, jot a few notes down, but never formalize them) have no legal weight and are not enforceable, no matter how fervent the intent behind them. And those updates are critical.

Deaths, births, or changes in ability; geographical moves; breaches of trust; changes in your relationships, such as divorce or estrangement—any of these can significantly impact plans you made just a year ago.

Historically, older adults and those who have been diagnosed with a serious illness such as cancer, HIV, or renal failure are most likely to put advance directives in place. But 2021's National Poll on Healthy Aging, which surveyed adults over the age of 50, found that only 46 percent had legally documented their advance-care preferences. The deadly COVID pandemic motivated only 7 percent of those polled to have conversations with their loved ones about their wishes, and a paltry 1 percent of those surveyed actually formalized those wishes by completing or updating advance directives.

Now might be a good time for a few key definitions. *Advance directive* is an umbrella term for legal documents that give instructions for your medical care in the event that you can't communicate your wishes. Advance directives allow you to spell out explicitly what you do or do not want to have done at what may be the end of your life. Standard advance directives are readily available on the internet. You can download and modify them to correspond to your precise wishes. They are binding, but not absolute. In other words, every decision you formalize can and will evolve as you do—assuming you update your advance directives as needed.

The three most common types of advance directives are:

- **Living Will**—tells doctors how you want to be treated in an emergency. This document typically stipulates which common medical treatments you would want or not want, and under which conditions your choices would apply. This may include your wishes about organ and tissue donation, decisions that can cause dissention and stress for your loved ones if left to them.

- **Durable Power of Attorney for Healthcare**—legally establishes your *healthcare proxy,* the person empowered to make healthcare decisions for you if you are unable to communicate them yourself. Your proxy should know you and your wishes well and should be trusted to advocate for you effectively under duress, even if their personal position differs from yours. It's their responsibility to ensure that the wishes expressed in your living will are carried out.

- **Do Not Resuscitate (DNR)/Allow Natural Death (AND) Order**—a legal document that puts all hospital or care-facility staff (including EMS) on notice that you do not want CPR, intubation, defibrillation, or other resuscitation measures to be attempted if your heartbeat or breathing stops. A DNR must become a part of your medical chart for it to be enforced. This requires an affirmative action by a hospital doctor who most likely doesn't know you and must be made aware of your wishes. Until that order is in your chart, you will be considered a "full code," which means that if your vital signs begin to fail, standard medical emergency practice (and oftentimes state law) will rule, and all life-support measures will automatically be taken.

Consider the What-Ifs

Many of the procedures that people consider to be "lifesaving" are, in reality, just prolonging death. And before you start calling me "Dr. Kevorkian," all I am advocating is that everyone should have the right to die a natural death if they so choose.

- *What if I change my mind about my advance directives?* I have a friend whose 90-year-old father with terminal cancer declined chemotherapy. When he found out his granddaughter was pregnant, he changed his mind. The few rounds of chemotherapy he ended up getting didn't change his ultimate outcome, but the treatments did give him and his loved ones a few extra meaningful months. As long as you are capable of making decisions for yourself, you can always change your mind—and your plans.

- *What if I'd rather keep my advance directives to myself until needed?* Just because these are highly personal decisions doesn't mean they should be kept private. In fact, in addition to legally documenting your plans and making sure they're easily accessible to those who you've empowered to use them, it's good to talk about them. Make your wishes for any significant decline and your end-of-life care and living conditions known, openly and often. Share updates and information or experiences that may have factored into your decisions. The more you do, the more comfortable you and your loved ones will be about the choices you make and their ability to see them through. You might also demystify the subject and inspire them to handle their own business.

- *What if I do nothing?* Without any advance directives, your state's laws will determine who will make medical decisions on your behalf. The responsibility will most likely fall to your spouse if you're married, your parents if you're single and they are accessible and able, or barring either of those, your children of adult age. If you are not legally married to your partner and you have not legally designated that person as your healthcare proxy, they might not even be consulted in the decision-making around your care, let alone be allowed to take the lead in it. It won't matter if you've been together for thirty years and they cared for you the last five.

- *What if my life is just . . . complicated?* It is important to note that the decisions you make in your advance directives should not be guided by anyone else's judgments or feelings but your own. News flash: A health proxy can be your adult children or spouse, but it need not be. This is not the way to compensate the child who always felt unseen or the old friend who felt stung when she didn't get to be your maid of honor. And as much as you may trust and love your spouse, if you worry that in a crisis their anguish might override your wishes, spare them that moral dilemma and choose someone else [♪ **"Lean on Me"**]. Remember: Your body, your choice.

Another very important piece of information here—just because you have a signed advance directive in your nightstand drawer or locked away in your safe-deposit box, doesn't mean that it automatically gets enacted. Your medical proxy should have their own copy of your living will and DNR or, at the very least, know where to find them. It is also imperative to have your emergency medical contact be the person who can legally execute your advance directive if they are not your next of kin.

In instances where you have no known family or friends to advocate on your behalf, the state may assign a physician to represent your interests. This person will most likely be a complete stranger.

The Best Time to Plan Ahead Is Right Now

In addition to my parents, I have lost three of my siblings, including two sisters who died prematurely and unexpectedly. My sister Vivian was strong and vibrant, and we were utterly unprepared to lose her when we did. But because Vivian had taken the time to execute her advance directives, when a stroke and subsequent surgery left her on life support, my family was never in doubt about what the correct course of action should be.

You can only imagine with seven siblings and two adult children how much confusion there could have been, but Vivian had left no room for that. Everyone may have had their own opinion, but at the end of the day, the only opinion that mattered was hers. And we all respected that.

The Takeaway: While the death of a loved one is never easy, advance planning can definitely help mitigate the trauma. And trauma is always worth mitigating, if you can.

As a doctor, I've also seen how empowering advance-care planning is to everyone, not just those who are old or very ill. At any age, a medical crisis could render you suddenly unable to speak or think clearly, making sound decisions impossible. Anticipating that possibility and documenting your wishes can give you a sense of control and the reassurance that your wishes will be at the core of any conversations around your treatment, whether you can participate directly in them or not. Advance directives don't presume that you will die, they just ensure that no matter what your condition is, your wishes are driving your care.

I often joke (if one can joke about death) that when I die, I'd like for it to be sad, not tragic. And I'd like for those I leave behind to be sad, not mad. To accomplish these goals, I try to take care of myself and my end-of-life business, so those I leave behind won't have to.

Toward that end, you know what's more important than your loved ones finding your bed made and toilet clean after you're gone? Their being able to find your will, your life insurance policies, recent tax filings, and the title to your car. If you've ever been an executor (the person appointed to carry out the terms of someone's will), you know what I'm talking about.

If you depart this life with your affairs in chaos, having to unravel that mess will almost surely take a few years off the life of the person charged with that responsibility. Talk about stress! Organizing that mess today will help your loved ones eventually, and you right now. On the other hand, you could have all of your ducks in a row—advance directives completed, funeral prearranged with all expenses prepaid, final outfit hanging in a garment bag on the far right side of your neat-as-a-pin closet—but if nobody knows you've done all of this, or where to find out if you have, you've probably wasted your time.

Handle-Your-Business Checklist

This isn't easy terrain to tackle, but it's also not as daunting as you might think. What might feel like an overwhelming task (both emotionally and practically) can be broken down into doable items that you can check off one by one. There are plenty of resources offering you step-by-step guides, questionnaires, and templates for estate planning, funeral arrangements, even writing your own obituary. Many are available online through organizations such as AARP and the Alzheimer's Association, as well as law firms that specialize in trusts and estates.

Funeral homes, hospices, financial institutions, and insurance providers usually offer similar guides that are easy to follow and booklets that you can fill out and physically leave with the appropriate people. For example, FreeWill.com offers a handy end-of-life planning checklist in a PDF version that you can print out and save. It outlines a dozen key documents you should gather in one safe place that you make known and accessible to your executor (who must be officially appointed in your will), as well as to those you most trust:

- Last will and testament

- Revocable living trust

- Beneficiary designations

- Durable financial power of attorney

- Durable medical power of attorney

- Living will

- Life insurance

- DNR (do not resuscitate) and POLST (physician orders for life-sustaining treatment) forms

- Pet trust

- End-of-life housing arrangements

- Instructions for your digital assets (including passwords)

- Funeral instructions and burial arrangements

Along with these documents, it can't hurt to keep copies of your birth certificate, social security card, passport, financial statements (including most recent tax filings), mortgage documents, titles, deeds, and miscellaneous insurance policies, such as for your home, health, or long-term care. There are apps you can use to facilitate this process.

Final Thoughts on Your Final Chapter

Elvin and Verna

My oldest brother is 88. He and his wife built their dream home when they retired from government service at 55. (I know, right? There was a time when you could retire after thirty years!)

They were thoughtful in the design. Everything was on one floor with a complete basement suite in case one of their kids moved back or they ever needed live-in care.

They included doorways wide enough for wheelchair access and installed grab bars and lipless showers in the bathrooms. Then they filled it with beautiful things, old and new, that they cherished. It was the perfect home to age in . . . or so they thought.

Verna, my sister-in-law, had a heart attack at 70 and survived, but her energy level never fully returned. Simple chores around the house (which was, in retrospect, too large) were burdensome. There was also a large yard to maintain. So, they made the bold decision to leave their dream house and downsize. They moved into a senior community that allowed for independent living, assisted living, or nursing care, depending on their care needs [♪ "Everything I Need"]. Parting with a lot of their stuff wasn't easy, but their two-bedroom flat had everything they needed and provided the peace of mind of knowing that, come what may, they were covered.

They had not been there for a year before Verna was diagnosed with terminal cancer. Elvin was able to get her everything she needed—nursing care, help with housekeeping, and meals right in their own home. Verna died peacefully in her own bed. After losing his partner of almost fifty years, Elvin was spared the immense task of clearing out a too-big house and having to move, alone. My brother was comforted by the community they had joined together, and more than fifteen years later he's still going strong in his right-sized home.

The Takeaway: Advance directives, wills, and medical proxies are important, but you need to also get your actual house in order. Many of us get too attached to things that none of us can take with us.

It helps to find a home where you can age in place easily [♪ "A
House Is Not a Home"] (or adapt your existing home to meet those
needs) before circumstances force you to. If you were to become incapacitated, even due to an injury or a surgery from which you fully expect to recover, could you do so comfortably in your home? Assuming
you live well into your 80s, or longer, how will you fare if your children
live two thousand miles away? What if you don't have children, or
anyone, to rely on? These are questions to be asked and answered when
you're 62, not 82.

Many of you have aging parents who categorically refuse to leave
their homes or discuss the things that you know would make the job
of caring for them and keeping them safe much easier. You may not be
able to change their minds, and I know you think that when the time
comes, you'll do better. I'm asking you not to wait. So, whether this
information is for you, your friend, or your aging parents, I'd like to
share a few common mistakes that people make as they age. Consider
it food for thought, grab a plate full, and dig in.

- **Make sure you have a trusted person as a joint tenant on
  your bank account.** Even if you've set up autopay for recur-
  ring bills and utilities, if you are temporarily incapacitated, *all*
  of your bills have to be paid. Once you're physically well, the
  last thing you want to have to recover from is a bad credit score.
  Have a person you trust (preferably the person who has your
  power of attorney) know where to find your important account
  information, including passwords. Again, hear me when I say
  trusted. If you have important papers or valuables in a safe-
  deposit box or household safe, make sure that person also
  knows where to find the key or combination.

- **Designate a trusty (secret) agent.** If something were to
  happen to you tomorrow, who would you want to be the first
  person in your house? Who would you trust enough to secure
  your valuables or to know where your most sensitive items are
  and what to do with them (including disposing of them, if

necessary) [♪ **"You Are My Friend"**]. Make a pact with that person that includes specific instructions. Make sure they have a key and the alarm code to your home. And put your wishes in writing, legibly signed by you, so they are covered in the event that your agent is ever questioned about their intentions.

- **Educate yourself about hospice care.** Hospice care is an option for patients whose diseases can no longer be cured or controlled by traditional medical care. The hospice care philosophy affirms the quality of a dying patient's life by focusing on the individual, rather than their disease. Either within one's home, a residential hospice, or a hospital setting, hospice care prioritizes a patient's wishes, pain management, comfort, and dignity. Hospice care also affirms death as the natural final stage of life. It does not seek to hasten death, but unlike contemporary medicine, it does not attempt to delay death either. American Cancer Society studies show that most people wait too long to engage hospice care, often because they view it as "giving up." Black people make up only 8 percent of hospice users, leaving us less well cared for, with poorer pain control, at a point in life when we most need it.

- **Write your own obituary.** Hear me out. An obituary is sort of the last word on your accomplishments. Who better to have that than you? If you write it in the full bloom of life, not only will it help you reflect on all that you've done so far, but it will also help center what you want to do with the time you've got left. What have you not yet seen or done that's important to you? What have you been putting off for years, for no good reason? How do you want to be remembered? What do you want people to say about you when you're gone? Don't think of it as your "obituary," think of it as your résumé for the afterlife, where nobody will know that you were a champion swimmer in college or a founding member of your sorority—unless you tell them. It may sound morbid, but trust me. Writing your own obit is like that old Alka-Seltzer commercial slogan from the 1970s: Try it, you'll like it! And attaching your favorite photo of yourself can't hurt.

- **It's never too soon to plan your funeral.** Maybe you think I'm taking this too far—or that I'm just a little bit of a control freak. You may not be wrong. But think about it: It is *your* funeral. And there are key decisions to be made here about your hereafter. Like, do you want to be cremated? Do you want a funeral or a memorial service or a great big ol' party? Do you have a family cemetery plot where you would like to be buried, or would being next door to your family for all of eternity be your worst nightmare? Maybe you hate a certain flower, or you love the idea of a white dove being released at your graveside. Whatever your wishes, write them down and give them to someone who will carry them out. Better yet, purchase your last bit of real estate and leave nothing to chance. Maybe that's a burial plot, or space in a mausoleum or columbarium. Or maybe you just need to direct your loved ones on where to spread your ashes, lest you end up in an urn gathering dust in a dark attic forever. Do you have insurance that will cover funeral costs? If not, get on that if you're able. I'm sure that you, like me, have had folks pass away and the burden of paying for funeral expenses has fallen to begrudging relatives. Remember, the goal is not just to make like you're at Burger King and have it your way, it's to let people be sad, not mad.

DR. SHARON'S RX FOR

Peace

The thought of death should not consume us. But peace is worth pursuing, and I don't want you to have to wait till you die to get it. So, for my final prescription, let's get you some of that!

1. Get your house in order (this includes your financial, metaphorical, and legal houses).

2. Consider long-term care insurance as well as a policy for funeral expenses, if you are not covered.

3. Designate your medical and legal proxy.

4. Make a will and other advance directives, and make sure that they are accessible.

5. Write your obituary or at least keep a current résumé so others will know what to write after you're gone.

6. Preserve your legacy. Label your pictures with names and dates. If you keep them on your phone, download your favorites to a CD or to a shared album so that family members can access them. Add your general and medical family trees to this—or details on where they can be found—because history begins at home and it's just as important to give your loved ones roots as it is to give them wings.

7. Discuss with anyone who wants to hear what your final wishes are. (Personally, I'm planning a dance party. You know I'm already working on my playlist.)

8. Relax. You'd be surprised how comforting it is to be ready for anything.

EPILOGUE

Dear Sis,

This book has truly been a labor of love. As a doctor for over thirty years, I have tried my level best to listen more than I have spoken, because that is how one truly gains experience. I have learned more from my patients than any textbook could have ever taught me. And I learned patience and common sense from my mother that are worth their weight in gold. These are the lessons I have shared with you.

I wrote this book as a road map that you can refer to on repeat because I know how difficult it is to navigate a healthcare system that is frustrating and perplexing even to those of us who work within it. I've spent countless hours with friends and family helping them negotiate this medical maze, and my goal was to give you the same sage advice I give them. It is the advice that I wish my mother, her mother, and the countless women who have felt left out of conversations about their most important asset—their health—had at their disposal. How different their lives might have been.

You now have it. So, grab those reins. Take control of your destiny. Realize the power you possess when you raise your voice. And keep our grown woman talk going, shamelessly, so that younger women benefit too. I have every confidence that you can truly chart a better course for yourself as you age. And remember, Sis, I'm not just talking to you, I am you—a sister, friend, daughter, auntie, mother, and wife. And a deejay, whose songs you will hopefully keep playing, a soundtrack for your long, healthy, and happy life.

xo, Dr. Sharon

People Make the World Go Round♪

Those who know me are well aware that one of my favorite sayings is "There are no accidents in the universe," and there is no better example of this sentiment than in the creation of this book. The unlikely series of events that led to it could not have happened merely by chance. There are so many people to thank.

First and foremost, I would like to thank Caroline Clarke, my collaborator and chief motivator in this project, who kept me on target, on time, and laser-focused on the task at hand. Her brilliance and expertise helped me craft the message I wanted to impart—coherently. With Caroline, I not only tapped into her immense talent, but I also gained a lifelong friend. I can thank my amazing agent, Gail Ross, for not only believing in this project but also for finding the perfect partner for me.

I would also like to thank my talented editor, Madhulika Sikka, and the entire team at Crown Publishing for taking a chance on a quirky medical memoir/advice book, complete with a musical soundtrack. I know there's not much of a template out there for this type of book, so thank you for understanding my vision.

They say that the devil is in the details, and no one out there can keep those details straight better than Ruth Mills, who was able to translate my less-than-organized record-keeping into a thing of beauty.

A very special thank you goes to David Walters, whose copyediting expertise caught the mistakes, big and small, that occur when the auto-correct in your brain blinds you.

To my able assistant, Jennifer Osias, thank you for always knowing where I'm supposed to be and when I'm supposed to be there and for helping me with the knowledge of technology that only the young possess.

And speaking of that "no accidents" thing, one lovely July day while the world was still in the midst of the COVID pandemic, my dear friend Michelle Obama invited me to be a guest on her newly minted podcast. By sharing her experiences with menopause, Michelle contributed greatly to removing the stigma associated with midlife women's health issues. There was absolutely "no shame in her menopause game." My appearances on her podcast transformed me from an obscure gynecologist with an interest in menopause and women's health to a slightly less-obscure gynecologist with a larger megaphone. For this and for the many years of friendship, laughter, fitness routines, and experiences of a lifetime, I am eternally grateful.

This selfsame eponymous podcast led my new partners at Alloy Women's Health, Anne Fulenwider and Monica Molenaar, to me and signaled the end of my lifelong career as a practicing physician. They gave me an exit strategy that I didn't even know I needed. Through my work with Alloy, I have met an amazing group of people, the menopause warriors—Jennifer Weiss-Wolf, Tamsen Fadal, Omisade Burney-Scott, Rachel Hughes, Kamili Wilson, and Donna Klassen. I would also like to acknowledge the OGs of menopause, those pioneering and persistent researchers who have been trying to set the record straight on menopause for years—Dr. Avrum Bluming, Dr. Howard Hodis, and Dr. Phil Sarrel. They have been generous with their time and expertise in helping me understand just exactly how the medical profession got so much of the story wrong when it comes to menopause and what we need to do to correct the record. To this next generation of menopause warriors, Dr. Rachel Rubin, Dr. Kelly Casperson, and Dr. Mary Claire Haver, thank you for your tireless efforts to provide accurate and sound medical advice in a sea of confusing and often-conflicting opinions. And I would be remiss if I did not thank the brilliant Dr. Lisa Mosconi, who is doing her best to figure out how menopause affects women's brains and their susceptibility to Alzheimer's. We simply cannot afford to ignore the many questions about women's brains that she is uniquely poised to answer.

To all the women with big voices who have shone a light on menopause and women's health—especially Maria Shriver, Oprah Winfrey, Gayle King, Tamron Hall, and Naomi Watts—please keep talking, because when you speak, people listen. You are all not only educating women but also providing examples of the productivity and vitality that women of a certain age possess.

Perhaps the biggest debt of gratitude is owed to my friends, patients, and family who have so graciously allowed me to share their stories. I would like to especially thank my friend Marilyn Milloy for being an early reader and for sharing her expertise and her journalist's eyes and ears. I would also like to thank my friend Michele Norris for her sage advice and her unlimited font of knowledge. To my girlfriends who have been there through thick and thin, my ride-or-dies, you know who you are and how much I love you [♪ **"My Old Friend"**].

I must thank my amazing sisters Joyce Malone Phillips and Margie Malone Tuckson, who have so graciously allowed me to share their stories. In my mother's absence, they provided me with living examples of everything I needed to become the grown woman I am today. I love you both more than you will ever know.

And last but certainly not least, to my husband, Eric, and my children, Maya, Brooke, and Eric III, who are the lights of my life, this journey has been made purposeful and more joyous with all of you in it. I love you to the moon and back [♪ **"Love, Love, Love"**].

PLAYLIST

Introduction

"Nuttin' But Love" (Heavy D & The Boyz)
"Both Sides Now" (Joni Mitchell)
"Beautiful Surprise" (India.Arie)
"You Are Not Alone" (Michael Jackson)
"Breathe" (Lalah Hathaway)
"Last Night a DJ Saved My Life" (Indeep)

Chapter 1
Solid: It's Time to Establish a Dependable Medical Home

"Solid" (Ashford & Simpson)
"Home" (Stephanie Mills)
"Wake Up Everybody" (Harold Melvin & the Blue Notes)
"Respect" (Aretha Franklin)
"No Scrubs" (TLC)

Chapter 2
Family Affair: Knowing Your History Helps You Build a Brighter Future

"Family Affair" (Sly and the Family Stone)
"A Song for Mama" (Boyz II Men)
"Grandma's Hands" (Bill Withers)

Chapter 3
In the Thick of It: Sick or Not-So-Sick? Be Ready and Make the Right Call

"In the Thick of It" (Brenda Russell)
"Superwoman" (Alicia Keys)
"Nobody Can Be You" (Steve Arrington)
"Alright" (Ledisi)

"Strength, Courage & Wisdom" (India.Arie)

"Mama Used to Say" (Junior)

"if you got a problem" (Joy Oladokun)

"Fever" (Ray Charles feat. Natalie Cole)

"Walk On By" (Dionne Warwick)

Chapter 4
Brave and Strong: What You Need to Know (and Do) About Cancer

"Brave & Strong" (Sly and the Family Stone)

"Cancer" (Joe Jackson)

"Inseparable" (Natalie Cole)

"Happy" (Pharrell Williams)

Chapter 5
Control: Chronic Stress, Weight Gain, and Diabetes: Tame Your Triple Threat

"Control" (Janet Jackson)

"Stressed Out" (Babyface)

"I Got You (I Feel Good)" (James Brown)

"Do Whatcha Gotta Do" (Phil Perry)

Chapter 6
Key to Your Heart: Guarding Against Cardiovascular Disease

"Key to My Heart" (The Emotions)

"With Each Beat of My Heart" (Stevie Wonder)

"Cleva" (Erykah Badu)

"Un-Break My Heart" (Toni Braxton)

"Please, Please, Please" (James Brown and the Famous Flames)

"How Can You Mend a Broken Heart" (Al Green)

Chapter 7
When It Don't Come Easy: Brain Health and Alzheimer's

"When It Don't Come Easy" (Patty Griffin)

"I Can't Write Left-Handed" (Bill Withers)

Chapter 8

I Will Survive: "Female Troubles" and Their Treatments

"I Will Survive" (Chantay Savage)

"I'm Every Woman" (Chaka Khan)

"Only Women Bleed" (Etta James)

"It's My Prerogative" (Bobby Brown)

"This Too Shall Pass" (Yolanda Adams)

"What Is Hip?" (Tower of Power)

"i tried everything" (Foster feat. Kailee Morgue & Zaini)

Chapter 9

Hot in Herre: Welcome to Puberty in Reverse

"Hot in Herre" (Nelly)

"Everything Must Change" (George Benson)

"(You Make Me Feel Like) A Natural Woman" (Aretha Franklin)

"How Will I Know" (Whitney Houston)

"Grown & Sexy" (Babyface)

"The Best Is Yet to Come" (Grover Washington, Jr.,
    feat. Patti LaBelle)

"Nick of Time" (Bonnie Raitt)

"Heat Wave" (Martha & the Vandellas)

Chapter 10

Finally!: Menopause and Beyond

"Finally" (CeCe Peniston)

"Always and Forever" (Heatwave)

"You Can't Always Get What You Want" (Aretha Franklin)

"Sisters Are Doin' It for Themselves" (The Eurythmics
    feat. Aretha Franklin)

"About Damn Time" (Lizzo)

"Love on Top" (Beyoncé)

"Bitch Better Have My Money" (Rihanna)

"The Weight" (Aretha Franklin)

"We Fall Down" (Donnie McClurkin)

"Help Me" (Joni Mitchell)

"Same Thing It Took" (The Impressions)

Chapter 11

Here Comes the Sun: Live Your *Best* Menopausal Life

"Here Comes the Sun" (Nina Simone)

"Ac-Cent-Tchu-Ate the Positive" (Al Jarreau)

"Beautiful Life" (Chuck Brown)

"Count on Me" (CeCe Winans and Whitney Houston)

"September" (Earth, Wind & Fire)

"That's What Friends Are For" (Dionne Warwick and Friends)

"Sexual Healing" (Marvin Gaye)

"I Ain't Gonna Stand for It" (Stevie Wonder)

"Never Stop" (The Brand New Heavies)

"Simply Beautiful" (Al Green)

"Sweetest Somebody I Know" (Stevie Wonder)

"Keep Your Head to the Sky" (Earth, Wind & Fire)

Chapter 12

Heaven Bound: Be a Benefactor, Not a Burden

"Heaven Bound" (Rufus & Chaka Khan)

"Lean on Me" (Bill Withers)

"Everything I Need" (Jarrod Lawson)

"A House Is Not a Home" (Luther Vandross)

"You Are My Friend" (Patti LaBelle)

Acknowledgments

People Make the World Go Round

"People Make the World Go Round" (The Stylistics)

"My Old Friend" (Al Jarreau)

"Love, Love, Love" (Donny Hathaway)

ADDITIONAL RESOURCES

Chapter 1
Solid: It's Time to Establish a Dependable Medical Home

1. How to find a good doctor: consumerreports.org/doctors/how-to-find-a-good-doctor

2. How to find out if a doctor is board-certified: certificationmatters.org

3. Information on the licensing, regulation, and discipline of physicians by state medical boards: fsmb.org/u.s.-medical-regulatory-trends-and-actions/guide-to-medical-regulation-in-the-united-states/about-physician-discipline

4. How to prepare for and make the most of a doctor's appointment, and what you should bring with you: nia.nih.gov/health/how-prepare-doctors-appointment

5. How to determine whether you should go to the ER or urgent care: acep.org/siteassets/sites/acep/media/advocacy/value-of-em/urgent-emergent-care.pdf

6. How to choose quality ambulatory care, quality hospice care, quality hospital care, and quality nursing care center services: jointcommission.org/resources/for-consumers

7. How to prevent medical and laboratory test mistakes: jointcommission.org/-/media/tjc/documents/resources/speak-up/speakup-medical-tests-5-15-2020.pdf

8. How to choose and name a medical proxy: nia.nih.gov/health/choosing-health-care-proxy

9. How to follow up on denied health insurance claims: propublica.org/article/find-out-why-health-insurance-claim -denied

10. Healthcare decision-making resources: americanbar.org/groups/ law_aging/resources/health_care_decision_making/power_atty _guide_and_form_2011

Chapter 2
Family Affair: Knowing Your History Helps You Build a Brighter Future

1. How to create a medical family health history: cbiit.github.io/ FHH/html/index.html

2. How to get copies of your medical records: verywellhealth.com/ how-to-get-copies-of-your-medical-records-2615505

3. Recommendations for immunizations for adults, by age: cdc.gov/vaccines/schedules/hcp/imz/adult.html

4. Information on what genetic testing is and who should get tested: cdc.gov/genomics/gtesting/genetic_testing.htm

Chapter 3
In the Thick of It: Sick or Not-So-Sick? Be Ready and Make the Right Call

1. How to determine if you should take a sick day; symptoms that may warrant staying home: verywellhealth.com/should-i-call-in -sick-770447

2. The difference between viruses and bacteria; when antibiotics are warranted: jointcommission.org/-/media/tjc/documents/ resources/speak-up/speak_up_infographic_antibiotics _2017pdf

3. Tips for when to go to urgent care: consumerreports.org/health -clinics/urgent-care-or-walk-in-health-clinic

4. When to use the emergency room: medlineplus.gov/ency/
    patientinstructions/000593.htm

5. How to use dietary supplements wisely: nccih.nih.gov/health/
    using-dietary-supplements-wisely

6. Pill trackers/medication reminders: apps.apple.com/us/
    app/mytherapy-medication-reminder/id662170995; also
    healthline.com/health/best-medication-reminders

Chapter 4

Brave and Strong: What You Need to Know (and Do) About Cancer

1. Early warning signs and symptoms of cancer: cancer.org/cancer/
    diagnosis-staging/signs-and-symptoms-of-cancer.html; also
    cancer.org/cancer/screening/american-cancer-society-guidelines
    -for-the-early-detection-of-cancer.html

2. Early detection of breast cancer: cancer.org/cancer/breast
    -cancer/screening-tests-and-early-detection/american-cancer
    -society-recommendations-for-the-early-detection-of-breast
    -cancer.html

3. How to find out about breast cancer trials: breastcancertrials
    .org/BCTIncludes/index.html?utm_source=BCO&utm
    _medium=site&utm_campaign=BDM

4. Breast cancer risk calculator: ibis-risk-calculator.magview.com

5. Facts and figures about cancer in African Americans: cancer.org/
    content/dam/cancer-org/research/cancer-facts-and-statistics/
    cancer-facts-and-figures-for-african-americans/cancer-facts-and
    -figures-for-african-americans-2019-2021.pdf

6. Information on trials for breast cancer in Black women:
    whenwetrial.org

7. How to sign up for a clinical trial: clinicaltrials.gov

Chapter 5
**Control: Chronic Stress, Weight Gain, and Diabetes:
Tame Your Triple Threat**

1. Dietary guidelines for Americans: dietaryguidelines.gov/sites/
   default/files/2021-03/Dietary_Guidelines_for_Americans-2020
   -2025.pdf

2. Information on diabetes: diabetes.org; also niddk.nih.gov/health
   -information/diabetes

3. What to know about body mass index and waist circumference:
   healthdirect.gov.au/body-mass-index-bmi-and-waist
   -circumference

4. Best sleep apps for tracking and improving sleep: verywellmind
   .com/best-sleep-apps-5114724

Chapter 6
Key to Your Heart: Guarding Against Cardiovascular Disease

1. Heart attack symptoms in women: heart.org/en/health-topics/
   heart-attack/warning-signs-of-a-heart-attack/heart-attack
   -symptoms-in-women

2. Stroke symptoms and FAST warning signs: stroke.org/en/about
   -stroke/stroke-symptoms

3. What is the Mediterranean diet? heart.org/en/healthy-living/
   healthy-eating/eat-smart/nutrition-basics/mediterranean-diet

4. How to find CPR training and first-aid training in your area:
   cpr.heart.org/en

Chapter 7
When It Don't Come Easy: Brain Health and Alzheimer's

1. Information on the Alzheimer's Association (for Alzheimer's and
   other types of dementia): alz.org/about

2. The National Institute on Aging's information on Alzheimer's disease and related dementias: nia.nih.gov/health/alzheimers

3. How to find and enroll in clinical trials for Alzheimer's and other dementias: alz.org/alzheimers-dementia/research _progress/clinical-trials/about-clinical-trials

4. How to participate in the discovery of treatments for brain diseases: brainhealthregistry.org

5. Research on women's brain diseases: neurology.weill.cornell .edu/research/womens-brain-initiative

Chapter 8
I Will Survive: "Female Troubles" and Their Treatments

1. Information on the diagnosis and treatment of fibroids: fibroidfoundation.org

2. Information on clinical trials for endometriosis: mayo.edu/ research/clinical-trials/diseases-conditions/endometriosis

3. Information about endometriosis: risk factors, symptoms, diagnosis of, and treatments for: nichd.nih.gov/health/topics/ endometriosis

Chapter 9
Hot in Herre: Welcome to Perimenopause, Fertility's Final Frontier

1. Information on IVF, egg-freezing statistics, and other topics related to advances in reproductive medicine: asrm.org

2. How to get relief from menopause symptoms: myalloy.com

3. Information on all aspects of menopause and after from the North American Menopause Society (NAMS): menopause.org/ for-women

4. Information from the American College of Obstetricians and Gynecologists (ACOG): acog.org/womens-health

Chapter 10
Finally!: Menopause and Beyond

1. Information on women's health topics from the National Institute on Aging department of the National Institutes of Health: nia.nih.gov/site-search/d29tZW4%3D

2. My favorite vibrator company: lovecrave.com

3. What you should know about preventing UTIs (urinary tract infections): ama-assn.org/delivering-care/public-health/what -doctors-wish-patients-knew-about-uti-prevention

4. How to prevent older adults from falling at home—a safety checklist: cdc.gov/steadi/pdf/check_for_safety_brochure-a.pdf

5. How to use the fall-detection feature on an Apple watch: support.apple.com/en-us/HT208944

6. How to use the fall-detection feature on a Google Pixel watch: blog.google/products/pixel/fall-detection-on-pixel-watch

Chapter 11
Here Comes the Sun: Live Your *Best* Menopausal Life

1. How to make friends as an adult: thecut.com/article/how-to -make-friends-as-an-adult.html

Chapter 12
Heaven Bound: Be a Benefactor, Not a Burden

1. A "life checklist" to prepare for death that covers your data and documents, your care, your possessions, and your legacy: deathwithdignity.org/wp-content/uploads/2021/12/life-file -checklist-web.pdf

2. How to start a conversation about end-of-life care: aarp.org/
    caregiving/basics/info-2020/end-of-life-talk-care-talk.html

3. Information on grief counseling: webmd.com/balance/grief
    -counseling

4. How to help your family plan your funeral far in advance:
    aarp.org/home-family/friends-family/info-2020/planning-your
    -own-funeral.html

5. How to access hospice care: hospicefoundation.org

Books I Recommend:

The XX Brain: The Groundbreaking Science Empowering Women to Maximize Cognitive Health and Prevent Alzheimer's Disease, by Lisa Mosconi, PhD

Estrogen Matters: Why Taking Hormones in Menopause Can Improve Women's Well-Being and Lengthen Their Lives—Without Raising the Risk of Breast Cancer, by Avrum Bluming, MD, and Carol Tavris, PhD

Being Mortal: Medicine and What Matters in the End, by Atul Gawande

The Complete Mediterranean Cookbook: 500 Vibrant, Kitchen-Tested Recipes for Living and Eating Well Every Day, edited by America's Test Kitchen

Weathering: The Extraordinary Stress of Ordinary Life in an Unjust Society, by Arline T. Geronimus

Under the Skin: The Hidden Toll of Racism on American Lives and on the Health of Our Nation, by Linda Villarosa

BIBLIOGRAPHY

Chapter 1
Solid: It's Time to Establish a Dependable Medical Home

ACOG [American College of Obstetricians and Gynecologists] Committee Opinion, Number 819, "Informed Consent and Shared Decision Making in Obstetrics and Gynecology," *Obstetrics & Gynecology,* January 21, 2021, journals .lww.com/greenjournal/Fulltext/2021/02000/Informed_Consent_and_Shared _Decision_Making_in.45.aspx

Orly Avitzur, "4 Ways to Find a Doctor Who's Right for You," *Consumer Reports,* May 23, 2016, consumerreports.org/doctors-hospitals/4-ways-to-find-the-right -doctor-for-you/

Lindsey Bever, "From heart disease to IUDs: How doctors ignore women's pain," *The Washington Post,* Dec. 13, 2022, washingtonpost.com/wellness/interactive/ 2022/women-pain-gender-bias-doctors/

Nathan Eddy, "Nearly 70% of U.S. physicians are employed by hospitals or corporate entities," *Healthcare Finance,* July 13, 2021, healthcarefinancenews .com/news/nearly-70-us-physicians-are-employed-hospitals-or-corporate-entities

Eden Health Team, "Concierge Costs: The Information You Need to Know," *edenhealth.com blog,* Sep. 13, 2021, edenhealth.com/blog/what-is-concierge -medicine/

Henry Ford Health, "Study: Role of Emergency Contact Is Mistaken for Advance Directive" (press release), Sep. 10, 2014, henryford.com/news/2014/09/study -role-of-emergency-contact-is-mistaken-for-advance-directive

Thomas J. Hwang, MD, and Otis W. Brawley, MD, "New Federal Incentives for Diversity in Clinical Trials," *New England Journal of Medicine,* Oct. 13, 2022, pp. 1347–1349, nejm.org/doi/full/10.1056/NEJMp2209043

Joel Keehn, "How to Find a Good Doctor: 9 Steps to Help You Find the Right Doctor for You and Your Family," *Consumer Reports,* Mar. 30, 2017, consumerreports.org/doctors/how-to-find-a-good-doctor/

Opinion letters responding to "A Crisis of Burnout Among Doctors," *The New York Times,* Oct. 17, 2022, nytimes.com/2022/10/17/opinion/letters/doctors-mental -health.html

Venkataraman Palabindala and Sohail Abdul Salim, "Era of Hospitalists," *Journal of Community Hospital Internal Medicine Perspectives* 8. no. 1, 2018, pp. 16–20, ncbi.nlm.nih.gov/pmc/articles/PMC5804680

Darrell Prescott, "Benign Neglect in Wilcox County," *The Harvard Crimson,* Dec. 14, 1970, thecrimson.com/article/1970/12/14/benign-neglect-in-wilcox -county-alabama

Eric Reinhart, "Doctors Aren't Burned Out from Overwork. We're Demoralized by Our Health Care System," *The New York Times,* Feb. 5, 2023, nytimes.com/ 2023/02/05/opinion/doctors-universal-health-care.html

Miranda Scott and Caitlin Dalzell, "St. Martin de Porres Hospital," *Clio: Your Guide to History,* Oct. 22, 2015, theclio.com/entry/19235

Sister Maria, R.S.M., "History of the St. Martin de Porres Hospital, Mobile, Alabama," *Journal of the National Medical Association* 56, no. 4, July 1964, pp. 303–306, ncbi.nlm.nih.gov/pmc/articles/PMC2610728/pdf/jnma00548 -0005.pdf

St. George's University School of Medicine, "What Is a Hospitalist? Learn What to Expect from Hospital Medicine," *St. George's University School of Medicine Medical School Blog,* June 16, 2022, sgu.edu/blog/medical/what-is-a-hospitalist/

Debra Wood, RN, "15 Surprising Facts About Hospitalists," *AMN Healthcare Staff Care,* Mar. 5, 2019, staffcare.com/locum-tenens-blog/news/15-surprising-facts -about-hospitalists-in-2020/

Chapter 2
Family Affair: Knowing Your History Helps You Build a Brighter Future

Reed Abelson, "Corporate Giants Buy Up Primary Care Practices at Rapid Pace," *The New York Times,* May 8, 2023, nytimes.com/2023/05/08/health/primary -care-doctors-consolidation.html

Association of American Medical Colleges, "AAMC Report Reinforces Mounting Physician Shortage" (press release), June 11, 2001, aamc.org/news/press-releases/ aamc-report-reinforces-mounting-physician-shortage

Leslie Bradford, MD, and Gretchen Glaser, MD, "Addressing Physician Burnout and Ensuring High-Quality Care of the Physician Workforce," *Obstetrics & Gynecology* 137, no. 1, January 2021, pp. 3–11, journals.lww.com/greenjournal/ Fulltext/2021/01000/Addressing_Physician_Burnout_and_Ensuring.2.aspx

CDC Staff, "Family Health History: The Basics," *CDC: Centers for Disease Control and Prevention,* May 5, 2023, cdc.gov/genomics/famhistory/famhist_basics.htm

Nathan Eddy, "Nearly 70% of U.S. physicians are employed by hospitals or corporate entities," *Healthcare Finance,* July 13, 2021, orthospinenews.com/ 2021/07/13/nearly-70-of-u-s-physicians-are-employed-by-hospitals-or-corporate -entities/

National Institutes of Health, "NIH Inclusion Outreach Toolkit: How to Engage, Recruit, and Retain Women in Clinical Research," *National Institutes of Health Office of Research on Women's Health,* orwh.od.nih.gov/toolkit/recruitment/ history

Nature Staff, "Women's health: End the disparity in funding," *Nature*, May 3, 2023, nature.com/articles/d41586-023-01472-5

Jecca R. Steinberg, MD, MSc, et al., "Analysis of Female Enrollment and Partici- pant Sex by Burden of Disease in US Clinical Trials Between 2000 and 2020," *JAMA [Journal of the American Medical Association] NetworkOpen 4, no. 6,* June 18, 2021, jamanetwork.com/journals/jamanetworkopen/fullarticle/2781192

Trisha Torrey, "How to Get Your Medical Records: Understanding the Process, Cost, and Your Rights," *VeryWellHealth.com,* May 11, 2023, verywellhealth.com/ how-to-get-copies-of-your-medical-records-2615505

University of Utah, "Family Health Histories: We Know They're Valuable, So Why Don't We Collect Them?" *healthcare.utah.edu,* May 8, 2015, healthcare.utah .edu/healthfeed/2015/05/family-health-histories-we-know-theyre-valuable-so -why-dont-we-collect-them

Chapter 3
In the Thick of It: Sick or Not-So-Sick? Be Ready and Make the Right Call

American College of Emergency Physicians, "Emergency Care, Urgent Care— What's the Difference?" *acep.org,* acep.org/siteassets/sites/acep/media/advocacy/ value-of-em/urgent-emergent-care.pdf

American Heart Association, "Cardiovascular deaths saw steep rise in U.S. during first year of the COVID-19 pandemic," *American Heart Association News,* Jan. 25, 2023, professional.heart.org/en/science-news/~/link.aspx?_id= C7CED782B3CB429FB1D4A417493DEAFE&_z=z

John J. B. Anderson, PhD, et al., "Calcium Intake from Diet and Supplements and the Risk of Coronary Artery Calcification and its Progression Among Older Adults: 10-Year Follow-up of the Multi-Ethnic Study of Atherosclerosis (MESA)," *Journal of the American Heart Association,* 5, no. 10, Oct. 2016, ncbi .nlm.nih.gov/pmc/articles/PMC5121484/

Kate M. Brett, PhD, and Catharine W. Burt, Ed.D., "Utilization of Ambulatory Care by Women: United States, 1997–98," *Vital and Health Statistics* 13, no. 149, July 2001, cdc.gov/nchs/data/series/sr_13/sr13_149.pdf

CDC, "Heart Disease Deaths (Health, United States, 2020–2021)," *CDC Centers for Disease Control and Prevention National Center for Health Statistics*, cdc.gov/ nchs/hus/topics/heart-disease-deaths.htm

Juanita J. Chinn, PhD, et al., "Health Equity Among Black Women in the United States," *Journal of Women's Health* 30, no. 2, February 2021, pp. 212–219, ncbi .nlm.nih.gov/pmc/articles/PMC8020496/

Bart M. Demaerschalk, MD, MSc, et al., "Assessment of Clinical Diagnostic Concordance with Video Telemedicine in the Integrated Multispecialty Practice at Mayo Clinic During the Beginning of COVID-19 Pandemic from March to June 2020," *JAMA NetworkOpen,* 5, no. 9, Sep. 2, 2022, jamanetwork.com/ journals/jamanetworkopen/fullarticle/2795871

Kristina Duda, RN, "Should I Take a Sick Day? Symptoms That May Warrant Staying Home," *VeryWellHealth.com,* May 7, 2023, verywellhealth.com/should-i -call-in-sick-770447

Editorial Board, "Opinion: Congress should not wait around for the end of the antibiotic era," *The Washington Post,* Jan. 18, 2023, washingtonpost.com/ opinions/2023/01/18/drug-resistant-bacteria-antibiotics-congress/

Steven Findlay, "When You Should Go to an Urgent Care or Walk-in Health Clinic," *Consumer Reports,* May 4, 2018, consumerreports.org/health-clinics/ urgent-care-or-walk-in-health-clinic/

Gianelli & Morris, "Anthem's Policy on Avoidable ER Visits: A Closer Look," May 13, 2021, gmlawyers.com/avoidable-er-visits-anthem-policy/

Sioban D. Harlow et al., "Disparities in Reproductive Aging and Midlife Health between Black and White Women: The Study of Women's Health Across the Nation (SWAN)," *Women's Midlife Health,* Feb. 8, 2022, p. 7.

Emily Ihara et al., "Prescription Drugs," The Center on an Aging Society, Georgetown University McCourt School of Public Policy Health Policy Institute, hpi.georgetown.edu/rxdrugs/

Jenny Jia, MD, MSc, et al., "Multivitamins and Supplements—Benign Prevention or Potentially Harmful Distraction?" *JAMA Network News,* June 21, 2022, jamanetwork.com/journals/jama/fullarticle/2793472

Kelvin Li et al., "The good, the bad, and the ugly of calcium supplementation: A review of calcium intake on human health," *Clinical Interventions in Aging,* 13, 2018, pp. 2443–2452, ncbi.nlm.nih.gov/pmc/articles/PMC 6276611/

The Lown Institute, "Medication Overload: America's Other Drug Problem: How the Drive to Prescribe Is Harming Older Adults," April 2019, lowninstitute.org/wp-content/uploads/2019/08/medication-overload-lown-web.pdf

JoAnn E. Manson, MD, "Ask a Doctor: How much vitamin D do I need? Should I take a supplement?" *The Washington Post,* Sep. 12, 2022, washingtonpost.com/wellness/2022/09/12/vitamin-d-supplement-deficiency-covid/

Mayo Clinic Staff, "Studies into video telemedicine diagnostic accuracy and patient satisfaction find positive trends," *Mayo Clinic News Network,* Dec. 2, 2022, newsnetwork.mayoclinic.org/discussion/studies-into-video-telemedicine -diagnostic-accuracy-and-patient-satisfaction-find-positive-trends/

National Institutes of Health, "Using Dietary Supplements Wisely," *National Center for Complementary and Integrative Health, U.S. Department of Health and Human Services, National Institutes of Health,* nccih.nih.gov/health/using-dietary -supplements-wisely

Jennifer O'Hara, "Mayo Clinic Q&A podcast: Study finds patients highly satisfied with telehealth," *Mayo Clinic News Network*, June 4, 2021, newsnetwork .mayoclinic.org/discussion/mayo-clinic-qa-podcast-study-finds-patients-highly -satisfied-with-telehealth/

Kristin Samuelson, "Vitamins, supplements are a 'waste of money' for most Americans," *Northwestern Now,* June 21, 2022, news.northwestern.edu/stories/2022/06/vitamins-supplements-are-a-waste-of-money-for-most-americans

Dana Sparks, "Nationwide survey finds physician satisfaction with telehealth," *Mayo Clinic News Network,* Jan. 21, 2021, newsnetwork.mayoclinic.org/discussion/nationwide-survey-finds-physician-satisfaction-with-telehealth/

Staff, "Fannie Lou Hamer (1917–1977)" profile, *University of Washington School of Public Health Department of Public Systems and Population Health,* obgyn.wustl.edu/black-history-month-week-2-fannie-lou-hamer/

Staff, "Helping you choose: Quality ambulatory care," *The Joint Commission: Association of Professionals in Infection Control and Epidemiology (APIC) and Centers for Disease Control and Prevention (CDC),* jointcommission.org/-/media/tjc/documents/resources/for-consumers/helping-you-choose-ambulatory.pdf

Staff, "J. Marion Sims," *Encyclopedia of Alabama,* encyclopediaofalabama.org/article/h-1099

Staff, "Speak Up™: Antibiotics," *The Joint Commission: Association of Professionals in Infection Control and Epidemiology (APIC) and Centers for Disease Control and Prevention (CDC)*, jointcommission.org/-/media/tjc/documents/resources/speak -up/speak_up_infographic_antibiotics_2017pdf.pdf

Staff, "Using Dietary Supplements Wisely," *National Center for Complementary and Integrative Health, U.S. Department of Health and Human Services National Institutes of Health*, January 2019, nccih.nih.gov/health/using-dietary -supplements-wisely

Connie Tsao, MD, MPH, FAHA, and Seth Martin, MD, MHS, FAHA, "Heart Disease and Stroke Statistics—2023 Update," *American Heart Association Professional Heart Daily*, Jan. 25, 2023, professional.heart.org/en/science-news/ heart-disease-and-stroke-statistics-2023-update

Linda J. Vorvick, MD, et al., "When to use the emergency room—adult," *National Library of Medicine MedLine Plus*, July 25, 2022, medlineplus.gov/ency/ patientinstructions/000593.htm

Robert B. Wallace et al., "Urinary tract stone occurrence in the Women's Health Initiative (WHI) randomized clinical trial of calcium and vitamin D supplements," *The American Journal of Clinical Nutrition* 94, no. 1, July 2011, pp. 270–277, ajcn.nutrition.org/article/S0002-9165(23)02300-6/fulltext

Audrey J. Weiss, PhD, et al., "Statistical Brief #174: Overview of Emergency Department Visits in the United States, 2011," *National Library of Medicine: National Center for Biotechnology Information*, June 2014, ncbi.nlm.nih.gov/ books/NBK235856/

Chapter 4
Brave and Strong: What You Need to Know (and Do) About Cancer

American Association for Cancer Research, "Disparities in the Burden of Preventable Cancer Risk Factors," *AACR Cancer Disparities Progress Report*, cancerprogressreport.aacr.org/disparities/cdpr22-contents/cdpr22-disparities-in -the-burden-of-preventable-cancer-risk-factors/

American Cancer Society, "American Cancer Society Recommendations for the Early Detection of Breast Cancer," Jan. 14, 2022, cancer.org/cancer/breast -cancer/screening-tests-and-early-detection/american-cancer-society -recommendations-for-the-early-detection-of-breast-cancer.html

American Cancer Society, "Breast Cancer Facts & Figures, 2019–2020, *cancer.org*, cancer.org/content/dam/cancer-org/research/cancer-facts-and -statistics/breast-cancer-facts-and-figures/breast-cancer-facts-and-figures-2019 -2020.pdf

American Cancer Society, "Cancer Facts and Figures for African Americans, 2019–2021," cancer.org/content/dam/cancer-org/research/cancer-facts-and -statistics/cancer-facts-and-figures-for-african-americans/cancer-facts-and-figures -for-african-americans-2019-2021.pdf

American Cancer Society, "Family Cancer Syndromes," *cancer.org*, Sep. 14, 2022, cancer.org/cancer/risk-prevention/genetics/family-cancer-syndromes.html

American Cancer Society, "Survival Rates for Colorectal Cancer," *cancer.org*, Mar. 1,

2023, cancer.org/cancer/types/colon-rectal-cancer/detection-diagnosis-staging/survival-rates.html

CDC Staff, "Hereditary Breast Cancer and BRCA Genes," *cdc.gov,* Mar. 21, 2023, cdc.gov/cancer/breast/young_women/bringyourbrave/hereditary_breast_cancer/index.htm

CDC Staff, "Lung Cancer Among People Who Never Smoked," *CDC Centers for Disease Control and Prevention,* cdc.gov/cancer/lung/nonsmokers/index.htm

CDC Staff, "Questions to Ask Your Doctor About Colorectal Cancer," *cdc.gov,* Feb. 23, 2023, cdc.gov/cancer/colorectal/basic_info/screening/questions.htm

CDC Staff, "QuickStats: Percentage of Women Aged ≥ 50 Years Who Have Had a Hysterectomy, by Race/Ethnicity and Year—National Health Interview Survey, United States, 2008 and 2018, *Morbidity and Mortality Weekly Report* 68, no. 41, Oct. 18, 2019, p. 935, cdc.gov/mmwr/volumes/68/wr/mm6841a3.htm #suggestedcitation

CDC Staff, "What are the risk factors for breast cancer?" *cdc.gov,* Sep. 26, 2022, cdc.gov/cancer/breast/basic_info/risk_factors.htm

David Chelmow, MD, et al., "Executive Summary of the Uterine Cancer Evidence Review Conference," *Obstetrics & Gynecology* 139, no. 4, April 2022, pp. 626–643, journals.lww.com/greenjournal/Fulltext/2022/04000/Executive_Summary_of_the_Uterine_Cancer_Evidence.21.aspx

Tianhui Chen, MD, PhD, et al., "Race and Ethnicity-Adjusted Age Recommendation for Initiating Breast Cancer Screening," *JAMA NetworkOpen* 6, no. 4, Apr. 19, 2023, jamanetwork.com/journals/jamanetworkopen/fullarticle/2803948

Rowan T. Chlebowski et al., "Breast Cancer Prevention: Time for Change," *JCO Oncolocy Practice* 17, no. 12, December 2021, pp. 709–716, pubmed.ncbi.nlm.nih.gov/34319769/

Rowan T. Chlebowski et al., "Long-term influence of estrogen plus progestin and estrogen alone use on breast cancer incidence: The Women's Health Initiative randomized trials," *San Antonio Breast Cancer Symposium,* Dec. 10–14, 2019, abstractsonline.com/pp8/#!/7946/presentation/2229

Beomyoung Cho et al., "Evaluation of Racial/Ethnic Differences in Treatment and Mortality Among Women with Triple-Negative Breast Cancer," *JAMA Oncology* 7, no. 7, May 13, 2021, jamanetwork.com/journals/jamaoncology/fullarticle/2780032

Megan A. Clarke, PhD, et al., "Hysterectomy-Corrected Uterine Corpus Cancer Incidence Trends and Differences in Relative Survival Reveal Racial Disparities and Rising Rates of Nonendometrioid Cancers," *Journal of Clinical Oncology* 37, no. 22, May 22, 2019, pp. 1895–1908, ncbi.nlm.nih.gov/pmc/articles/PMC6675596/

Megan A. Clarke, PhD, et al., "Racial and Ethnic Differences in Hysterectomy-Corrected Uterine Corpus Cancer Mortality by Stage and Histologic Subtype," *JAMA Oncology* 8, no. 6, May 5, 2022, jamanetwork.com/journals/jamaoncology/article-abstract/2792010

Megan A. Clarke, PhD, "Uterine cancer deaths are rising in the United States, and are highest among Black women," *cancer.gov,* May 5, 2022, cancer.gov/news-events/press-releases/2022/uterine-cancer-deaths-black-women

Angelena Crown, MD, FACS, et al., "Disparity in Breast Cancer Care: Current State of Access to Screening, Genetic Testing, Oncofertility, and Reconstruction," *Journal of the American College of Surgeons* 236, no. 6, June 2023, pp. 1233–1239, journals.lww.com/journalacs/Abstract/2023/06000/Disparity _in_Breast_Cancer_Care__Current_State_of.32.aspx

Carol E. DeSantis, MPH, et al., "Breast Cancer Statistics, 2019," *CA: A Cancer Journal for Clinicians,* Oct. 2, 2019, acsjournals.onlinelibrary.wiley.com/doi/full/ 10.3322/caac.21583

Kemi M. Doll and Aaron N. Winn, "Assessing endometrial cancer risk among US women: Long-term trends using hysterectomy-adjusted analysis," *American Journal of Obstetrics and Gynecology* 221, no. 4, May 22, 2019, pubmed.ncbi.nlm .nih.gov/31125544/

Yvonne L. Eaglehouse, PhD, MPH, et al., "Racial-Ethnic Comparison of Guideline-Adherent Gynecologic Cancer Care in an Equal-Access System," *Obstetrics & Gynecology* 137, no. 4, April 2021, pp. 629–640, journals.lww.com/ greenjournal/Fulltext/2021/04000/Racial_Ethnic_Comparison_of_Guideline _Adherent.11.aspx

Erik Eckhert, MD, MS, et al., "Breast Cancer Diagnosis, Treatment, and Outcomes of Patients from Sex and Gender Minority Groups," *JAMA Oncology* 9, no. 4, May 1, 2023, pp. 473–480, jamanetwork.com/journals/jamaoncology/article -abstract/2800989

Neha Goel, MD, et al., "Neighborhood Disadvantage and Breast Cancer-Specific Survival," *JAMA NetworkOpen* 6, no. 4, Apr. 21, 2023, jamanetwork.com/ journals/jamanetworkopen/fullarticle/2804100

Nada Hassanein, "Black women make up majority of new HIV cases among women. But they aren't getting care," *USA Today,* Nov. 21, 2022, usatoday.com/ story/news/health/2022/11/21/hiv-cases-black-women-treatment-prevention/ 8303299001/

Marci A. Landsmann, "Why Do African Americans Have Increased Breast Cancer Mortality?" *Cancertoday,* Nov. 13, 2020, cancertodaymag.org/cancer-talk/Why -Do-African-Americans-Have-Increased-Breast-Cancer-Mortality/

Marissa B. Lawson, MD, et al., "Multilevel Factors Associated with Time to Biopsy After Abnormal Screening Mammography Results by Race and Ethnicity," *JAMA Oncology* 8, no. 8, June 23, 2022, pp. 1115–1126, jamanetwork.com/ journals/jamaoncology/fullarticle/2793713?resultClick=1

Jack J. Lee, PhD, "Rising endometrial cancer rates spur new approaches to prevention," *cancer.gov,* June 28, 2022, prevention.cancer.gov/news-and-events/blog/ rising-endometrial-cancer-rates-spur-new-approaches-prevention

Jonathan M. Loree, MD, et al., "disparity of race reporting and representation in clinical trials leading to cancer drug approvals from 2008 to 2018," *JAMA Oncology* 5, no. 10, Aug. 15, 2019, jamanetwork.com/journals/jamaoncology/ fullarticle/2748395

Anne Marie McCarthy et al., "Relationship of established risk factors with breast cancer subtypes," *Cancer Medicine,* Aug. 31, 2021, onlinelibrary.wiley.com/doi/ 10.1002/cam4.4158

Megan A. Mullins and Michele L. Cote, "Beyond Obesity: The Rising Incidence and Mortality Rates of Uterine Corpus Cancer," *Journal of Clinical Oncology* 37, no. 22, Aug. 1, 2019, pp. 1851–1853, pubmed.ncbi.nlm.nih.gov/31232669/

Dawn Mussallem, "Lifestyle and Breast Cancer Risk Reduction," *The North American Menopause Society Practice Pearl,* Mar. 17, 2022, menopause.org/docs/default-source/professional/practice-pearl-mussallem-lifestyle-and-breast-cancer-risk-reduction.pdf

Anna Najor, MD, et al., "Systematic Scoping Literature Review of Disparities of Stage in Endometrial Cancer," *Obstetrics & Gynecology* 139, May 2022, pp. 92S-93S, journals.lww.com/greenjournal/Abstract/2022/05001/Systematic_Scoping_Literature_Review_of.318.aspx

National Cancer Institute, "Cancer stat facts: lung and bronchus cancer," *cancer.gov,* seer.cancer.gov/statfacts/html/lungb.html

National Cancer Institute, "Cancer Statistics," *cancer.org,* Sep. 25, 2020, cancer.gov/about-cancer/understanding/statistics

Lisa A. Newman, MD, MPH, "Race and Ethnicity as a Sociopolitical Construct That Is Biologically Relevant in Breast Cancer," *JAMA Surgery* 158, no. 6, Apr. 12, 2023, jamanetwork.com/journals/jamasurgery/article-abstract/2803001

Samilia Obeng-Gyasi, MD, MPH, et al., "Association of Allostatic Load with All-Cause Mortality in Patients with Breast Cancer," *JAMA NetworkOpen* 6, no. 5, May 18, 2023, jamanetwork.com/journals/jamanetworkopen/fullarticle/2805017

OCRA (Ovarian Cancer Research Alliance) Staff, "Ovarian Cancer Statistics," *OCRAhope.org,* ocrahope.org/get-the-facts/statistics

Jesse J. Plascak, PhD, et al., "Association Between Residence in Historically Redlined Districts Indicative of Structural Racism and Racial and Ethnic Disparities in Breast Cancer Outcomes," *JAMA NetworkOpen* 5, no. 7, July 8, 2022, jamanetwork.com/journals/jamanetworkopen/fullarticle/2794026

Roni Caryn Rabin, "Uterine Cancer Is on the Rise, Especially Among Black Women," *The New York Times,* June 17, 2022, nytimes.com/2022/06/17/health/uterine-cancer-black-women.html

Gelareh Sadigh, MD, et al., "Assessment of Racial Disparity in Survival Outcomes for Early Hormone Receptor-Positive Breast Cancer After Adjusting for Insurance Status and Neighborhood Deprivation," *JAMA Oncology* 8, no. 4, Feb. 17, 2022, pp. 579–586, jamanetwork.com/journals/jamaoncology/fullarticle/2789162

Dana Shively et al., "Racial Disparities in Survival Outcomes of Colorectal Cancer Patients After Surgical Resection," *Cureus* 14, no. 2, Feb. 9, 2022, ncbi.nlm.nih.gov/pmc/articles/PMC8916922/

Staff, "The Sister Study," National Institutes of Health: U.S. Department of Health and Human Services, sisterstudy.niehs.nih.gov/English/new.htm

U.S. Cancer Statistics Working Group, "Leading Cancer Cases and Deaths, All Races and Ethnicities, Male and Female, 2020," *cdc.gov,* June 2023, gis.cdc.gov/Cancer/USCS/#/AtAGlance/

U.S. Cancer Statistics Working Group, "U.S. Cancer Statistics Data Visualizations Tool, 1999–2020," *U.S. Department of Health and Human Services, Centers for Disease Control and Prevention and National Cancer Institute*; June 2023, gis.cdc.gov/Cancer/USCS/#/AtAGlance/

Weill Cornell Medicine Staff, "Early Detection Is Important in Breast Cancer Care," *weillcornell.org,* Oct. 5, 2021, weillcornell.org/news/early-detection-is-important -in-breast-cancer-care

Weill Cornell Medicine Staff, "Reducing Breast Cancer Risks in African American Communities," *weillcornell.org,* Feb. 10, 2021, weillcornell.org/news/reducing -breast-cancer-risks-in-african-american-communities

Sara Whetstone, MD, MHS, et al., "Health Disparities in Uterine Cancer," *Obstetrics & Gynecology* 139, no. 4, April 2022, pp. 645–659, journals.lww.com/ greenjournal/Fulltext/2022/04000/Health_Disparities_in_Uterine_Cancer_ _Report_From.22.aspx

David R. Williams, PhD, MPH, et al., "Understanding and Effectively Addressing Breast Cancer in African American Women: Unpacking the Social Context," *Cancer* 122, no. 14, July 15, 2016, pp. 2138–2149, ncbi.nlm.nih.gov/pmc/ articles/PMC5588632/

Clement G. Yedjou et al., "Health and Racial Disparity in Breast Cancer," *Advances in Experimental Medicine and Biology,* Aug. 28, 2019, ncbi.nlm.nih.gov/pmc/ articles/PMC6941147/

Chapter 5
Control: Chronic Stress, Weight Gain, and Diabetes: Tame Your Triple Threat

Ann Smith Barnes, MD, MPH, "The Epidemic of Obesity and Diabetes," *The Texas Heart Institute Journal* 38, no. 2, 2011, pp. 142–144, ncbi.nlm.nih.gov/pmc/ articles/PMC3066828/

Sarah L. Becker, BA, and JoAnn E. Manson, MD, DrPH, NCMP, "Menopause, the gut microbiome, and weight gain: Correlation or causation?" *Menopause* 28, no. 3, March 2021, pp. 327–331, journals.lww.com/menopausejournal/pages/ articleviewer.aspx?year=2021&issue=03000&article=00014&type=Abstract

Marialaura Bonaccio et al., "Joint association of food nutritional profile by Nutri-Score front-of-pack label and ultra-processed food intake with mortality: Moli-sani prospective cohort study," *The BMJ,* Aug. 31, 2022, bmj.com/content/378/ bmj-2022-070688

Alice Callahan, "Ask Well: Why Do Women Gain Belly Fat in Midlife?" *The New York Times,* Jan. 11, 2022, nytimes.com/2022/01/11/well/move/belly-fat-women .html; swanstudy.org/wps/wp-content/uploads/2022/01/NewYorkTimesArticle -WhyDoWomenGainBellyFatInMidlife.pdf

CDC Staff, "A Snapshot: Diabetes in the United States," *cdc.gov,* Aug. 11, 2022, cdc.gov/diabetes/library/socialmedia/infographics/diabetes.html

CDC Staff, "Adult Obesity Facts," *cdc.gov,* May 17, 2022, cdc.gov/obesity/data/ adult.html

CDC Staff, "Diabetes and Women," *cdc.gov,* June 20, 2022, cdc.gov/diabetes/ library/features/diabetes-and-women.html

CDC Staff, "Prevalence of Childhood Obesity in the United States," *cdc.gov,* May 17, 2022, cdc.gov/obesity/data/childhood.html

CDC Staff, "Unfit to Serve: Obesity and Physical Inactivity Are Impacting National

Security," *cdc.gov,* July 2022, cdc.gov/physicalactivity/downloads/unfit-to-serve
-062322-508.pdf

Christopher D. Cooper et al., "Sleep deprivation and obesity in adults: A brief
narrative review," *BMJ Open Sport & Exercise Medicine* 4, no. 1, Oct. 4, 2018,
ncbi.nlm.nih.gov/pmc/articles/PMC6196958/

Dana DeSilva, PhD, RD, and Dennis Anderson-Villaluz, MBA, RD, LDN, FAND,
"Nutrition as We Age: Healthy Eating with the Dietary Guidelines," *health.gov,*
July 20, 2021, health.gov/news/202107/nutrition-we-age-healthy-eating-dietary
-guidelines

Lilian Golzarri-Arroyo, MS, et al., "What's New in Understanding the Risk
Associated with Body Size and Shape? Pears, Apples, and Olives on Toothpicks,"
JAMA NetworkOpen 2, no. 7, July 24, 2019, jamanetwork.com/journals/
jamanetworkopen/fullarticle/2738617

Tianna Hicklin, PhD, "Factors contributing to higher incidence of diabetes for
black Americans," *NIH Research Matters,* Jan. 9, 2018, nih.gov/news-events/
nih-research-matters/factors-contributing-higher-incidence-diabetes-black
-americans

Rachel Hosie, "One chart shows why exercise only plays a tiny role in weight loss,"
Insider.com, Jan. 14, 2023, insider.com/why-exercise-doesnt-help-you-lose
-weight-chart-fat-loss-2023-1

Michael G. Knight, MD, MSHP, et al., "Weight Regulation in Menopause,"
Menopause 28, no. 8, May 24, 2021, pp. 960–965, ncbi.nlm.nih.gov/pmc/
articles/PMC8373626/

Gina Kolata, "These Sisters with Sickle Cell Had Devastating, and Preventable,
Strokes," *The New York Times,* May 23, 2021, nytimes.com/2021/05/23/health/
sickle-cell-black-children.html

Luisa Lampignano et al., "Cross-sectional relationship among different anthropo-
metric parameters and cardiometabolic risk factors in a cohort of patients with
overweight or obesity," *PLOSOne,* Nov. 5, 2020, journals.plos.org/plosone/
article?id=10.1371/journal.pone.0241841

G. L. Mills et al., "Low-density lipoproteins in patients homozygous for familial
hyperbetalipoproteinaemia," *Clinical Science and Molecular Medicine* 27, no. 5,
May 2017, pp. 1137–1144.

D. V. Monaco-Ferreira and V. A. Leandro-Methi, "Weight Regain 10 Years
After Roux-en-Y Gastric Bypass," *Obesity Surgery* 27, no. 5, May 2017,
pp. 1137–1144.

Dariush Mozaffarian, "Perspective: Obesity—an unexplained epidemic," *The
American Journal of Clinical Nutrition* 115, no. 6, June 2022, pp. 1445–1450,
sciencedirect.com/science/article/pii/S0002916522002684

Anahad O'Connor, "The best foods to feed your gut microbiome," *washingtonpost
.com,* Sep. 20, 2022, washingtonpost.com/wellness/2022/09/20/gut-health
-microbiome-best-foods/

Anahad O'Connor, "What are ultra-processed foods? And what should I eat
instead?" *washingtonpost.com,* Sep. 27, 2022, washingtonpost.com/wellness/
2022/09/27/ultraprocessed-foods/

Office of Minority Health Staff, "Obesity and African Americans," *U.S. Department*

of Health and Human Services, minorityhealth.hhs.gov/omh/browse.aspx?lvl
=4&lvlid=25

PCNA [Preventive Cardiovascular Nurses Association] Staff, "New Hypertension
Recommendations and Guidelines: PCNA Statement," *PCNA.net,* Nov. 13,
2017, pcna.net/new-hypertension-guidelines-pcna-statement/

Diana Sonntag et al., "Beyond Food Promotion: A Systematic Review on the
Influence of the Food Industry on Obesity-Related Dietary Behaviour Among
Children," *Nutrients,* Oct. 16, 2015, mdpi.com/2072-6643/7/10/5414

Norbert Stefan et al., "Causes, Characteristics, and Consequences of Metabolically
Unhealthy Normal Weight Gain in Humans," *Cell Metabolism* 26, no. 2, Aug. 1,
2017, pp. 292–300, sciencedirect.com/science/article/pii/S1550413117304291

Thomas Unger et al., "2020 International Society of Hypertension Global Hypertension Guidelines," *Hypertension* 75, no. 6, May 6, 2020, pp. 1334–1357,
www.ahajournals.org/doi/full/10.1161/HYPERTENSIONAHA.120.15026

USDA Staff, "Dietary Guidelines for Americans, 2020–2025," *Dietaryguidelines.gov,*
December 2020, dietaryguidelines.gov/sites/default/files/2021-03/Dietary
_Guidelines_for_Americans-2020-2025.pdf

Eline S. Van der Valk et al., "Stress and Obesity: Are There More Susceptible
Individuals?" *Current Obesity Reports,* Apr. 16, 2018, pp. 193–203, link.springer
.com/article/10.1007/s13679-018-0306-y

Angélica T. Vieira et al., "Influence of Oral and Gut Microbiota in the Health of
Menopausal Women," *Frontiers in Microbiology,* Sep. 28, 2017, ncbi.nlm.nih
.gov/pmc/articles/PMC5625026/

"Weight gain after surgery," https://pubmed.ncbi.nih.gov/183929W07

Yafeng Wang et al., "Sex differences in the association between diabetes and risk of
cardiovascular diabetes and risk of cardiovascular disease, cancer, and all-cause
and cause-specific mortality: A systematic review and meta-analysis of 5,162,654
participants," *BMC Medicine* 17, no. 136, July 12, 2019, bmcmedicine
.biomedcentral.com/articles/10.1186/s12916-019-1355-0

Chapter 6
Key to Your Heart: Guarding Against Cardiovascular Disease

Haim A. Abenhaim, MD, MPH, et al., "Menopausal Hormone Therapy Formulation and Breast Cancer Risk," *Obstetrics & Gynecology* 139, no. 6, June 2022, pp.
1103–1110, journals.lww.com/greenjournal/Abstract/2022/06000/Menopausal
_Hormone_Therapy_Formulation_and_Breast.16.aspx

American Heart Association, "Heart Attack, Stroke, and Cardiac Arrest Symptoms,"
heart.org, heart.org/en/about-us/heart-attack-and-stroke-symptoms

American Heart Association Editorial Staff, "Heart Attack Symptoms in Women,"
heart.org, Dec. 5, 2022, heart.org/en/health-topics/heart-attack/warning-signs-of
-a-heart-attack/heart-attack-symptoms-in-women

American Heart Association Editorial Staff, "Heart Disease and Stroke in Black
Women," *goredforwomen.org,* goredforwomen.org/en/about-heart-disease-in
-women/facts/heart-disease-in-african-american-women

Mercedes R. Carnethon et al., "Cardiovascular Health in African Americans: A

Scientific Statement from the American Heart Association," *Circulation* 136, no. 21, Oct. 23, 2017, pp. e393–e423, www.ahajournals.org/doi/10.1161/CIR .0000000000000534

CDC Staff, "Leading Causes of Death," *CDC/National Center for Health Statistics,* Jan. 18, 2023, cdc.gov/nchs/fastats/leading-causes-of-death.htm

CDC Staff, "Women and Stroke," *cdc.gov,* May 4, 2023, cdc.gov/stroke/women.htm

Cleveland Clinic, "Silent Heart Attack," *my.clevelandclinic.org,* July 28, 2021, my.clevelandclinic.org/health/diseases/21630-silent-heart-attack

Imo Ebong, MD, MS, and Khadijah Breathett, MD, MS, "The Cardiovascular Disease Epidemic in African American Women: Recognizing and Tackling a Persistent Problem," *Journal of Women's Health* 29, no. 7, July 2020, pp. 891–893, ncbi.nlm.nih.gov/pmc/articles/PMC7371547/

Ramón Estruch, MD, PhD, et al., "Primary Prevention of Cardiovascular Disease with a Mediterranean Diet," *New England Journal of Medicine,* Apr. 4, 2013, pp. 1279–1290, nejm.org/doi/10.1056/NEJMoa1200303

Stephanie S. Faubion, MD, et al., "Statin Therapy: Does Sex Matter?" *Menopause* 26, no. 12, December 2019, pp. 1425–1435, ncbi.nlm.nih.gov/pmc/articles/ PMC7664983/

Grishma Hirode, MAS, and Robert J. Wong, MD, MS, "Trends in the Prevalence of Metabolic Syndrome in the United States, 2011–2016," *JAMA Network* 323, no. 24, June 23, 2020, pp. 2526–2528, ncbi.nlm.nih.gov/pmc/articles/ PMC7312413/

Howard N. Hodis and Wendy J. Mack, "Menopausal Hormone Replacement Therapy and Reduction of All-Cause Mortality and Cardiovascular Disease: It Is About Time and Timing," *Cancer* 28, no. 3, May–June 2022, pp. 208–223, pubmed.ncbi.nlm.nih.gov/35594469/

National Cancer Institute, "Oral contraceptives and cancer risk," *cancer.gov,* Feb. 22, 2018, cancer.gov/about-cancer/causes-prevention/risk/hormones/oral -contraceptives-fact-sheet

National Center for Chronic Disease Prevention and Health Promotion, Division for Heart Disease and Stroke Prevention, "Stroke Signs and Symptoms," *Centers for Disease Control and Prevention,* May 4, 2022, cdc.gov/stroke/signs_symptoms .htm

National Center for Chronic Disease Prevention and Health Promotion, Division for Heart Disease and Stroke Prevention, "Women and Heart Disease," *Centers for Disease Control and Prevention,* May 15, 2023, cdc.gov/heartdisease/women .htm

National Center for Health Statistics, "Age-Adjusted Death Rates of Heart Disease and Cancer, by Sex—United States, 2010–2020," *Morbidity and Mortality Weekly Report* 71, no. 15, Apr. 15, 2022, cdc.gov/mmwr/volumes/71/wr/pdfs/ mm7115a4-H.pdf

Hannah Nichols and Vincent J. Tavella, DVM, MPH, "What are the leading causes of death in the U.S.?" *medicalnewstoday.com,* July 4, 2019, medicalnewstoday .com/articles/282929

Sanne A. E. Peters et al., "Sex Differences in the Prevalence of, and Trends in, Cardiovascular Risk Factors, Treatment, and Control in the United States,

2001 to 2016," *Circulation* 139, no. 8, Feb. 19, 2019, pp. 1025–1035, www.ahajournals.org/doi/10.1161/CIRCULATIONAHA.118.035550

Tiffany M. Powell-Wiley et al., "Obesity and Cardiovascular Disease: A Scientific Statement from the American Heart Association," *Circulation* 143, no. 21, Apr. 22, 2021, pp. e984-e1010, www.ahajournals.org/doi/10.1161/CIR .0000000000000973

Brooke C. Schneider et al., "Association of vascular risk factors with cognition in a multiethnic sample," *The Journals of Gerontology, Series B, Psychological Sciences and Social Sciences,* May 12, 2014, pubmed.ncbi.nlm.nih.gov/24821298/

Connie W. Tsao et al., "Heart Disease and Stroke Statistics—2023 Update: A Report from the American Heart Association," *American Heart Association Journals,* Jan. 25, 2023, www.ahajournals.org/doi/10.1161/CIR .0000000000001123

U.S. Department of Health and Human Services, "Heart Disease and African Americans," *U.S. Department of Health and Human Services Office of Minority Health,* Mar. 9, 2023, minorityhealth.hhs.gov/heart-disease-and-african-americans

Chapter 7
When It Don't Come Easy: Brain Health and Alzheimer's

Alzheimer's Association, "2023: Alzheimer's Disease Facts & Figures," *alz.org,* alz.org/media/Documents/alzheimers-facts-and-figures.pdf

Alzheimer's Association, "Why Participate in a Clinical Trial?" *alz.org,* alz.org/ alzheimers-dementia/research_progress/clinical-trials/why-participate

Alzheimer's Association, "Women and Alzheimer's," *alz.org,* alz.org/alzheimers -dementia/what-is-alzheimers/women-and-alzheimer-s

Nicholas Bakalar, "5 Measures That May Lower Your Alzheimer's Risk," *The New York Times,* June 23, 2020, nytimes.com/2020/06/23/well/mind/5-measures-that -may-lower-your-alzheimers-risk.html

Clarissa Brincat and Jill Seladi-Schulman, PhD, "Alzheimer's: Healthy lifestyle linked to slower memory decline, regardless of genetic risk," *Medical News Today,* Feb. 5, 2023, medicalnewstoday.com/articles/healthy-diet-lifestyle-slower -memory-decline-alzheimers-dementia

Sybil L. Crawford, PhD, "Contributions of oophorectomy and other gynecologic surgeries to cognitive decline and dementia," *Menopause* 29, no. 5, May 2022, pp. 499–501, journals.lww.com/menopausejournal/Citation/2022/05000/ Contributions_of_oophorectomy_and_other.1.aspx

Klodian Dhana et al., "Healthy lifestyle and the risk of Alzheimer dementia," *Neurology* 95, no. 4, June 17, 2020, n.neurology.org/content/95/4/e374

Judith Garber, "A tale of two drugs: Accountability and evidence in Alzheimer's treatments," *LownInstitute.org,* Jan. 20, 2023, lowninstitute.org/a-tale-of-two -drugs-accountability-and-evidence-in-alzheimers-treatments/

Kristen M. George et al., "Impact of Cardiovascular Risk Factors in Adolescence, Young Adulthood, and Midlife on Late-Life Cognition: Study of Health Aging in African Americans," *The Journals of Gerontology, Series A, Biological Sciences and Medical Sciences,* Aug. 13, 2021, pubmed.ncbi.nlm.nih.gov/34387334/

Andrew Gregory, "HRT 'potentially important' in reducing women's dementia risk," *theguardian.com*, Jan. 13, 2023, theguardian.com/society/2023/jan/14/hrt -potentially-important-in-reducing-womens-dementia-risk

Robert Langreth and Madeline Campbell, "Alzheimer's Trials Exclude Black Patients at 'Astonishing' Rate," *Bloomberg.com*, Apr. 19, 2022, bloomberg.com/news/ articles/2022-04-19/drug-trials-are-more-likely-to-admit-white-people

Usha Lee McFarling, "Brains of Black Americans age faster, study finds, with racial stressors a likely factor," *STATNews.com*, Nov. 14, 2022, statnews.com/2022/11/ 14/aging-black-adults-brains/

Aarti Mishra et al., "A tale of two systems: Lessons learned from female mid-life aging with implications for Alzheimer's prevention & treatment," *Ageing Research Reviews* 74, February 2022, pubmed.ncbi.nlm.nih.gov/34929348/

Lisa Mosconi et al., "Menopause impacts human brain structure, connectivity, energy metabolism, and amyloid-beta deposition," *Scientific Reports*, June 9, 2021, ncbi.nlm.nih.gov/pmc/articles/PMC8190071/

NCCIH Staff, "7 Things to Know About Dietary Supplements for Cognitive Function, Dementia, and Alzheimer's Disease," *U.S. Department of Health and Human Services, National Institutes of Health*, June 21, 2023, nccih.nih.gov/ health/tips/things-to-know-about-dietary-supplements-for-cognitive-function -dementia-and-alzheimers-disease

Rasha N. M. Saleh et al., "Hormone replacement therapy is associated with improved cognition and larger brain volumes in at-risk *APOE4* women: Results from the European Prevention of Alzheimer's Disease (EPAD) cohort," *Alzheimer's Research & Therapy* 15, no. 10, Jan. 9, 3023, alzres.biomedcentral.com/ articles/10.1186/s13195-022-01121-5

Dana G. Smith, "How to Know If You Have a Genetic Risk for Alzheimer's," *The New York* Times, Nov. 23, 2022, nytimes.com/2022/11/23/well/alzheimers -disease-genetic-risk.html

Indira C. Turney, PhD, et al., "Brain Aging Among Racially and Ethnically Diverse Middle-Aged and Older Adults," *JAMA Neurology*, Nov. 14, 2022, jamanetwork .com/journals/jamaneurology/article-abstract/2798587

WebMD Staff and Melinda Ratini, MS, DO, "Alcohol and the Aging Process," *webmd.com*, Nov. 6, 2022, webmd.com/mental-health/addiction/ss/slideshow -alcohol-aging

Karen G. Wooten, MA, et al., "Racial and Ethnic Differences in Subjective Cognitive Decline—United States, 2015–2020," *Morbidity and Mortality Weekly Report* 72, no. 10, Mar. 10, 2023, pp. 249–255, cdc.gov/mmwr/volumes/72/wr/ mm7210a1.htm

Kristine Yaffe et al., "Cardiovascular Risk Factors Across the Life Course and Cognitive Decline: A Pooled Cohort Study," *Neurology*, Apr. 27, 2021, pubmed .ncbi.nlm.nih.gov/33731482/

Chapter 8
I Will Survive: "Female Troubles" and Their Treatments

ACOG Staff, "Management of Acute Abnormal Uterine Bleeding in Nonpregnant Reproductive-Aged Women," *Obstetrics & Gynecology* 121, no. 4, April 2013, pp. 891–896, journals.lww.com/greenjournal/Fulltext/2013/04000/Committee_Opinion_No__557__Management_of_Acute.42.aspx

ACOG Staff, "Management of Symptomatic Uterine Leiomyomas," *Obstetrics & Gynecology* 137, no. 6, June 2021, pp. e100–e115, journals.lww.com/greenjournal/Abstract/2021/06000/Management_of_Symptomatic_Uterine_Leiomyomas__ACOG.36.aspx

Moon Kyoung Cho, "Use of Combined Oral Contraceptives in Perimenopausal Women," *Chonnam Medical Journal* 54, no. 3, Sep. 27, 2018, pp. 153–158, ncbi.nlm.nih.gov/pmc/articles/PMC6165915/

Kelly M. Hoffman et al., "Racial bias in pain assessment and treatment recommendations, and false beliefs about biological differences between Blacks and whites," *PNAS (Proceedings of the National Academy of Sciences of the United States of America)* 113, no. 16, Apr. 4, 2016, pnas.org/doi/full/10.1073/pnas.1516047113

Patricia G. Moorman et al., "Comparison of characteristics of fibroids in African American and white women undergoing premenopausal hysterectomy," *Fertility and Sterility* 99, no. 3, Mar. 1, 2013, pp. 768–776, pubmed.ncbi.nlm.nih.gov/23199610/

Camran Nezhat, MD, et al., "Optimal Management of Endometriosis and Pain," *Obstetrics & Gynecology 134(4)*, October 2019, pp. 834–839, journals.lww.com/greenjournal/Fulltext/2019/10000/Optimal_Management_of_Endometriosis_and_Pain.25.aspx

Robert Pokras, MA, and Vicki Georges Hufnagel, MD, "Hysterectomy in the United States, 1965–84," *American Journal of Public Health* 78, no. 7, July 1988, pp. 852–853, ncbi.nlm.nih.gov/pmc/articles/PMC1350353/pdf/amjph00246-0102.pdf

Ema Sagner, "More States Move to End 'Tampon Tax' That's Seen as Discriminating Against Women," *npr.org*, Mar. 25, 2018, npr.org/2018/03/25/564580736/more-states-move-to-end-tampon-tax-that-s-seen-as-discriminating-against-women

Mara Ulin, MD, et al., "Uterine fibroids in menopause and perimenopause," *Menopause* 27, no. 2, February 2020, pp. 238–242, journals.lww.com/menopausejournal/Abstract/2020/02000/Uterine_fibroids_in_menopause_and_perimenopause.17.aspx

Kedra Wallace, PhD, et al., "Comparative effectiveness of hysterectomy versus myomectomy on one-year health-related quality of life in women with uterine fibroids," *Fertility and Sterility* 113, no. 3, March 2020, pp. 618–626, fertstert.org/action/showPdf?pii=S0015-0282%2819%2932498-7

Chapter 9
Hot in Herre: Perimenopause: Fertility's Final Frontier

Dani Blum and Nicole Stock, "What to Know Before You Freeze Your Eggs," *The New York Times,* Dec. 23, 2022, nytimes.com/2022/12/23/well/family/egg-freezing-risks-cost.html

S. J. Chua et al., "Age-related natural fertility outcomes in women over 35 years: A systematic review and individual participant data meta-analysis," *Human Reproduction* 35, no. 8, August 2020, pp. 1808–1820, academic.oup.com/humrep/article/35/8/1808/5874626

Sarah Druckenmiller Cascante et al., "Fifteen years of autologous oocyte thaw outcomes from a large university-based fertility center," *Fertility and Sterility* 118, no. 1, July 2022, pp. 158–166, pubmed.ncbi.nlm.nih.gov/35597614/

Amber Ferguson, "America has a Black sperm donor shortage. Black women are paying the price," *The Washington Post,* Oct. 20, 2022, washingtonpost.com/business/2022/10/20/black-sperm-donors/

Harris Williams Staff, "Fertility Services: Strong Demand with Room to Grow," *harriswilliams.com,* Sep. 11, 2019, harriswilliams.com/our-insights/fertility-services-strong-demand-room-grow

Gina Kolata, " 'Sobering' Study Shows Challenges of Egg Freezing," *The New York Times,* Sep. 23, 2022, nytimes.com/2022/09/23/health/egg-freezing-age-pregnancy.html

Joyce A. Martin, MPH, et al., "Births: Final Data for 2019," *National Vital Statistics Reports* 70, no. 2, Mar. 23, 2021, cdc.gov/nchs/data/nvsr/nvsr70/nvsr70-02-508.pdf

Joyce A. Martin, MPH, et al., "Births in the United States, 2019," *National Center for Health Statistics Data Brief* 387, October 2020, cdc.gov/nchs/products/databriefs/db387.htm

Anne Morse, "Stable Fertility Rates 1990–2019 Mask Distinct Variations by Age," *United States Census Bureau,* Apr. 6, 2022, census.gov/library/stories/2022/04/fertility-rates-declined-for-younger-women-increased-for-older-women.html

Pew Trusts, "The Long-Term Decline in Fertility—and What It Means for State Budgets," *pewtrusts.org,* Dec. 5, 2022, pewtrusts.org/en/research-and-analysis/issue-briefs/2022/12/the-long-term-decline-in-fertility-and-what-it-means-for-state-budgets

The Practice Committee of the American Society for Reproductive Medicine, "Evidence-based outcomes after oocyte cryopreservation for donor oocyte in vitro fertilization and planned oocyte cryopreservation: A guideline," *Fertility and Sterility* 116, no. 1, July 2021, pp. 36–47, fertstert.org/article/S0015-0282(21)00142-4/fulltext

Amira Yashruti and Sachiyo Yagi, "Event Review: A Decade of Egg Freezing—Experiences, Ethics, Expectations," *progress.org,* Nov. 7, 2022, progress.org.uk/event-review-a-decade-of-egg-freezing-experiences-ethics-expectations/

Chapter 10
Finally!: Menopause and Beyond

Haim Aire Abenhaim, MD, MPH, et al., "Bioidentical, Synthetic, and Animal Based Hormone Replacement Therapies and Risk of Breast Cancer [1M]," *Obstetrics & Gynecology* 129, no. 5, May 8, 2017, p. S132, journals.lww.com/greenjournal/Abstract/2017/05001/Bioidentical,_Synthetic,_and_Animal_Based_Hormone.473.aspx

Haim Aire Abenhaim, MD, MPH, et al., "Menopausal Hormone Therapy Formulation and Breast Cancer Risk," *Obstetrics & Gynecology* 139, no. 6, June 2022, pp. 1103–1110, journals.lww.com/greenjournal/Abstract/2022/06000/Menopausal_Hormone_Therapy_Formulation_and_Breast.16.aspx

ACOG Staff, "Management of Menopausal Symptoms," *ACOG [The American College of Obstetricians and Gynecologists] Practice Bulletin* 141, January 2014, acog.org/clinical/clinical-guidance/practice-bulletin/articles/2014/01/management-of-menopausal-symptoms

Niki Bezzant, " 'She will not become dull and unattractive': The charming history of menopause and HRT," *theguardian.com,* Jan. 17, 2022, theguardian.com/world/2022/jan/18/she-will-not-become-dull-and-unattractive-the-charming-history-of-menopause-and-hrt

Nardy Baezel Bickel, "25 years of research shows insidious effect of racism on Black women's menopausal transition, health," *University of Michigan School of Public Health News,* Feb. 23. 2022, sph.umich.edu/news/2022posts/insidious-effect-of-racism-on-black-womens-menopausal-transition.html

Juan E. Blumel, MD, PhD, et al., "Health screening of middle-aged women: What factors affect longevity?" *Menopause* 29, no. 9, September 2022, pp. 1008–1013, journals.lww.com/menopausejournal/Fulltext/2022/09000/Health_screening_of_middle_aged_women__what.3.aspx

Avrum Zvi Bluming, "Hormone Replacement Therapy After Breast Cancer: It Is Time," *Cancer* 28, no. 3, May–June 2022, pp. 183–190, pubmed.ncbi.nlm.nih.gov/35594465/

Avrum Bluming, "Should estrogen therapy be used by breast cancer survivors?" *Endocrine Today,* Mar. 16, 2023, healio.com/news/endocrinology/20230307/should-estrogen-therapy-be-used-by-breast-cancer-survivors

Trudy L. Bush, PhD, MHS, et al., "Hormone Replacement Therapy and Breast Cancer," *Obstetrics & Gynecology* 98, no. 3, September 2001, pp. 498–508.

Brenda W. Campbell Jenkins et al., "Association of the joint effect of menopause and hormone replacement therapy and cancer in African American women: The Jackson Heart Study," *International Journal of Environmental Research and Public Health* 8, no. 6, June 23, 2011, pubmed.ncbi.nlm.nih.gov/21776241/

Rowan T. Chlebowski, MD, PhD, et al., "Association of Menopausal Hormone Therapy with Breast Cancer Incidence and Mortality During Long-term Follow-up of the Women's Health Initiative Randomized Clinical Trials," *JAMA* 324, no. 4, July 28, 2020, pp. 369–380, jamanetwork.com/journals/jama/fullarticle/2768806

Rowan T. Chlebowski, MD, PhD, and Aaron K. Aragaki, MS, "The Women's Health Initiative randomized trials of menopausal hormone therapy and breast cancer: Findings in context," *Menopause* 30, no. 4, April 2023, pp. 454–461, journals.lww.com/menopausejournal/Abstract/2023/04000/The_Women_s _Health_Initiative_randomized_trials_of.16.aspx

Carolyn J. Crandall, MD, MS, FACP, et al., "Safety of vaginal estrogens: A systematic review," *Menopause* 27, no. 3, March 2020, pp. 339–360, journals .lww.com/menopausejournal/Abstract/2020/03000/Safety_of_vaginal_estrogens __a_systematic_review.14.aspx

Jeff Craven, "Older Black women have worse outcomes after fragility fracture," *MDedge.com/endocrinology,* Sep. 26, 2019, mdedge.com/endocrinology/article/ 208903/osteoporosis/older-black-women-have-worse-outcomes-after-fragility

Sybil L. Crawford, PhD, et al., "Menopausal hormone therapy trends before versus after 2002: Impact of the Women's Health Initiative Study results," *Menopause* 26, no. 6, June 2019, pp. 588–597, journals.lww.com/menopausejournal/ Abstract/2019/06000/Menopausal_hormone_therapy_trends_before_versus.5 .aspx

Christine M. Derzko, MD, FRCSC, et al., "Does age at the start of treatment for vaginal atrophy predict response to vaginal estrogen therapy? Post hoc analysis of data from a randomized clinical trial involving 205 women treated with 10 µg estradiol vaginal tablets," *Menopause* 28, no. 2, February 2021, pubmed.ncbi .nlm.nih.gov/33038141/

Samar R. El Khoudary, PhD, MPH, FAHA, et al., "The menopause transition and women's health at midlife: A progress report from the Study of Women's Health Across the Nation (SWAN)," *Menopause* 26, no. 10, October 2019, pp. 1213–1227, ncbi.nlm.nih.gov/pmc/articles/PMC6784846/

Ellen W. Freeman, PhD, et al., "Duration of Menopausal Hot Flushes and Associated Risk Factors," *Obstetrics & Gynecology* 117, no. 5, May 2011, pp. 1095–1104, pubmed.ncbi.nlm.nih.gov/21508748/

E. W. Freeman, PhD, et al., "Premenstrual Syndrome as a Predictor of Menopausal Symptoms," *Obstetrics & Gynecology* 103, no. 5, May 2004, pp. 960–966, pubmed.ncbi.nlm.nih.gov/15121571/

Kate A. Fox, BS, et al., "Evaluation of systemic estrogen for preventing urinary tract infections in postmenopausal women," *Menopause* 28, no. 7, July 2021, journals .lww.com/menopausejournal/Abstract/9000/Evaluation_of_systemic_estrogen _for_preventing.96957.aspx

Jay Furst, "Mayo Clinic puts price tag on cost of menopause symptoms for women in the workplace," *Mayo Clinic News Network,* Apr. 26, 2023, newsnetwork .mayoclinic.org/discussion/mayo-clinic-study-puts-price-tag-on-cost-of -menopause-symptoms-for-women-in-the-workplace/

Csaba Gajdos, MD, et al., "Breast Cancer Diagnosed During Hormone Replace- ment Therapy," *Obstetrics & Gynecology* 95, no. 4, April 2000, pp. 513–518, pubmed.ncbi.nlm.nih.gov/10725482/

Margery L. S. Gass, MD, FACOG, NCMP, et al., "NAMS supports judicious use of systemic hormone therapy for women aged 65 years and older," *Menopause* 22, no. 7, 2015, menopause.org/docs/default-source/2015/nams-editorial-on -judicious-use-of-ht-65.pdf

Argyri Gialeraki, PhD, et al., "Oral Contraceptives and HRT Risk of Thrombosis,"

Clinical and Applied Thrombosis/Hemostasis 24, no. 2, March 2018, pp. 217–225, ncbi.nlm.nih.gov/pmc/articles/PMC6714678/

Steven R. Goldstein, MD, FACOG, CCD, NCMP, "Appropriate evaluation of postmenopausal bleeding," *Menopause* 25, no. 12, December 2018, pp. 1476–1478, journals.lww.com/menopausejournal/Abstract/2018/12000/Appropriate_evaluation_of_postmenopausal_bleeding.12.aspx

Steven R. Goldstein, MD, NCMP, CCD, FACOG, FRCOG(H), "Sarcopenic obesity: A double whammy," *Menopause* 29, no. 6, June 2022, pp. 644–645, journals.lww.com/menopausejournal/Citation/2022/06000/Sarcopenic_obesity__a_double_whammy.3.aspx

Tara Haelle, "Better Training for Menopausal Management Urgently Needed," *Medscape Medical News,* Mar. 4, 2016, medscape.com/viewarticle/859847#vp_3

Benjamin S. Harris, MD, MPH, et al., "Hormonal management of menopausal symptoms in women with a history of gynecologic malignancy," *Menopause* 27, no. 2, February 2020, pp. 243–248, journals.lww.com/menopausejournal/Abstract/2020/02000/Hormonal_management_of_menopausal_symptoms_in.18.aspx

Howard N. Hodis, MD, et al., "Menopausal Hormone Therapy and Breast Cancer: What Is the Evidence from Randomized Trials?" *Climacteric* 21, no. 6, Oct. 9, 2018, pp. 521–528, ncbi.nlm.nih.gov/pmc/articles/PMC6386596/

Sheryl A. Kingsberg, PhD, et al., "Clinical Effects of Early or Surgical Menopause," *Obstetrics & Gynecology* 135, no. 4, April 2020, pp. 853–868, journals.lww.com/greenjournal/Abstract/2020/04000/Clinical_Effects_of_Early_or_Surgical_Menopause.15.aspx

Juliana M. Kling, MD, MPH, et al., "Menopause Management Knowledge in Postgraduate Family Medicine, Internal Medicine, and Obstetrics and Gynecology Residents: A Cross-Sectional Survey," *Mayo Clinic Proceedings* 94, no. 2, February 2019, pp. 242–253, mayoclinicproceedings.org/article/S0025-6196(18)30701-8/fulltext

Grace E. Kohn et al., "The History of Estrogen Therapy," *Sexual Medicine Reviews* 7, no. 3, July 2019, pp. 416–421, ncbi.nlm.nih.gov/pmc/articles/PMC7334883/

R. D. Langer, "The evidence base for HRT: What can we believe?" *Climacteric* 20, no. 2, April 2017, pp. 91–96, pubmed.ncbi.nlm.nih.gov/28281363/

Beth Levine and Kacy Church, MD, "What Experts Want Women of Color to Know About Menopause," *Everydayhealth.com,* Jan. 13, 2022, everydayhealth.com/menopause/what-experts-want-bipoc-women-to-know-about-menopause/

Roger A. Lobo, "Where Are We 10 Years After the Women's Health Initiative?" *The Journal of Clinical Endocrinology & Metabolism* 98, no. 5, May 1, 2013, pp. 1771–1780, academic.oup.com/jcem/article/98/5/1771/2536695

JoAnn E. Manson, MD, DrPH, NCMP, et al., "The Women's Health Initiative trials of menopausal hormone therapy: Lessons learned," *Menopause* 27, no. 8, August 2020, pp. 918–928, journals.lww.com/menopausejournal/Abstract/2020/08000/The_Women_s_Health_Initiative_trials_of_menopausal.14.aspx

Jane V. R. Marsh, MS, et al., "Racial Differences in Hormone Replacement Therapy Prescriptions," *Obstetrics & Gynecology* 93, no. 6, June 1999, pp. 999–1003,

journals.lww.com/greenjournal/Fulltext/1999/06000/Racial_Differences_in
_Hormone_Replacement_Therapy.21.aspx

Virginia M. Miller, PhD, et al., "The Kronos Early Estrogen Prevention Study
(KEEPS): What have we learned?" *Menopause* 26, no. 9, September 2019,
pp. 1071–1084, pubmed.ncbi.nlm.nih.gov/31453973/

Michael Monostra, "Early initiation of menopausal HT reduces all-cause mortality,
CHD events in women," *Endocrinology,* Dec. 3, 2020, healio.com/news/
endocrinology/20201203/early-initiation-of-menopausal-ht-reduces-allcause
-mortality-chd-events-in-women

NAMS, "Understanding the Controversy: Hormone Testing and Bioidentical
Hormones," *North American Menopause Society 17th Annual Meeting,*
Oct. 11, 2006, menopause.org/docs/default-document-library/
pg06monogrpahC2AF519C07F6.pdf?sfvrsn=daa4c306_2

The NAMS 2020 GSM Position Statement Editorial Panel, "The 2020 genitourinary syndrome of menopause position statement of The North American
Menopause Society," *Menopause* 27, no. 9, September 2020, pp. 976–992,
pubmed.ncbi.nlm.nih.gov/3285244

Rossella E. Nappi, MD, PhD, et al., "The burden of vulvovaginal atrophy on
women's daily living: Implications on quality of life from a face-to-face real-life
survey," *Menopause* 26, no. 5, May 2019, pp. 485–491, journals.lww.com/
menopausejournal/Abstract/2019/05000/The_burden_of_vulvovaginal_atrophy
_on_women_s.8.aspx

National Cancer Institute, "Breast cancer risk in American women," *cancer.gov,*
Dec. 16, 2020, cancer.gov/types/breast/risk-fact-sheet

National Institute of Arthritis and Musculoskeletal and Skin Diseases (NIAMS),
"Calcium and Vitamin D: Important for Bone Health," *National Institutes of
Health: National Institute of Arthritis and Musculoskeletal and Skin Diseases,* May
2023, niams.nih.gov/health-topics/calcium-and-vitamin-d-important-bone
-health

National Institute on Aging, "Falls and Fractures in Older Adults: Causes and
Prevention," *nia.nih.gov,* Sep. 12, 2022, nia.nih.gov/health/falls-and-fractures
-older-adults-causes-and-prevention

National Institute on Aging, "Research explores the impact of menopause on
women's health and aging," *nia.nih.gov,* May 6, 2022, nia.nih.gov/news/research
-explores-impact-menopause-womens-health-and-aging

The North American Menopause Society (NAMS), "NAMS Position Statement:
Management of osteoporosis in postmenopausal women: The 2021 position
statement of The North American Menopause Society," *Menopause* 28, no. 9,
2021, pp. 993–997, menopause.org/docs/default-source/professional/2021
-osteoporosis-position-statement.pdf

The North American Menopause Society (NAMS), "The 2022 hormone therapy
position statement of The North American Menopause Society," *Menopause* 29,
no. 7, July 2022, pp. 767–794, journals.lww.com/menopausejournal/Abstract/
2022/07000/The_2022_hormone_therapy_position_statement_of_The.4.aspx

Matthew Nudy, MD, et al., "The severity of individual menopausal symptoms,
cardiovascular disease, and all-cause mortality in the Women's Health Initiative

Observational Cohort," *Menopause* 29, no. 12, December 2022, pp. 1365–1374, journals.lww.com/menopausejournal/Abstract/2022/12000/The_severity_of _individual_menopausal_symptoms,.5.asp

Anita Pershad, BS, et al., "Racial and Ethnic Disparities in Menopausal Hormone Therapy Acceptance [A134]," *Obstetrics & Gynecology* 139, May 2022, p. 39S, journals.lww.com/greenjournal/abstract/2022/05001/racial_and_ethnic _disparities_in_menopausal.132.aspx

David D. Rahn, MD, et al., "Vaginal Estrogen for Genitourinary Syndrome of Menopause," *Obstetrics & Gynecology* 124, no. 6, December 2014, pp. 1147–1156, journals.lww.com/greenjournal/Abstract/2014/12000/ Vaginal_Estrogen_for_Genitourinary_Syndrome_of.12.aspx

Louise Lind Schierbeck et al., "Effect of hormone replacement therapy on cardiovascular events in recently postmenopausal women: Randomized trial," *BMJ*, Oct. 9, 2012, bmj.com/content/345/bmj.e6409

Margaret Sherburn, MWH, et al., "Is Incontinence Associated with Menopause?" *Obstetrics & Gynecology* 98, no. 4, October 2001, pp. 628–633

Talia H. Sobel, MD, NCMP, and Wen Shen, MD, MPH, "Transdermal estrogen therapy in menopausal women at increased risk for thrombotic events: A scoping review," *Menopause* 29, no. 4, April 2022, pp. 483–490, journals.lww.com/ menopausejournal/Abstract/2022/04000/Transdermal_estrogen_therapy_in _menopausal_women.14.aspx

Yu-jia Song et al., "The Effect of Estrogen Replacement Therapy on Alzheimer's Disease and Parkinson's Disease in Postmenopausal Women: A Meta-Analysis," *Frontiers in Neuroscience* 14, no. 157, Mar. 10, 2020, ncbi.nlm.nih.gov/pmc/ articles/PMC7076111/

Cynthia A. Stuenkel, MD, NCMP, "Compounded bioidentical hormone therapy: New recommendations from the 2020 National Academies of Sciences, Engineering, and Medicine," *Menopause* 28, no. 5, May 2021, journals.lww.com/ menopausejournal/Fulltext/2021/05000/Compounded_bioidentical_hormone _therapy__new.15.aspx

Leslie M. Swanson et al., "Associations between sleep and cognitive performance in a racially/ethnically diverse cohort: The Study of Women's Health Across the Nation," *Sleep* 44, no. 2, February 2021, ncbi.nlm.nih.gov/pmc/articles/ PMC7879413/

Vikram Sinai Talaulikar, "Hormone Replacement Therapy for Menopausal Symptoms—A Summary of Current Scientific Evidence," *EC Gynaecology* 11, no. 9, Aug. 22, 2022, pp. 39–45, ecronicon.net/assets/ecgy/pdf/ECGY-11-00784.pdf

Gim Gee Teng, MD, et al., "Mortality and osteoporotic fractures: Is the link causal, and is it modifiable?" *Clinical and Experimental Rheumatology* 26, no. 5, Sep–Oct 2008, pp. S125–S137, ncbi.nlm.nih.gov/pmc/articles/PMC4124750

Holly N. Thomas, MD, MS, et al., "'I want to feel like I used to feel': A qualitative study of causes of low libido in postmenopausal women," *Menopause* 27, no. 3, March 2020, pp. 289–294, journals.lww.com/menopausejournal/Abstract/2020/ 03000/_I_want_to_feel_like_I_used_to_feel___a.7.aspx

Rebecca C. Thurston et al., "Vasomotor Symptoms and Accelerated Epigenetic Aging in the Women's Health Initiative (WHI)," *The Journal of Clinical Endocri-*

nology and Metabolism 104, no. 4, Apr. 1, 2020, pp. 1221–1227, pubmed.ncbi
.nlm.nih.gov/32080740/

Ana M. Valdes et al., "Role of the gut microbiota in nutrition and health," *The BMJ,*
June 13, 2018, bmj.com/content/361/bmj.k2179

Sarah Vander Schaaff, "Black women's health problems during menopause haven't
been a focus of medicine. Experts and activists want to change that," *The
Washington Post,* Mar. 6, 2021, washingtonpost.com/health/black-women
-menopause-hot-flashes/2021/03/05/97a02c44-7b8a-11eb-a976-c028a4215c78
_story.html

Makeba Williams, MD, et al., "A review of African American women's experiences
in menopause," *Menopause* 29, no. 11, November 2022, pp. 1331–1337,
journals.lww.com/menopausejournal/Citation/2022/11000/A_review_of
_African_American_women_s_experiences.16.aspx

Rena R. Wing, PhD, et al., "Weight Gain at the Time of Menopause," *Archives of
Internal Medicine* 151, no. 1, January 1991, pp. 97–102, jamanetwork.com/
journals/jamainternalmedicine/article-abstract/614449

Nicole C. Wright et al., "Racial Disparities Exist in Outcomes After Major Fragility
Fractures," *Journal of the American Geriatrics Society* 68, no. 8, August 2020,
pp. 1803–1810, pubmed.ncbi.nlm.nih.gov/32337717/

Writing Group for the Women's Health Initiative Investigators, "Risks and Benefits
of Estrogen Plus Progestin in Healthy Postmenopausal Women," *JAMA Network*
288, no. 3, July 17, 2002, pp. 321–333, jamanetwork.com/journals/jama/
fullarticle/195120

Chapter 11
Here Comes the Sun: Live Your *Best* Menopausal Life

CDC, "Loneliness and Social Isolation Linked to Serious Health Conditions," *CDC
Alzheimer's Disease and Health Aging,* April 29, 2021, cdc.gov/aging/publications/
features/lonely-older-adults.html

Daniel A. Cox, "The State of American Friendship: Change, Challenges, and Loss,"
American Enterprise Institute Survey Center on American Life, June 8, 2021,
americansurveycenter.org/research/the-state-of-american-friendship-change
-challenges-and-loss/

Margaret Darby, "Studies show friendships for middle-aged men are dwindling,"
deseret.com, Feb. 3, 2023, deseret.com/23574827/studies-friendships-middle
-aged-men-no-friends

Lynne C. Giles et al., "Effect of social networks on 10-year survival in very old
Australians: The Australian longitudinal study of aging," *Journal of Epidemiology
and Community Health* 59, no. 7, June 17, 2005, jech.bmj.com/content/59/7/574

Natalie M. Golaszewski, PhD, et al., "Evaluation of Social Isolation, Loneliness, and
Cardiovascular Disease Among Older Women in the US," *JAMA NetworkOpen*
5, no. 2, 2022, jamanetwork.com/journals/jamanetworkopen/fullarticle/
2788582

National Council on Aging Staff, "Get the Facts on Older Americans," Dec. 12,
2022, ncoa.org/article/get-the-facts-on-older-americans

National Institutes of Health, "Social isolation, loneliness in older people pose health risks," *National Institute on Aging,* April 23, 2019, nia.nih.gov/news/social -isolation-loneliness-older-people-pose-health-risks.

K. Orth-Gomer et al., "Lack of social support and incidence of coronary heart disease in middle-aged Swedish men," *Psychosomatic Medicine* 55, no. 1, January 1993, pp. 37–43, journals.lww.com/psychosomaticmedicine/Citation/1993/ 01000/Lack_of_social_support_and_incidence_of_coronary.7.aspx

Loren Stein, "Sex and Seniors: The 70-Year Itch," *Health Day,* Jan. 18, 2022, consumer.healthday.com/encyclopedia/aging-1/misc-aging-news-10/sex-and -seniors-the-70-year-itch-647575.html

Magdalene J. Taylor, "Have More Sex, Please!" *The New York Times,* Feb. 13, 2023, nytimes.com/2023/02/13/opinion/have-more-sex-please.html

UCLA Staff, "The pain of chronic loneliness can be detrimental to your health," *UCLA Health News & Insights,* Dec. 22, 2016, uclahealth.org/news/the-pain-of -chronic-loneliness-can-be-detrimental-to-your-health

United States Census Bureau, "Older People Projected to Outnumber Children for First Time in U.S. History" (press release), Mar. 13, 2018, census.gov/ newsroom/press-releases/2018/cb18-41-population-projections.html

Chapter 12
Heaven Bound: Be a Benefactor, Not a Burden

Nancy Aldrich and William F. Benson, "Advance Care Planning: Ensuring Your Wishes Are Known and Honored If You Are Unable to Speak for Yourself," *Critical Issue Brief, Centers for Disease Control and Prevention,* 2012, cdc.gov/aging/ pdf/advanced-care-planning-critical-issue-brief.pdf

The American Cancer Society Medical and Editorial Content Team, "What is hospice care?" *cancer.org,* May 10, 2019, cancer.org/cancer/end-of-life-care/ hospice-care/what-is-hospice-care.html

Bruce Horovitz, "Pandemic Isn't Spurring Older Adults to Discuss, Record Advance Health Care Wishes," *AARP,* Apr. 6, 2021, aarp.org/caregiving/financial-legal/ info-2021/poll-many-have-no-advance-directives.html

C. Perumalswami et al., "Older Adults' Experiences with Advance Care Planning," *University of Michigan National Poll on Aging,* April 2021, healthyagingpoll.org/ reports-more/report/older-adults-experiences-advance-care-planning

Tim Pittman, "Hospice Use Lower Among African Americans," *Duke Health,* Jan. 15, 2018, physicians.dukehealth.org/articles/hospice-use-lower-among -african-americans

READING GROUP GUIDE

1. What is your biggest takeaway from this book? Is there something you learned that you didn't know before? In what ways did it affirm your understanding?

2. What reasons keep women, especially Black women, from seeking medical help? Why is it important to understand how history has influenced these reasons?

3. Women's pain has historically been diminished or discounted; Black women's pain has practically been ignored. What are some misconceptions surrounding women's suffering? Are there any you may have believed? How can society—and the healthcare industry—change these biases?

4. After reading *Grown Woman Talk,* do you feel empowered to take care of your own health? What are your next steps?

5. Dr. Sharon asks you to get familiar with the term *health span*. What does health span mean to you? How does it differ from lifespan?

6. What's on your wellness wish list?

7. How familiar are you with your family's health and medical history? How much do you know about your own health history? How does knowing help you in your health journey?

8. Was there a particular chapter that spoke to you (heart disease, cancer, diabetes, women's issues, etc.)? Do you feel more informed and empowered after reading it?

9. What does self-care mean to you? How is self-care important to your health?

10. How can stress affect your health? While some stress is systemic and outside your control, some stressors are manageable. What steps can you take to better deal with stress and possibly prevent greater health problems?

11. When it comes to racial disparities in health, why is it important to look deeper than the headlines? What sort of information matters? What stories do the statistics really tell about illness and wellness?

12. Why is a book like this important? How does it differ from other books on health? Who would you give it to?

READER NOTES

INDEX

ABOUT THE AUTHOR

SHARON MALONE, M.D., is a board-certified OB/GYN and a certified menopause practitioner who has practiced medicine in the nation's capital for more than thirty years. She is the chief medical advisor of Alloy Women's Health and a passionate advocate for improved research and education around women's health in midlife. She lives in Washington, D.C., with her husband, Eric Holder.